ACCESS TO SURGERY: 500 SINGLE BEST ANSWER QUESTIONS IN GENERAL & SYSTEMIC PHYSIOLOGY

PasTest

Dedicated to your success

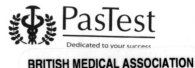

To my wife, Irfana, for her patience, strength and support.

ACCESS TO SURGERY: 500 SINGLE BEST ANSWER QUESTIONS IN GENERAL & SYSTEMIC PHYSIOLOGY

Shahzad G. Raja

BSc, MBBS, MRCS

Specialist Registrar Cardiothoracic Surgery

Department of Cardiothoracic Surgery

Western Infirmary

Glasgow

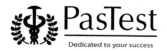

PasTest

Dedicated to your success

© 2007 PASTEST LTD

Egerton Court
Parkgate Estate
Knutsford
Cheshire
WA16 8DX

Telephone: 01565 752000

First published 2007

ISBN: 1 905635 28 1

ISBN: 978 1 905635 28 3

A catalogue record for this book is available from the British Library.

PasTest Revision Books and Intensive Courses

PasTest has been established in the field of postgraduate medical education since 1972, providing revision books and intensive study courses for doctors preparing for their professional examinations.

Books and courses are available for the following specialties:

MRCGP, MRCP Parts 1 and 2, MRCPCH Parts 1 and 2, MRCPsych, MRCS, MRCOG Parts 1 and 2, DRCOG, DCH, FRCA, PLAB Parts 1 and 2.

For further details contact:

PasTest, Freepost, Knutsford, Cheshire WA16 7BR

Tel: 01565 752000   Fax: 01565 650264

www.pastest.co.uk   enquiries@pastest.co.uk

Text prepared by Carnegie Book Production, Lancaster, UK

Printed and bound in the UK by Athenaeum Press Ltd, Gateshead

CONTENTS

PREFACE

Recent reforms in medical education in the United Kingdom have prompted replacement of multiple-choice questions (MCQs) with single best answer questions. **Access to Surgery: 500 Single Best Answer Questions in General & Systemic Physiology** is the first book of its kind that provides 500 practice single best answer questions in General & Systemic Physiology for candidates taking the surgical examinations. As the title indicates, it is primarily written for surgical trainees, with emphasis mainly on surgical aspects of human physiology. However, it can be used as a practice tool by undergraduate medical students as well as trainees in other medical disciplines for whom physiology can be a major examination hurdle.

Each question has been carefully formulated to cover a given topic in physiology. All major aspects of physiology are dealt with, being organised in sequence under the headings General Physiology, Cardiovascular Physiology, Respiratory Physiology, Fluids, Electrolytes and Acid–Base Physiology, Renal Physiology, Gastrointestinal Physiology, Neurophysiology, Endocrine Physiology and Reproductive Physiology. The questions also cover the complete MRCS applied physiology syllabus and are expected to be useful for the specialty FRCS candidates as well. This book contains a substantial number of patient-based questions or clinical vignettes that will enable prospective candidates to test their ability to integrate key basic physiological concepts with relevant clinical problems. In addition, factual recall questions have also been included that probe for basic recall of facts. Detailed and comprehensive explanations, rather than just brief answers, to questions have been provided so that the candidates do not have to consult textbooks for clarification, as is the case with most other MCQs books.

The questions in this book can be used in a number of ways: (i) as a diagnostic tool (pretest); (ii) as a guide and focus for further study; and (iii) for self-assessment. The least effective use of these questions is to 'study' them by reading them one at a time and then looking at the correct response. These 500 practice questions are intended to be an integral part of a well-planned review as well as an isolated resource. If used appropriately, these questions can provide self-assessment information beyond a numeric score. Furthermore, the questions have been planned in such a way that this book can be used as companion to any textbook of physiology.

I am hopeful that this book will prove a useful revision and self-assessment tool for all those involved in learning physiology.

Shahzad G. Raja

2007

ABBREVIATIONS

ABP	androgen-binding protein
ACE	angiotensin-converting enzyme
ACh	acetylcholine
ACTH	adrenocorticotrophic hormone
ADH	antidiuretic hormone
ADHD	attention deficit hyperactivity disorder
ADP	adenosine diphosphate
AF	atrial fibrillation
AIDS	acquired immune deficiency syndrome
APC	antigen-presenting cell
ALT	alanine transaminase
Apo	apoplipoprotein
aPTT	activated partial thromboplastin time
ARDS	acute (or adult) respiratory distress syndrome
ARF	acute renal failure
ARR	aldosterone-to-renin ratio
ASD	atrial septal defect
AST	aspartate aminotransferase
ATN	acute tubular necrosis
ATP	adenosine triphosphate
AV	atrioventricular
BBB	blood–brain barrier
BE	base excess
BFU-E	erythroid burst-forming units
BMR	basal metabolic rate
BP	blood pressure
BSA	body surface area
BT shunt	Blalock–Taussig shunt
BUN	blood urea nitrogen
C_AO_2	oxygen concentration of arterial blood
cAMP	cyclc adenosine monophosphate
CAH	congenital adrenal hyperplasia
CCK	cholecystokinin
CF	cystic fibrosis

CFU-E	erythroid colony-forming units
cGMP	cyclic guanosine monophosphate
CI	cardiac index
CLIP	corticotrophin-like intermediate lobe peptide
CN	cranial nerve
CNS	central nervous system
CO	cardiac output
CoA	coenzyme A
COPD	chronic obstructive pulmonary disease
CRF	chronic renal failure
CRH	corticotrophin-releasing hormone
CSF	cerebrospinal fluid
CT	computed tomography
C_vO_2	oxygen concentration of venous blood
DAG	diacyl glycerol
DBP	diastolic blood pressure
DCML	dorsal column-medial lemniscus system
DCT	distal convoluted tubule
DDAVP	1-desamino-8-D-arginine vasopressin
DHEA	dehydroepiandrosterone
DHT	dihydrotestosterone
DIC	disseminated intravascular coagulation
DKA	diabetic ketoacidosis
DL_{CO}	diffusing capacity for carbon monoxide
DNA	deoxyribonucleic acid
DPG	2,3-diphosphoglycerate
DVT	deep venous thrombosis
EBV	Epstein–Barr virus
ECF	extracellular fluid
ECG	electrocardiogram
EDRF	endothelium-derived relaxing factor
EDTA	ethylenediamine tetra-acetic acid
EDV	end-diastolic volume
EEG	electroencephalogram
EF or Ef	ejection fraction
ENaC	epithelial Na^+ channel
EPO	erythropoietin

ER	endoplasmic reticulum
ERCP	endoscopic resonance cholangiopancreatography
ESV	end-systolic volume
FA	fatty acid
F_ACO_2	fraction of alveolar CO_2
$FADH_2$	reduced fluorine adenine dinucleotide
FBC	full blood count
FDP	fibrin degradation product
FEV	forced expiratory volume
FEV_1	forced expiratory volume in the first second
F_IO_2	fraction of inspired air that is O_2
FSH	follicle-stimulating hormone
FVC	forced vital capacity
FXa	activated factor X
G1P	glucose-1-phosphate
GABA	gamma-aminobutyric acid
GBS	Guillain–Barré syndrome
GFR	glomerular filtration rate
GGT	γ-glutamyl transpeptidase
GH	growth hormone
GHRH	growth hormone releasing hormone
GI	gastrointestinal
GLA	gamma-carboxyglutamate
GLUT	glucose transporter
GN	glomerulonephritis
GnRH	gonadotrophin-releasing hormone
GTD	gestational trophoblastic diseases
Hb	haemoglobin
HBV	hepatitis B virus
HC	haptocorrin
hCG	human chorionic gonadotrophin
Hct	haematocrit
HDL	high-density lipoprotein
HDN	haemolytic disease of the newborn
HELLP	haemolysis, elevated liver enzymes, low platelets
HHV	human herpes virus
HIT	heparin-induced thrombocytopenia

HITT	heparin-induced thrombocytopenia and thrombosis
HIV	human immunodeficiency virus
HLA	human leukocyte antigen
HMWK	high-molecular-weight kininogen
hPL	human placental lactogen
HPV	hypoxic pulmonary vasoconstriction
HR	heart rate
HRT	hormone replacement therapy
3b-HSD	3b-hydroxysteroid dehydrogenase
5HT	5-hydroxytryptophen
ICF	intracellular fluid
ICP	Intrahepatic cholestasis of pregnancy
ICU	intensive care unit
IDL	Intermediate-density lipoprotein
IF	intrinsic factor
IFCR	intrinsic factor complex receptor
I_f	inward 'funny' current
Ig	immunoglobulin
IGF 1	insulin-like-growth-factor-1
IL	interleukin
I_K	inward K^+
IM	intramuscular
I_{Na}	inward Na^+
INF	interferon
INR	international normalised ratio
IP_3	inosito triphosphate
IRS-1	insulin receptor substrate 1
IV	intravenous
JG cells	juxtaglomerular
JGA	juxtaglomerular apparatus
K_a	acid disassociation constant
LAP	left atrial pressure
LCHAD	long-chain 3-hydroxyacyl-coenzyme A dehydrogenase
LDL	low-density lipoprotein
L-DOPA	L-hydroxyphenyl alanine
LGN	lateral genic-ulate nucleus
LH	luteinising hormone

LMN	lower motor neurone
LMWH	low-molecular-weight heparin
LP	lumbar puncture
β-LPH	lipotrophin
LPL	lipoprotein lipase
LR	living-related
LUR	living-unrelated
M	motor
MAC	membrane attack complex
MAP	mean arterial pressure
MCH	mean corpuscular haemoglobin
MCHC	mean corpuscular haemoglobin concentration
MCQs	multiple-choice questions
MCV	mean corpuscular volume
MHC	major histocompatibility complex
MN	motor neurone
MPAP	mean pulmonary artery pressure
MRCP	magnetic resonance cholangiopancreatography
MRI	magnetic resonance imaging
MSH	melanocyte-stimulating hormone
MW	molecular weight
NADH	reduced nicontinamide adenine dinucleotide
NK	natural killer
NK1R	neurokinin 1 receptor
NOS	nitric oxide synthase
NSAID	non-steroidal anti-inflammatory drug
NTS	nucleus of the tractus solitarius
17OHP	17-hydroxyprogesterone
OVLT	organum vasculosum of the lamina terminalis
PADP	Pulmonary artery diastolic pressure
PAF	platelet activating factor
PABA	para-aminobenzoic acid
$p_A(CO_2)$	alveolar CO_2 pressure
$p_a(CO_2)$	arterial CO_2 pressure
PAI	Plasminogen activator inhibitor
$p_A(O_2)$	alveolar O_2 pressure
$p_a(O_2)$	arterial O_2 pressure

PAH	para-aminohippuric acid
PAP	pulmonary artery pressure
PASP	Pulmonary artery systolic pressure
PAWP	pulmonary artery wedge pressure
PCML	posterior column-medial lemniscus
PCOS	polycystic ovarian syndrome
PCR	polymerase chain reaction
PCT	proximal convoluted tubule
PE	pulmonary embolism
PEEP	positive end-expiratory pressure
$p_E(CO_2)$	expired CO_2 tension
PF4	platelet factor 4
PG	prostaglandin
PGO	pons, geniculate, occipital (wave)
PIVKA	proteins formed in vitamin K absence
PKU	phenylkenoturia
p_{LA}	left atrial pressure
POMC	pro-opiomelanocortin
PP	pulse pressure
PPH	post-partum haemorrhage
p_{pl}	intrapleural pressure
PPV	pulse pressure variation
PR	prothrombin ratio
PRA	plasma renin activity
PRU	peripheral resistance units
PT	prothrombin time
PTH	parathyroid hormone
PTT	partial thromboplastin time
PV	polycythaemia vera
PVR	pulmonary vascular resistance
PVRI	pulmonary vascular resistance index
Q	cardiac output
RAP	right atrial pressure
RBC	red blood cell
RBF	renal blood flow
rCBF	regional cerebral blood flow
REM	rapid eye movement

Rh	Rhesus
RNA	ribonucleic acid
RPF	renal plasma flow
RPL	recurrent pregnancy loss
RVDP	right ventricular diastolic pressure
RVP	right ventricular pressure
RVSP	right ventricular systolic pressure
S	sensory
SA	sinoatrial
$Sa(O_2)$	arterial oxygen saturation
SBC	standard bicarbonate
SBE	standard base excess
SBP	systolic blood pressure
SCN	suprachiasmatic nucleus
SGLT	sodium–glucose co-transporter
SHO	senior house officer
SIADH	syndrome of inappropriate antidiuretic hormone secretion
SIRS	systemic inflammatory response syndrome
SLE	systemic lupus erythematosus
SP	systolic pressure
SPV	systolic pressure variation
SR	sarcoplasmic reticulum
SRD5A	steroid 5α-reductase
SV	stroke volume
SVI	stroke volume index
SVR	systemic vascular resistance
SVRI	systemic vascular resistance index
SVV	stroke volume variation
T_3	tri-iodothyronine
T_4	thyroxine
TBW	total body water
TC II	transcobalamin II
TCT	thrombin clotting time
TeBG	testosterone-binding globulin
TF	tissue factor
TFPI	tissue factor pathway inhibitors

TGF	transforming growth factor
T_m	transport maximum
TNF	tumour necrosis factor
TOF	tetralogy of fallot
TPA	tissue plasminogen activator
TPN	total parenteral nutrition
TPR	total peripheral resistance
TRH	thryrotropin-releasing hormone
TSAb	thyroid-stimulating antibodies
TSH	thyroid-stimulating hormone
TSI	thyroid-stimulating immunoglobulin
TT	thrombin time
UDP	uridine diphosphate
UDPG	uridine diphosphate glucose
UFH	unfractionated heparin
ULN	upper limit of normal
V_A	alveolar ventilation
VO_2	whole-body oxygen consumption
VPL	ventral posterolateral (nucleus)
VPM	ventral posteromedial (nucleus)
VSD	ventricular septal defect
vWD	von Willebrand's disease
vWF	von Willebrand factor
WBC	white blood cell
ZPI	protein-Z-dependent protease inhibitor

QUESTIONS

SECTION 1:
GENERAL PHYSIOLOGY –
QUESTIONS

For each question given below choose the ONE BEST option.

1.1 **A fluorescent dye that cannot cross cell membranes is used to label several contiguous cells. One cell in the middle is experimentally bleached with light that destroys the dye, but the cell soon recovers dye fluorescence. This recovery is best explained by the presence of which of the following structures between the bleached cell and its fluorescent neighbours?**

    A Basal lamina

    B Desmosomes

    C Gap junctions

    D Glycosaminoglycans

    E Tight junctions

1.2 **During pregnancy the uterus increases considerably in size. After delivery, the regression of uterine size is brought about by which of the following cellular organelles?**

    A Endoplasmic reticulum

    B Golgi apparatus

    C Mitochondria

    D Lysosomes

    E Nucleus

1.3 **During an experiment a poison is injected into the cell that specifically destroyed the rough endoplasmic reticulum. This will result in no:**

O A Synthesis of glycogen

O B Synthesis of proteins

O C Glycosylation of protein and carbohydrate moieties

O D Synthesis of lipids

O E Autolysis of proteins

1.4 **Myoglobin is released from damaged muscle tissue (rhabdomyolysis), which has very high concentrations of myoglobin. In a skeletal muscle, myoglobin:**

O A Acts like haemoglobin and binds with O_2

O B Is found in fast fibres only

O C Releases O_2 only at high $p(O_2)$

O D Forms sigmoid dissociation curve (similar to haemoglobin)

O E Is devoid of iron

1.5 **A person standing in the upright position begins to lean to one side. The postural muscles that are closely connected to the vertebral column on the side will stretch. Because of this, stretch receptors in those muscles contract to correct posture. Which of the following statements regarding the stretch reflex is CORRECT?**

O A It is monosynaptic

O B It is polysynaptic

O C It is initiated by stimulation of Golgi tendon organ

O D It involves type II fibres

O E It involves higher centres

1.6 An organelle is a discrete structure of a cell having specialised functions. There are many types of organelles, particularly in the eukaryotic cells of higher organisms. What is the organelle that regenerates and replicates spontaneously?

○ A Golgi apparatus
○ B Mitochondrion
○ C Smooth endoplasmic reticulum
○ D Rough endoplasmic reticulum
○ E Vacuole

1.7 Atractyloside is an inhibitor of the electron transport chain. It would be expected to have little or no effect on the functioning of which of the following cell types?

○ A Cardiac muscle cells
○ B Parietal cells of the stomach
○ C Parotid duct cells
○ D Proximal convoluted tubule cells
○ E Red blood cells

1.8 Action potentials can be created by many types of cells, but are used most extensively by the nervous system for communication between neurones and to transmit information from neurones to other body tissues such as muscles and glands. During the activation of a nerve cell membrane:

○ A Chloride ions flow outward
○ B Potassium ions flow inward
○ C Potassium ions flow outward
○ D Sodium ions flow inward
○ E Sodium ions flow outward

general

1.9 **Skeletal muscle fibres can be divided into two basic types, type I (slow-twitch fibres) and type II (fast-twitch fibres). Fast muscle fibres:**

○ A Use anaerobic metabolism

○ B Have lots of myoglobin

○ C Are shorter for great strength of contraction

○ D Have relatively high endurance

○ E Have numerous mitochondria

1.10 **A patient developed a stitch granuloma following surgery. Which leukocyte in the peripheral blood will become an activated macrophage in this granuloma?**

○ A Basophil

○ B Eosinophil

○ C Lymphocyte

○ D Monocyte

○ E Neutrophil

1.11 **A 36-year-old man with end-stage renal disease who is undergoing haemodialysis has normocytic normochromic anaemia. Which of the following is the most appropriate therapy?**

○ A Erythropoietin

○ B Ferrous sulphate

○ C Folate

○ D Vitamin B_6

○ E Vitamin B_{12}

1.12 A blood sample taken from the umbilical artery of a newborn was subjected to electrophoresis to detect antibodies (immunoglobulins). Which of the following antibodies will have the highest percentage in a newborn?

○   A   IgA
○   B   IgD
○   C   IgE
○   D   IgG
○   E   IgM

1.13 A 58-year-old male patient needed a blood transfusion after repair of an abdominal aortic aneurysm. His blood was sent to the laboratory. The technician, while checking for this patient's blood group, said that the patient's blood agglutinates with antisera anti-A and anti-D, while the patient's serum agglutinates cells of blood group B. What is the blood group of this patient?

○   A   A positive
○   B   B positive
○   C   A negative
○   D   B negative
○   E   O positive

1.14 In humans there are five types of antibody: IgA, IgD, IgE, IgG and IgM. Which of the following statements regarding IgM is CORRECT?

○   A   It binds to allergens
○   B   It functions mainly as an antigen receptor on B cells
○   C   It is the largest immunoglobulin molecule
○   D   It is the most abundant immunoglobulin
○   E   It is a tetramer of four subunits

general

7

1.15 **The lack of normal factor VIII causes haemophilia A, an inherited bleeding disorder. Factor VIII is synthesised predominantly in:**

- ○ A Hepatocytes
- ○ B Histiocytes
- ○ C Kupffer cells
- ○ D Platelets
- ○ E Vascular endothelium

1.16 **A 45-year-old woman, with a past history of easy bruising and heavy menstrual periods, was admitted for elective cholecystectomy and was diagnosed with von Willebrand's disease on routine preoperative investigations. von Willebrand's disease is:**

- ○ A Autosomal dominant
- ○ B Characterised by decreased bleeding time
- ○ C Characterised by decreased factor VII
- ○ D Characterised by decreased platelets
- ○ E X-linked

1.17 **A 68-year-old woman complaining of easy fatigability and shortness of breath after abdominal aortic aneurysm repair was diagnosed with iron-deficiency anaemia and prescribed an oral iron preparation. Which of the following statements about iron metabolism is CORRECT?**

- ○ A Ferritin is a plasma protein that transports iron in the blood
- ○ B Haemosiderin is a product of haemoglobin degradation
- ○ C Iron is more efficiently absorbed in the ferrous state (Fe^{2+}) than in the ferric state (Fe^{3+})
- ○ D Most iron in the body is stored as haemosiderin
- ○ E The gastrointestinal rate of iron absorption is extremely high

general

1.18 **A 45-year-old man on warfarin for a mechanical mitral valve was admitted in the Accident and Emergency Department with persistent bleeding following dental extraction. He was told that his coagulation was deranged. Which of the following statements about blood coagulation is CORRECT?**

○ A Absence of Ca^{2+} promotes blood coagulation

○ B Disseminated intravascular coagulation (DIC) results in depletion of fibrin split products

○ C Patients with haemophilia A usually have a normal bleeding time

○ D von Willebrand factor suppresses platelet adhesion

○ E von Willebrand factor suppresses blood coagulation

1.19 **Nerve gas (organophosphate) is a weapon of chemical warfare that kills by causing respiratory and cardiovascular failure. The expected effect of organophosphate poisoning on the heart would be:**

○ A Decrease the force of myocardial contractions by potentiating the vagal tone to the ventricular muscle

○ B Decrease the rate of rhythmicity of the sinoatrial (SA) node by inducing hyperpolarisation

○ C Depolarise cells of the SA node by closing potassium channels under the control of the muscarinic acetylcholine receptor

○ D Increase the rate of rhythmicity of the SA node by increasing the upward drift in membrane potential caused by sodium leakage

○ E Increase conductivity at the atrioventricular (AV) junction by inducing depolarisation

general

1.20 **The resting membrane potential of a neuronal cell body is −60 mV. Opening chloride channels in the neuronal membrane will most likely cause:**

A Depolarisation to about −30 mV

B Depolarisation to about +30 mV

C Hyperpolarisation to about −70 mV

D Initiation of an action potential

E No change in membrane potential

1.21 **Chloride ions are associated with changes in neuronal membrane potential. Which of the following statements most accurately describes the response of a neurone to a decrease in the conductance of the cell membrane to chloride ions?**

A The cell will depolarise if its membrane potential is positive with respect to the equilibrium potential for chloride ions

B The cell will hyperpolarise if its membrane potential is positive with respect to the equilibrium potential for chloride ions

C The cell will hyperpolarise if the external chloride concentration is greater than the internal chloride concentration

D The cell will hyperpolarise if the external chloride concentration is less than the internal chloride concentration

E No change in membrane potential will occur if the external and internal chloride ion concentrations are equal

1.22 The stimulation of nerve endings in the Golgi tendon organs leads directly to:

- A Contraction of extrafusal muscle fibres
- B Contraction of intrafusal muscle fibres
- C Increased gamma-efferent discharge
- D Increased activity in group II afferent fibres
- E Reflex inhibition of motor neurones

1.23 Miniature endplate potentials that can be recorded from a muscle fibre are believed to represent:

- A The opening of a single receptor ion channel in the muscle membrane
- B The opening of multiple ion channels in the muscle membrane caused by spontaneous release of a small amount of neurotransmitter
- C The opening of multiple ion channels in the postsynaptic membrane in response to a single presynaptic action potential
- D The postsynaptic action of a single neurotransmitter molecule released from the presynaptic terminal
- E The spontaneous opening of ion channels in the muscle membrane in the absence of presynaptically released transmitter

general

1.24 In pacemaker tissue the gradual depolarisation between action potentials is mainly the result of:

O   A   A combination of gradual inactivation outward I_K along with the presence of an inward 'funny' current (I_f) due to opening of channels permeable to both Na^+ and K^+ ions

O   B   A gradual change in the ratio of extracellular to intracellular ion concentration across the cell membrane

O   C   A gradual increase in inward Na^+ (I_{Na}) channels current through fast Na^+ channels

O   D   An increase in the 'delayed rectifier' current due to outward movement of inward K^+ (I_K)

O   E   Changes in permeability of cells to the principal extracellular anions, Cl^- and HCO_3^-

1.25 The extra energy required by skeletal muscle fibres of an athlete for a burst of vigorous physical activity lasting between 20 and 100 s comes from:

O   A   Gluconeogenesis

O   B   Oxidative reactions

O   C   The breakdown of adenosine triphosphate in muscle cells

O   D   The breakdown of creatine phosphate

O   E   The breakdown of glycogen to lactic acid

1.26 A 52-year-old man presented for elective inguinal hernia repair. Shortly after induction of anaesthesia with halothane, the patient developed circulatory instability, tachypnoea and a sharp rise in body temperature (malignant hyperthermia). What is the cause of fever in this patient?

○ A Decreased convectional heat loss
○ B Increased blood levels of interleukin-1
○ C Increased heat production by skeletal muscle
○ D Increased hypothalamic temperature set point
○ E Increased sweat production

1.27 A 60-year-old man was seen in the surgical out-patient clinic following a prolonged ICU stay after right hemicolectomy for carcinoma of caecum, which was complicated by anastomotic leak and sepsis. He complained of chronic fatigue. A full blood count revealed: haematocrit = 30%, erythrocytes = $4 \times 10^6/\mu l$, haemoglobin level = 8 g/dl. To determine the likely cause of his anaemia, red blood cell indices were calculated by the Coulter counter. Which of the following red blood cell indices is CORRECT?

○ A MCHC = haemoglobin concentration × 10/erythrocyte number
○ B MCHC = haemoglobin concentration/haematocrit
○ C MCV = haematocrit × 1000/haemoglobin
○ D MCV = haemoglobin concentration × 10/erythrocyte number
○ E MCV = haemoglobin concentration/haematocrit

general

1.28   A patient with a low cardiac output was administered adrenaline, which stimulates the β-receptors. Stimulation of β-receptors:

○ A   Decreases glucagon secretion by pancreatic β-cells

○ B   Decreases insulin secretion by pancreatic β-cells

○ C   Promotes glycogen synthesis in liver cells

○ D   Promotes glycogen synthesis in muscle cells

○ E   Promotes lipolysis

1.29   Aspirin, a non-steroidal anti-inflammatory agent, inhibits the formation of prostaglandins (PGS), which are important mediators of inflammation. Which of the following statements about the role of prostaglandins during inflammatory processes is CORRECT?

○ A PGE_2 contracts bronchial smooth muscle

○ B PGE_2 sensitises nociceptive nerve endings, causing pain

○ C $PGF_{2\alpha}$ and PGE_2 relax uterine smooth muscle

○ D $PGF_{2\alpha}$ relaxes bronchial smooth muscle

○ E   Thromboxane A_2 inhibits platelet aggregation

general

1.30 **A 45-year-old patient was seen in the Accident and Emergency Department within half an hour of the onset of severe chest pain. Based on his electrocardiogram (ECG) finding he was diagnosed with acute myocardial infarction. The attending consultant decided to treat this patient with streptokinase, a fibrinolytic agent. Fibrinolysis in this patient will be:**

○ A Due to activation of tissue plasminogen activator by streptokinase

○ B Due to hydrolysis of fibrin by plasmin

○ C Due to hydrolysis of fibrin by streptokinase

○ D Inhibited by plasmin

○ E Inhibited by streptokinase

1.31 **Cytokines are produced by a wide variety of cell types (both haemopoietic and non-haemopoietic) and can have effects on nearby cells or throughout the organism. Sometimes these effects are strongly dependent on the presence of other chemicals and cytokines. Which of the following cytokines is produced by T cells and induces MHC-II (major histocompatibility) proteins?**

○ A α-Interferon

○ B β-Interferon

○ C γ-Interferon

○ D Interleukin-1

○ E Tumour necrosis factor

general

1.32 **A 58-year-old man with complaint of increasing fatigability and shortness of breath had a full blood count, which showed microcytic anaemia, low ferritin serum level and low transferrin saturation. Which of the following statements correctly describes intestinal iron absorption in this patient?**

○ A Dietary iron is more readily absorbed when ferritin stores of the intestinal epithelium are low

○ B Free iron is more readily absorbed than iron bound to organic molecules

○ C Intestinal iron absorption depends on intrinsic factor

○ D Iron is mainly absorbed in the distal ileum

○ E Iron is more readily absorbed in the ferric state (Fe^{3+}) than in the ferrous state (Fe^{2+})

1.33 **In an experiment a drug blocked the transmembrane proteins mainly responsible for the resting membrane potential of vascular smooth muscle cells. Which of the following transmembrane proteins was blocked by the drug?**

○ A Cl^- channels

○ B K^+ channels

○ C Na^+/K^+ pump

○ D Na^+ channels

○ E Non-selective cation channels

1.34 A 26-year-old female patient had a full blood
count that showed RBC count = 3.0 × 10⁶/μl,
haematocrit = 27% and haemoglobin = 11 g/dl.
Normal values (woman): haemoglobin = 12–16 g/dl,
mean corpuscular volume (MCV) = 80–100 fl, mean
corpuscular haemoglobin concentration (MCHC) =
31–37 g/dl. This patient's erythrocytes have:

  A Decreased MCV
  B Decreased MCHC
  C Increased cell diameter
  D Normal MCHC
  E Normal MCV

1.35 A 26-year-old female patient had a full blood
count that showed RBC count = 3.0 × 10⁶/μl,
haematocrit = 27% and haemoglobin = 11 g/dl,
mean corpuscular volume (MCV) = 90 fl, mean
corpuscular haemoglobin concentration (MCHC)
= 41 g/dl. Further laboratory examination of
this patient's blood sample revealed increased
osmotic fragility of the erythrocytes. Which of
the following is a likely cause of this patient's
findings?

  A Iron-deficiency anaemia
  B Liver disease
  C Sickle cell anaemia
  D Spherocytosis
  E Thalassaemia

general

1.36 **A 32-year-old woman was prescribed vitamin B$_{12}$ and folic acid by her GP. She asked him the reason for this prescription. The GP told her that vitamin B$_{12}$ or folic acid deficiency causes:**

A Erythroblastic cells of the bone marrow to become smaller than normal

B The adult red blood cell to be smaller than normal

C The adult red blood cell to have a thicker membrane than normal

D The adult red blood cell to have an ovoid shape rather than the usual biconcave disc shape

E The adult red blood cells to exhibit increased osmotic fragility

1.37 **An 18-year-old girl was prescribed iron supplement by her GP as she was thought to be taking a diet deficient in iron. Lack of iron in the diet often causes:**

A Erythraemia

B Hypochromic anaemia

C Pernicious anaemia

D Megaloblastic anaemia

E Polycythaemia

1.38 **Which of the following conditions is most likely to be associated with a depression of the normal coagulation system and excessive bleeding after surgery?**

A Gastrointestinal disease

B Heart disease

C Kidney disease

D Liver disease

E Pulmonary disease

1.39 **Failure to absorb vitamin B_{12} from the gastrointestinal tract results in a syndrome called:**

○ A Erythraemia

○ B Hypochromic anaemia

○ C Pernicious anaemia

○ D Polycythaemia

○ E Thalassaemia

1.40 **Platelet activating factor can cause life-threatening inflammation of the airways. Which of the following statements regarding the platelet-activating factor is CORRECT?**

○ A It is a cholesterol derivative

○ B It is involved in platelet degranulation

○ C It is a potent vasoconstrictor

○ D It is present in platelet granules

○ E It functions as a soluble signal messenger

1.41 **C5a is a complement component. It is a potent:**

○ A Anaphylotoxin

○ B Cytokine

○ C Kinin

○ D Opsonin

○ E Platelet-activating factor

general

1.42 **Which of the following structural proteins enables the erythrocyte to withstand the stress on its plasma membrane as it presses through narrow capillaries?**

- A Actin
- B Integrin
- C Myosin
- D Spectrin
- E Tubulin

1.43 **The serum of a patient admitted for oesophagectomy showed low levels of the lightest plasma protein in terms of weight. In terms of weight, the lightest plasma protein is:**

- A Albumin
- B Beta-globulin
- C Ceruloplasmin
- D Gamma-globulin
- E Transferrin

1.44 **A 27-year-old multiple trauma victim was brought to the Accident and Emergency Department in shock due to massive blood loss. His blood group was unknown but in the transfusion laboratory his blood coagulated when mixed with serum containing anti-B antibodies and similarly coagulated when his serum was mixed with A +ve blood. The blood most suitable to be transfused to him is:**

- A A +ve
- B AB +ve
- C B +ve
- D O −ve
- E O +ve

1.45 Over the past 8 weeks, a 65-year-old man with altered bowel habits has had worsening of his shortness of breath and exertional chest pains. Examination shows pallor and jugular venous distension. Test of the stool for occult blood is positive. Laboratory studies show:

Haemoglobin 7.4 g/dl

Mean corpuscular volume 70 fl

Leukocyte count 5400/mm³

Platelet count 580 000/mm³

Erythrocyte sedimentation 33 mm/h

A blood smear shows hypochronic, microcytic RBCs with moderate poikilocytosis. Which of the following is the most likely diagnosis?

○ A   Anaemia of chronic disease
○ B   Autoimmune haemolytic anaemia
○ C   Folate deficiency anaemia
○ D   Iron deficiency anaemia
○ E   Microangiopathic haemolytic anaemia

1.46 A 62-year-old man with poorly controlled diabetes leading to renal failure presents for haemodialysis. He is found to be anaemic and is given a dose of erythropoietin along with his usual vitamin and mineral supplements. Which of the following intermediates in haematopoiesis will be stimulated by erythropoietin?

○ A   Basophilic erythroblasts
○ B   Erythroid burst-forming units (BFU-E)
○ C   Erythroid colony-forming units (CFU-E)
○ D   Multipotential stem cells
○ E   Reticulocytes

general

1.47 A patient is diagnosed with anaemia secondary to destruction of red blood cells. Which of the following conditions can lead to anaemia characterised by destruction of circulating red blood cells?

- A Bone marrow aplasia
- B Living at high altitude
- C Presence of haemoglobin S
- D Total gastrectomy
- E Vitamin B$_{12}$ deficiency

1.48 You have donated a unit of blood. Which one of the following anticoagulants will the blood bank technician prefer for storage of your donated blood?

- A Citrate
- B Coumarin
- C Enoxaparin
- D Heparin
- E Oxalate

1.49 The signal passes through the neuromuscular junction via the neurotransmitter acetylcholine. After release from the skeletal muscle neuromuscular junction, acetylcholine:

- A Activates presynaptic potassium channels
- B Causes postsynaptic depolarisation
- C Enters the sarcoplasmic reticulum
- D Is triggered by acetylcholinesterase
- E Suppresses noradrenaline secretion

1.50 **In an experiment a drug was used that selectively poisoned a protein involved in skeletal muscle contraction but not smooth muscle contraction. Which of the following proteins is involved in skeletal muscle contraction but not smooth muscle contraction?**

○ A Actin

○ B ATPase

○ C Calmodulin

○ D Troponin

○ E Tropomyosin

1.51 **At the neuromuscular junction, binding of transmitter to postsynaptic receptors leads to:**

○ A A decreased permeability of the postsynaptic membrane to anions

○ B An increased permeability of the postsynaptic membrane to Ca^{2+}

○ C An increased permeability of the presynaptic membrane to Ca^{2+}

○ D An increased permeability of the postsynaptic membrane to small cations

○ E An increased permeability of the postsynaptic membrane to anions

general

23

1.52 **Extracellular calcium plays an important role in neuromuscular transmission. Decreasing the extracellular concentration of calcium:**

○ A Acts like increased magnesium to facilitate release of vesicles at all types of synapses

○ B Activates acetylcholinesterase

○ C Facilitates destruction of transmitter at cholinergic synapses

○ D Inhibits destruction of transmitter at cholinergic synapses

○ E Inhibits release of vesicles at all types of synapses

1.53 **A polytrauma patient with multiorgan failure developed disseminated intravascular coagulation associated with low fibrinogen levels. Fibrinogen:**

○ A Is a naturally occurring fibrinolytic

○ B Is a polypeptide produced by platelets

○ C Is crosslinked by factor XIII to form a clot

○ D Is made from zymogen fibrin

○ E Normally has a concentration between 1.5–4.0 g/l in blood plasma

1.54 **A 26-year-old man experienced haemolysis following a mismatched transfusion. The plasma level of which of the following substances is likely to be raised in this patient?**

○ A Bilirubin

○ B Ferritin

○ C Haemosiderin

○ D Melanin

○ E Transferrin

1.55 **A 45-year-old woman following a complex abdominal aortic aneurysm repair was transfused four units of packed red cells as her postoperative haematocrit was 17%. Which of the following statements regarding the red blood cells is CORRECT?**

○ A Red blood cells are the largest human cell
○ B Red blood cell count of men is more than that of women
○ C Red blood cells collectively store about 1.0 g of iron
○ D Reticulocytes comprise about 10% of circulating red blood cells
○ E The blood types of humans are due to variations in nuclear glycoproteins of red blood cells

1.56 **The immune system protects organisms from infection with layered defences of increasing specificity. Which of the following associations concerning body defence mechanisms against infections is CORRECT?**

○ A First line of defence → lymphocytes
○ B Non-specific cellular mechanism → B lymphocytes
○ C Non-specific humoral mechanism → T lymphocytes
○ D Specific cellular mechanism → cytotoxic T cells
○ E Specific humoral mechanism → complement complex

general

1.57 **The coagulation of blood is a complex process, during which blood forms solid clots. Which of the following statements regarding coagulation is CORRECT?**

○ A Extrinsic pathway activation follows contact of blood with collagen

○ B Tissue factor pathway inhibitor inhibits factor VIIIa-related activation of factor IX and factor X after its original initiation

○ C Prekallikrein is converted to kallikrein during activation of tissue factor pathway

○ D Thrombin converts fibrinogen to fibrin

○ E Vitamin K is an essential co-factor for hepatic synthesis of factor VIII

1.58 **A 26-year-old woman with Rh –ve blood group, delivered an Rh +ve baby. To prevent the Rh incompatibility in subsequent pregnancy, the most appropriate measure is:**

○ A Abortion

○ B Amniocentesis

○ C Blood transfusion

○ D Corticosteroids

○ E Immunoglobulin D

1.59 **Which of the following cell types if selectively destroyed will affect antibody production?**

○ A Eosinophils

○ B Macrophages

○ C Neutrophils

○ D Plasma cells

○ E T lymphocytes

1.60 **A 22-year-old previously healthy woman developed anaemia following blood loss after a road traffic accident. She is most likely to have:**

○ A   A decreased heart rate

○ B   A decreased respiratory rate

○ C   A high reticulocyte count

○ D   A low cardiac output

○ E   A low $p(O_2)$ in arterial blood

1.61 **A previously fit and healthy 28-year-old man after returning from a trip to the Himalayas, having spent 6 months there, arrived in the Accident and Emergency Department complaining of headache and peripheral cyanosis of his fingers. The most probable cause for his complaints is:**

○ A   Anaemia

○ B   Methaemoglobinaemia

○ C   Physiological polycythaemia

○ D   Polycythaemia vera

○ E   Primary polycythaemia

1.62 **If natural killer cells are selectively destroyed by irradiation then:**

○ A   Adaptive immunity will be affected

○ B   Lyses of tumour cells will be accelerated

○ C   Host rejection of tumour cells will be impaired

○ D   Host rejection of cells infected with bacteria will be impaired

○ E   The affected person becomes highly susceptible to fungal infections

general

1.63 **A 62-year-old patient with obstructive jaundice, secondary to inoperable carcinoma of head of pancreas, presented in the Accident and Emergency Department with spontaneous nose bleeding and easy bruisability. The most probable underlying cause for bleeding is:**

   A Iron-deficiency anaemia

   B Low platelet count

   C Vitamin B_{12} deficiency

   D Vitamin C deficiency

   E Vitamin-K-dependent clotting factors deficiency

1.64 **A 10-year-old Somalian boy presented in the surgical outpatient clinic with enlargement of the lower jaw. His blood film showed blast cells and macrophages. The most likely cause for this child's condition is:**

   A Coxsackie B virus

   B Cytomegalovirus

   C Epstein–Barr virus

   D Hepatitis B virus

   E Hepatitis C virus

1.65 **A blood sample from a patient with polycythaemia vera is sent for laboratory analysis. Which of the following abnormalities is most likely to be reported?**

   A High platelet count

   B Low neutrophil count

   C Low total white blood cell count

   D Low red blood cell count

   E Low haematocrit

general

1.66 **Tissue factor is an important coagulation factor necessary for the initiation of thrombin formation from the zymogen prothrombin. Tissue factor:**

○ A Is also known as factor V

○ B Is the cell surface receptor for the serine protease factor VIa

○ C Complexes with factor VIIa to catalyse the conversion of factor X

○ D Is an important component of the intrinsic coagulation pathway

○ E Is normally expressed by endothelial cells

1.67 **Factor V is a protein of the coagulation system. Factor V:**

○ A Like most other coagulation factors is enzymatically active

○ B Deficiency leads to predisposition for thrombosis

○ C Is able to bind to activated platelets

○ D Is inactivated by thrombin

○ E Is activated by activated protein C

1.68 **A 56-year-old man who was bleeding heavily after a prolonged cardiac surgical operation was prescribed recombinant factor VII to control bleeding that was unresponsive to routine measures. Factor VII:**

○ A Is a co-factor in the coagulation cascade

○ B Initiates the process of coagulation in conjunction with tissue factor

○ C Is vitamin K independent

○ D Is produced by platelets

○ E Deficiency is common

general

1.69 **A 23-year-old woman with deep venous thrombosis was diagnosed with protein C deficiency. Protein C:**

   A Is a major physiological anticoagulant

   B Is a vitamin-K-independent serine protease enzyme

   C Is activated by prothrombin into activated protein C

   D In its activated form degrades factor VII

   E Is a break down product of C-reactive protein

1.70 **A 42-year-old woman admitted for elective cholecystectomy revealed that she has factor IX deficiency. Factor IX:**

   A Is a co-factor in the coagulation cascade

   B Is activated by factor V

   C Requires prostacyclin for its activity

   D Acts by hydrolysing one arginine–isoleucine bond in factor X to form factor Xa

   E Deficiency causes haemophilia A

1.71 **A 36-year-old man admitted for elective thyroidectomy revealed that he has a bleeding tendency due to deficiency of factor XI. Factor XI:**

   A Is produced by platelets

   B Is a member of the tissue factor (extrinsic) coagulation pathway

   C Activates factor X

   D Has a plasma half-life of approximately 60 min

   E Deficiency causes haemophilia C

1.72 Factor VIII (FVIII) is an essential clotting factor. The lack of normal FVIII causes haemophilia A, an inherited bleeding disorder. Factor VIII:

○ A Is a serine protease
○ B Is mainly synthesised by the vascular endothelium
○ C Is activated by von Willebrand factor
○ D Is a co-factor to factor X
○ E Is proteolytically inactivated by von Willebrand factor

1.73 Streptokinase was used for thrombolysis of a clot blocking the right branch pulmonary artery in a patient with acute pulmonary embolism. The mechanism of action of streptokinase involves:

○ A Formation of an active complex with plasminogen
○ B Depletion of α2 antiplasmin
○ C Direct conversion of plasminogen to plasmin
○ D Proteolytic activation of fibrinogen
○ E Proteolytic breakdown of fibrin

1.74 In humans there are five types of antibody namely IgA, IgD, IgE, IgG and IgM. Which of the following is a feature of IgA?

○ A It binds to allergens and triggers histamine release from mast cells
○ B It can be found in areas containing mucus
○ C It functions mainly as an antigen receptor on B cells
○ D It provides the majority of antibody-based immunity against invading pathogens
○ E It is expressed on the surface of B cells

general

general

1.75 **In humans there are five types of antibody namely IgA, IgD, IgE, IgG and IgM. Which of the following is a feature of IgE?**

○ A It binds to allergens and triggers histamine release from mast cells

○ B It can be found in areas containing mucus

○ C It functions mainly as an antigen receptor on B cells

○ D It provides the majority of antibody-based immunity against invading pathogens

○ E It is expressed on the surface of B cells

1.76 **A 49-year-old man following elective inguinal hernia repair bled excessively. Investigations suggested that he had a defect of primary haemostasis. Deficiency of which of the following is most likely to cause a defect of primary haemostasis?**

○ A Factor V

○ B Factor VII

○ C Factor IX

○ D Platelets

○ E Protein C

1.77 **A 38-year-old woman presenting with deep venous thrombosis was diagnosed with deficiency of protein S. Which of the following is a feature of protein S?**

○ A It is synthesised by the endothelium

○ B Its synthesis requires vitamin C

○ C It functions as a co-factor to protein C

○ D It is involved in the inactivation of factor IXa

○ E It is involved in the inactivation of factor Xa

1.78 **High-molecular-weight kininogen (HMWK) is a protein from the blood coagulation system. Which of the following is a feature of HMWK?**

A It functions as a co-factor for bradykinin

B It is a strong activator of cysteine proteases

C It is enzymatically active

D It is necessary for the activation of factor XI by factor XIIa

E It is one of the early participants of the extrinsic pathway of coagulation

1.79 **Antithrombin III is a serine protease inhibitor with an important role in haemostasis. Which of the following substances enhances antithrombin III activity?**

A Aspirin

B Citrate

C Coumarin

D Heparin

E Warfarin

1.80 **The coagulation factors are generally serine proteases. However, there are some exceptions. Which of the following coagulation factors is not a serine protease?**

A Factor I

B Factor II

C Factor IX

D Factor XII

E Factor XIII

general

1.81 T helper cells are a subgroup of lymphocytes that play an important role in establishing and maximizing the capabilities of the immune system. Which of the following is a feature of T helper cells?

   ○ A They activate other immune cells

   ○ B They are increased in HIV infection

   ○ C They express the surface protein CD3

   ○ D They have cytotoxic activity

   ○ E They have phagocytic activity

1.82 Dendritic cells are immune cells. Which of the following organs is most likely to have dendritic cells?

   ○ A Heart

   ○ B Kidney

   ○ C Muscle

   ○ D Skin

   ○ E Stomach

1.83 Cytotoxic T cells are a component of the adaptive immune system. Which of the following is a feature of the cytotoxic T cells?

   ○ A They activate other immune cells

   ○ B They belong to a subgroup of B lymphocytes

   ○ C They express the surface protein CD4

   ○ D They have a pathogenetic role in HIV infection

   ○ E They have cytotoxic activity

1.84 **A patient admitted for elective coronary artery bypass surgery was noted to have prolonged activated partial thromboplastin time. The most likely cause is:**

○ A Heparin therapy

○ B Liver disease

○ C Malabsorption of vitamin K

○ D Poor factor VII synthesis

○ E Warfarin therapy

1.85 **A patient admitted for elective cholecystectomy is noted to have prolonged prothrombin time. The most likely cause is:**

○ A Antiphospholipid antibody

○ B Haemophilia

○ C Heparin therapy

○ D Liver disease

○ E von Willebrand factor deficiency

1.86 **A 38-year-old man being haemofiltered in the intensive care unit for acute renal failure following polytrauma was diagnosed with heparin-induced thrombocytopaenia secondary to administration of unfractionated heparin. Which of the following is a feature of heparin-induced thrombocytopaenia?**

○ A It develops 4 weeks after the administration of heparin

○ B It is a thrombotic disorder

○ C It is best treated by administration of low-molecular-weight heparin

○ D It is characterised by increased bleeding

○ E It is cured by administration of protamine sulphate

1.87   **Low-molecular-weight heparin (LMWH) permits outpatient treatment of conditions such as deep vein thrombosis. Which of the following is a feature of LMWH?**

○   A   It has an average molecular weight of 20 kDa

○   B   It has to be administered as a continuous infusion

○   C   It has a very high risk of osteoporosis following prolonged use

○   D   It has a smaller risk of heparin-induced thrombocytopaenia

○   E   It is mandatory to monitor LMWH with aPTT three times a day

1.88   **A 43-year-old woman admitted for elective cholecystectomy was noted to have prolonged bleeding time. Which of the following is the most likely cause for prolonged bleeding time in this woman?**

○   A   Factor II deficiency

○   B   Factor VII deficiency

○   C   Factor IX deficiency

○   D   Haemophilia

○   E   Thrombocytopaenia

1.89   **D-dimer assay of a patient revealed a value exceeding 500 ng/ml. What is the most likely cause of this positive assay?**

○   A   Aspirin therapy

○   B   Deep venous thrombosis

○   C   Thrombocytopaenia

○   D   von Willebrand's disease

○   E   Warfarin therapy

1.90 **The thrombin clotting time result of a patient is outside the reference interval. What is the most likely cause for this abnormal result?**

○ A Aspirin therapy
○ B Heparin therapy
○ C Thrombocytopaenia
○ D von Willebrand's disease
○ E Warfarin therapy

general

SECTION 2: CARDIOVASCULAR PHYSIOLOGY – QUESTIONS

For each question given below choose the ONE BEST option.

2.1 **Ventricular filling occurs due to delay in which part of the cardiac conducting system?**

- ○ A SA node
- ○ B AV node
- ○ C Purkinje system
- ○ D Bundle branches
- ○ E Atrial muscle

2.2 **A 37-year-old man suffering from severe haemorrhage caused by a motorcycle accident has a blood pressure of 70/33 mmHg, a heart rate of 140 beats/min, and a weak pulse. Immediately following transfusion of 3 l of blood, his blood pressure rises to 100/70 mmHg and his heart rate slows to 90 beats/min. Which of the following is decreased due to transfusion of the blood?**

- ○ A Cardiac output
- ○ B Right atrial pressure
- ○ C Stroke volume
- ○ D Total peripheral resistance
- ○ E Pulmonary artery pressure

39

cardiovascular

2.3 **A 35-year-old man has a 30% decrease in cardiac output following a haemorrhage in which he lost an estimated 20–30% of his blood volume. Which of the following changes in pulmonary vascular resistance (PVR) and pulmonary artery pressure (PAP) would be most likely to result from the decrease in cardiac output?**

	PVR	PAP
A	Decrease	Decrease
B	Decrease	Increase
C	Increase	Decrease
D	Increase	Increase
E	No change	No change

2.4 **A 24-year-old man arrived in the Accident and Emergency Department with a stab in right side of chest. X-ray chest confirmed haemothorax. It was estimated that about 20% blood volume had been lost due to acute haemorrhage. It is true to say that in this patient:**

A Coronary arteries are constricted due to catecholamines

B Plasma adrenaline stimulates hypothalamic thirst centre

C Plasma vasopressin is increased in response to reduced ECF volume

D Plasma aldosterone increase will lead to retention of potassium

E The major acid–base abnormality will be hyperkalaemic alkalosis

2.5 **An 18-year-old man comes to casualty with a fracture of right femoral shaft. It is estimated that about 500 ml of blood volume has been lost due to acute haemorrhage, It is true to say that in this patient:**

O A The brain blood flow will be reduced
O B The mesenteric blood flow is increased
O C The lactic acid production will be reduced
O D The skin vessels are constricted
O E Veins are dilated

2.6 **Which of the following compensatory factors is responsible for increasing the blood pressure in a 35-year-old patient who is in shock with blood pressure of 50 mmHg?**

O A Atrial stretch receptors
O B Baroreceptor reflex
O C Bainbridge reflex
O D Carotid body chemoreceptors
O E Ischaemic brain response

2.7 **Which of the following peptides can increase blood pressure acutely and cause hypokalaemia chronically?**

O A Angiotensin II
O B Atrial natriuretic factor
O C Desmopressin
O D Endorphin
O E Oxytocin

cardiovascular

2.8 **A 32-year-old man suffering from severe haemorrhage caused by a road traffic accident has a blood pressure of 70/30 mmHg, a heart rate of 140 beats/min and a weak pulse. Immediately following infusion of 3 l of blood, his blood pressure rises to 100/70 mmHg and his heart rate slows to 90 beats per minute. Which of the following is most likely to decrease due to infusion of the blood?**

○ A Baroreceptor discharge
○ B Cardiac output
○ C Right atrial pressure
○ D Stroke volume
○ E Total peripheral resistance

2.9 **A 36-year-old woman presented in the Accident and Emergency Department with irregularly irregular pulse. On ECG, there were absent P-waves with irregularity of RR interval. The woman most likely had:**

○ A Atrial fibrillation
○ B Atrial flutter
○ C Atrial tachycardia
○ D Ventricular fibrillation
○ E Ventricular tachycardia

2.10 **The electrocardiogram (ECG) of a 35-year-old man shows small or low-voltage QRS complexes. The patient most likely has:**

○ A Atrial fibrillation
○ B Myocardial infarction
○ C Pericardial effusion
○ D Thyrotoxicosis
○ E Ventricular tachycardia

2.11 **The electrocardiogram (ECG) of a patient on surgical ward shows flattened (notched) T-waves. The patient is most likely to have:**

○ A Hypokalaemia

○ B Hyperkalaemia

○ C Hypocalcaemia

○ D Myocardial infarction

○ E Thyrotoxicosis

2.12 **The electrocardiogram (ECG) of a patient on the surgical ward shows prominent U-waves. The most likely condition associated with this ECG finding is:**

○ A Hypokalaemia

○ B Hypocalcaemia

○ C Hyponatraemia

○ D Hypertension

○ E Myxoedema

2.13 **The electrocardiogram (ECG) of a patient shows prolonged PR interval. The normal duration of PR interval is:**

○ A 0.001–0.002 s

○ B 0.12–0.20 s

○ C 0.25–0.35 s

○ D 0.35–0.45 s

○ E 0.45–0.50 s

cardiovascular

2.14 **The electrocardiogram (ECG) of a patient shows a prolonged QT interval. A normal QT interval is usually about:**

○ A 0.10 s

○ B 0.20 s

○ C 0.30 s

○ D 0.40 s

○ E 0.50 s

2.15 **A patient with chest pain had ST depression on his electrocardiogram (ECG). ST segment ordinarily lasts about:**

○ A 0.02 s

○ B 0.04 s

○ C 0.08 s

○ D 0.16 s

○ E 0.8 s

2.16 **During a street fight a young man immediately fainted on receiving a direct stroke to his left carotid sinus. Which of the following occurred during this event?**

○ A Decreased pressure at the carotid sinus baroreceptors

○ B Decreased firing rate of the carotid sinus fibres

○ C Decreased firing rate of cardiac sympathetic fibres

○ D Decreased firing rate of the vagus nerve efferents

○ E Increased heart rate

2.17 **While investigating a 34-year-old man with essential hypertension it was noticed that he had blood renin level of 5 ng/ml per hour (normal 1–2.5 ng/ml per hour). Which of the following could be a major stimulus for the release of renin from the juxtaglomerular apparatus in this patient?**

○ A Dilatation of renal arteries
○ B Hypertension
○ C Increased delivery of sodium to the distal tubules
○ D Increased sympathetic activity via renal nerves
○ E Overhydration

2.18 **The autonomic nervous system (or visceral nervous system) is the part of the nervous system that controls homeostasis or the constancy of the 'milieu intérieur'. It does so mostly by controlling cardiovascular, digestive and respiratory functions. Which of the following statements correctly describes effects of autonomic nervous activity on the cardiovascular system in a healthy subject?**

○ A Inhibition of parasympathetic nerves increases heart rate
○ B Inhibition of parasympathetic nerves increases total peripheral resistance
○ C Inhibition of parasympathetic nerves decreases total peripheral resistance
○ D Stimulation of parasympathetic nerves decreases the strength of cardiac ventricular contractions
○ E Stimulation of sympathetic nerves decreases the strength of cardiac ventricular contractions

cardiovascular

2.19 **A patient with cardiac arrest is resuscitated and now shows shortened, irregular QT intervals on his ECG. Which of the following ion channels is responsible for the plateau phase of the cardiac action potential that is reflected by the QT interval?**

- A Cl^- channels
- B K^+ channels
- C Na^+ channels
- D   L-type Ca^{2+} channels
- E   T-type Ca^{2+} channels

2.20 **Total peripheral resistance refers to the cumulative resistance of the thousands of arterioles in the body. If a patient at rest has a systolic/diastolic blood pressure of 130/70 mmHg and a cardiac output of 5 l/min, what is his total peripheral resistance?**

- A   18 mmHg × min/l
- B   20 mmHg × min/l
- C   22 mmHg × min/l
- D   0.05 l/min × mmHg
- E   20 l/min × mmHg

2.21 **A 35-year-old man with congenital aortic stenosis is admitted for cardiac function testing. O_2 consumption (measured by analysis of mixed expired gas) in this patient is 300 ml/min, arterial O_2 content is 20 ml/100 ml blood, pulmonary arterial O_2 content is 15 ml/100 ml blood and his heart rate is 60/min. His cardiac stroke volume is:**

- A 1 ml
- B 10 ml
- C 60 ml
- D 100 ml
- E 200 ml

2.22 **Which of the following conditions is most likely to increase the resistance to blood flow in the cerebral circulation of humans?**

- A Reduction of $p_a(O_2)$ to < 50 mmHg
- B Inhalation of a gas mixture enriched with CO_2
- C Reduction in haematocrit to < 0.30 by isovolaemic exchange transfusion
- D Elevation in systemic arterial pressure from 100 to 130 mmHg
- E Epileptic seizure

cardiovascular

2.23 **Acute vasodilatation usually results if sympathetic nerve fibres that supply blood vessels in the arms or legs are cut. The acute vasodilatation is due to:**

○ A Compensatory increase of adrenaline release from the adrenal medulla

○ B Compensatory increase of noradrenaline release from the adrenal medulla

○ C Development of hypersensitivity to circulating catecholamines

○ D Loss of sympathetic tone

○ E Parasympathetic fibres dilating blood vessels

2.24 **A 65-year-old woman with aortic stenosis was investigated in the cardiac catheterisation laboratory. The following measurements were made: oxygen uptake 200 ml/min, oxygen concentration in peripheral vein 7 vol% (7 ml oxygen/100 ml blood), oxygen concentration in pulmonary artery 10 vol% (10 ml oxygen/100 ml blood), oxygen concentration in aorta 15 vol% (15 ml oxygen/100 ml blood). What will be the cardiac output of this patient?**

○ A 1333 ml/min

○ B 2000 ml/min

○ C 2500 ml/min

○ D 3000 ml/min

○ E 4000 ml/min

2.25 **Under resting conditions a marathon runner compared to untrained people will have a higher:**

○ A Cardiac output

○ B Cardiac stroke volume

○ C Heart rate

○ D Oxygen consumption

○ E Respiratory rate

2.26 **A 36-year-old man was brought to the Accident and Emergency Department following an automobile accident in which he suffered a pelvic fracture with significant internal blood loss resulting in haemorrhagic shock. Which of the following organs is especially vulnerable during the shock phase in this patient?**

○ A Brain

○ B Heart muscle

○ C Kidneys

○ D Skin

○ E Skeletal muscle

2.27 **A 56-year-old man suffered a myocardial infarction following which the velocity of impulse conduction through the atrioventricular (AV) node decreased. This patient will have:**

○ A Atrial fibrillation

○ B Decreased PR interval

○ C Disappearance of the T-wave

○ D Increased heart rate

○ E Increased PR interval

cardiovascular

2.28 **Purkinje fibres (or Purkyne tissue) are located in the inner ventricular walls of the heart, just beneath the endocardium. These fibres are specialised myocardial fibres that conduct an electrical stimulus or impulse that enables the heart to contract in a co-ordinated fashion. The rate of conduction of action potentials in Purkinje fibres is about:**

○   A   0.2–1.1 m/s
○   B   1.5–4.0 m/s
○   C   5.0–8.5 m/s
○   D   9.0–12.5 m/s
○   E   15.0–18.5 m/s

2.29 **Electrocardiogram of a patient with chest pain showed inverted T-waves. The T-wave of the normal electrocardiogram is caused by:**

○   A   Atrial repolarisation
○   B   Atrial depolarisation
○   C   Bundle of His depolarisation
○   D   Ventricular depolarisation
○   E   Ventricular repolarisation

2.30 **Cardiac cycle is the term used to describe the sequence of events that occur as the heart works to pump blood through the body. The opening of the atrioventricular (AV) valves occurs at about the same time in the cardiac cycle as the:**

○   A   Beginning of diastole
○   B   Beginning of systole
○   C   End of isovolumic contraction
○   D   First heart sound
○   E   QRS complex of the electrocardiogram

2.31 **Cardiac cycle is the term used to describe the sequence of events that occur as the heart works to pump blood through the body. Closure of the atrioventricular (AV) valves occurs at about the time in the cardiac cycle as the:**

○ A Beginning of diastole

○ B End of isovolumic relaxation

○ C First heart sound

○ D Second heart sound

○ E T complex in the electrocardiogram

2.32 **In the laboratory, a cardiac catheterisation is done in a 35-year-old healthy man. The blood sample withdrawn from the catheter shows 70% oxygen saturation, and the pressure recording shows oscillations from a maximum of 24 mmHg to a minimum of 12 mmHg. Where was the catheter tip located?**

○ A Ductus arteriosus

○ B Foramen ovale

○ C Left atrium

○ D Pulmonary artery

○ E Right atrium

2.33 The following cardiac catheterisation data are obtained during evaluation of a 19-year-old man:

	Pressure (mmHg)	O_2 saturation (%)
Right atrium	7 (N = 5)	90 (N = 75)
Right ventricle	35/7 (N = 25/5)	90 (N = 75)
Pulmonary artery	35/8 (N = 25/15)	90 (N = 75)
Left atrium	7 (N = 9)	95 (N = 95)
Left ventricle	110/7 (N = 110/9)	95 (N = 95)
Aorta	110/75 (N = 110/75)	95 (N = 95)

N = Normal value

Which of the following is the most likely diagnosis?

O   A   Atrial septal defect

O   B   Mitral stenosis

O   C   Patent ductus arteriosus

O   D   Pulmonary stenosis

O   E   Tricuspid insufficiency

2.34 The procedure for measuring cardiac output using the Fick principle involves measuring oxygen uptake by the lungs and measuring the arterial-to-venous oxygen tension difference. Because of differences in the oxygen content of blood emerging from different organs, which of the following is the best source of venous blood for this measurement?

O   A   Jugular vein

O   B   Pulmonary artery

O   C   Pulmonary vein

O   D   Saphenous vein

O   E   Superior vena cava

2.35 A 2-week-old male baby was brought to the paediatric emergency department by his parents because his lips had turned blue on three occasions during feeding; he also sweated during feeding. He was born at 38 weeks' gestation and weighed 2466 g (5 lb 7 oz); he currently weighs 2778 g (6 lb 2 oz). On examination his temperature was 37.8°C (100°F), blood pressure was 75/45 mmHg, pulse was 170/min, and respiratory rate was 44/min. A grade 3/6 harsh systolic ejection murmur was heard at the left upper sternal border. An X-ray film of the chest showed a small boot-shaped heart and decreased pulmonary vascular markings. Which of the following is the most likely diagnosis?

- A Anomalous left coronary artery
- B Atrial septal defect
- C Endocardial fibroelastosis
- D Tetralogy of Fallot
- E Total anomalous pulmonary venous return

2.36 Cardiac index is a derived haemodynamic parameter. Cardiac index:

- A Increases with disease
- B Is related to body surface area
- C Is about 5–6 l/min
- D Increases with age
- E Is related to body weight

2.37 **A 25-year-old man was brought into the Accident and Emergency Department following an automobile accident in which he sustained steering wheel injury. His blood pressure was 120/90 mmHg. When he inhaled his systolic blood pressure dropped to 100 mmHg. This man is most likely to have:**

- A Pulsus alternans
- B Pulsus bisferiens
- C Pulsus paradoxus
- D Pulsus parvus
- E Pulsus tardus

2.38 **Carotid bodies are located at the bifurcation of common carotid arteries. Stimulation of these causes:**

- A Decrease in depth of respiration
- B Decreased discharge in the IXth cranial nerve
- C Increased discharge in the Xth cranial nerve
- D Increase in blood pressure
- E Stimulation of respiratory centre

2.39 **A 28-year-old man is involved in an exercise, which involves isometric muscle contractions. Which of the following circulatory changes is most likely to happen during this type of exercise?**

- A Blood flow to the contracting muscles is increased
- B Diastolic pressure rises
- C Heart rate decreases
- D Systolic pressure decreases
- E Stroke volume increases markedly

2.40 **A 58-year-old woman suffered a left ventricular infarct that affected her left ventricular function. Which of the following parameters would best indicate that the functioning capability of his heart is less than optimum?**

○ A Stroke volume (SV) = 40 ml, end-diastolic volume (EDV) = 95 ml, end-systolic volume (ESV) = 55 ml, ejection fraction (EF) = 40%

○ B SV = 32 ml, EDV = 150 ml, ESV = 118 ml, EF = 21%

○ C SV = 45 ml, EDV = 175 ml, ESV = 130 ml, EF = 42%

○ D SV = 50 ml, EDV = 195 ml, ESV = 145 ml, EF = 42%

○ E SV = 70 ml, EDV = 125 ml, ESV = 55 ml, EF = 50%

2.41 **The proportions of substrates utilised vary greatly with the nutritional status. Under normal (basal) conditions, most of the energy used by cardiac muscle comes from metabolism of:**

○ A Fatty acids

○ B Glucose

○ C Ketoacids

○ D Lactate

○ E Pyruvate

2.42 **The Frank–Starling law of the heart states that:**

○ A Blood entering the atria is pumped immediately into the ventricles

○ B Cardiac output is controlled entirely by the activity of the heart

○ C Heart rate controls cardiac output during exercise

○ D The heart can pump a certain amount of blood and no more

○ E Within physiological limits, the heart pumps all the blood that comes to it

cardiovascular

2.43 **In an experiment set up to measure resistance to flow in an artery the pressure at one end of the artery is 60 mmHg, the pressure at the other end of the artery is 20 mmHg and the flow through the artery is 200 ml/min. What is the resistance of the artery expressed in the above units?**

- A 0.05
- B 0.1
- C 0.2
- D 0.4
- E 0.6

2.44 **Poiseuille–Hagen formula can be used for determining the relation between the resistance of a blood vessel and its diameter. If the resistance of a blood vessel is 16 PRU then doubling the vessel diameter would change the resistance to:**

- A 1 PRU
- B 2 PRU
- C 4 PRU
- D 8 PRU
- E 10 PRU

2.45 **A patient is administered a sympathetic agonist. One of the expected effects of this drug is a rise in total peripheral resistance. Sympathetic stimulation of which vessels causes the greatest increase in total peripheral resistance?**

- A Arteries
- B Arterioles
- C Capillaries
- D Veins
- E Venules

2.46 The sinoatrial node is the pacemaker for the heart because the SA node:

○ A Has the highest rate of automatic discharge
○ B Has the most stable transmembrane potential
○ C Is the most richly enervated structure in the heart
○ D Is the only structure in the heart capable of generating action potentials
○ E Is the cardiac cell least sensitive to catecholamines

2.47 An independence of the P-waves and the QRS complexes of the electrocardiogram (ECG) indicates:

○ A A conduction block in the left bundle branch
○ B A failure of the atrioventricular (AV) node to conduct
○ C An early repolarisation of ventricular fibres
○ D Depression of the sinoatrial node
○ E Slowing of conduction at the atrioventricular node

2.48 If the end-diastolic ventricular volumes are increased (within physiological limits):

○ A Cardiac output would be decreased
○ B The force of cardiac contraction would be decreased
○ C The output of the right ventricle would exceed the output of the left ventricle
○ D The stroke volume would be increased
○ E Venous pressure would be decreased

cardiovascular

2.49 Digoxin is a positive inotropic agent. Positive inotropism refers to:

O A Decreased stroke volume

O B Decreased end-diastolic volume

O C Increased contractility of the heart

O D Movement of blood elements related to a change in chemical gradient

O E Repolarisation of the SA node

2.50 Usually, the resting pulse pressure in healthy adults, in sitting position, it is about 40 mmHg. Pulse pressure is:

O A Determined by the stroke volume

O B Decreased when arterial resistance decreases

O C The highest pressure measured in the arteries

O D The lowest pressure measured in the arteries

O E The time averaged pressure in the arteries

2.51 The following values were obtained in a normal male patient:

Heart rate	70 beats/min
Arterial [O_2]	0.24 ml O_2/min
Venous [O_2]	0.16 ml O_2/min
Whole body O_2 consumption	500 ml/min
Pulmonary diastolic pressure	15 mmHg
Pulmonary systolic pressure	25 mmHg
Wedge pressure	5 mmHg

cardiovascular

What is the cardiac output?

O   A   1.65 l/min
O   B   4.55 l/min
O   C   5.00 l/min
O   D   6.25 l/min
O   E   8.00 l/min

2.52 The following values were obtained in a normal male patient:

Heart rate	70 beats/min
Arterial [O_2]	0.24 ml O_2/min
Venous [O_2]	0.16 ml O_2/min
Whole body O_2 consumption	500 ml/min
Pulmonary diastolic pressure	15 mmHg
Pulmonary systolic pressure	25 mmHg
Wedge pressure	5 mmHg

What is the stroke volume?

O   A   75 ml
O   B   80 ml
O   C   85 ml
O   D   90 ml
O   E   95 ml

2.53 The following values were obtained in a normal male patient:

Heart rate	70 beats/min
Arterial [O_2]	0.24 ml O_2/min
Venous [O_2]	0.16 ml O_2/min
Whole body O_2 consumption	500 ml/min
Pulmonary diastolic pressure	15 mmHg
Pulmonary systolic pressure	25 mmHg
Wedge pressure	5 mmHg

What is the pulmonary vascular resistance?

- A   1.5 resistance units (mmHg/l per min)
- B   2.0 resistance units (mmHg/l per min)
- C   2.5 resistance units (mmHg/l per min)
- D   3.0 resistance units (mmHg/l per min)
- E   3.5 resistance units (mmHg/l per min)

2.54 An electrocardiogram of a patient with tachycardia revealed a pattern consistent with a small ventricular posteroseptal infarct resulting from inadequate blood supply. Despite the rapid heartbeat, its regularity indicates that the infarct has involved only:

- A   A localised region of ventricular myocardium
- B   Atrioventricular bundle
- C   Atrioventricular node
- D   Both atrioventricular node and bundle
- E   Sinoatrial node

2.55 The effect of parasympathetic nervous stimulation on the heart is:

○ A Slowing of the heart
○ B Increased activity of the sinoatrial (SA) node
○ C Increased activity of the atrioventricular (AV) node
○ D Increased conduction velocity through bundle of His
○ E Increased force of contraction

2.56 A 45-year-old man, with ischaemic heart disease and good left ventricular function, admitted for elective coronary artery bypass surgery, had oxygen consumption = 300 ml/min, arterial oxygen content = 20 ml/100 ml blood, pulmonary arterial oxygen content = 15 ml/100 ml blood and heart rate = 100 beats/min on preoperative assessment. What is the stroke volume in this patient?

○ A 1 ml
○ B 10 ml
○ C 60 ml
○ D 100 ml
○ E 200 ml

2.57 If the blood supply (flow) to a given tissue bed is maintained constant and tissue metabolism is altered, oxygen levels in venous blood will change in an appropriate and predictable way. Which of the following factors is most likely to decrease oxygen extraction by tissue?

○ A Fever
○ B Hyperthyroidism
○ C Infusion of adrenaline
○ D Ingestion of thyroxine tablets
○ E Tissue cooling

cardiovascular

2.58 **The brain is the least tolerant of all the body organs to ischaemia. Interruption of cerebral blood flow for as little as 5 s may cause fainting (syncope), while even transient decreases in blood flow result in dizziness. What percentage of cardiac output is received by brain?**

○ A 1%
○ B 15%
○ C 35%
○ D 50%
○ E 75%

2.59 **The angioarchitecture and physiology of the myocardium result in several unique aspects of the coronary circulation. One of these is the anatomical considerations of the blood supply itself. The left coronary flow:**

○ A Does not exhibit reactive hyperaemia
○ B Is independent of the oxygen needs of the myocardium
○ C Is the same as the right coronary flow
○ D Peak in early systole
○ E Peak in early diastole

2.60 **The primary function of the skin circulation is to help maintain body temperature. Blood vessels constrict to prevent heat loss and dilate to facilitate transfer of heat from the body core to the body surface. What percentage of cardiac output is received by skin?**

○ A 2%
○ B 12%
○ C 20%
○ D 50%
○ E 70%

SECTION 3:
RESPIRATORY PHYSIOLOGY –
QUESTIONS

For each question given below choose the ONE BEST option.

3.1   **A 65-year-old coal miner with decades of work-related exposure to dust is examined for pulmonary fibrosis. His FEV$_1$ is 75% (normal > 65%) and his arterial oxygen saturation is 92%. His alveolar ventilation is 6000 ml/min at a tidal volume of 600 ml and a breathing rate of 12 breaths/min. Pathological changes in lung compliance and residual volume are also documented in this patient. Which of the following best describes this patient's lung compliance measured under static conditions?**

○ A Change in distending pressure $(p_{alv} - p_{pl})$ divided by change in lung volume

○ B Change in distending pressure $(p_{alv} - p_{pl})$ minus the change in lung volume

○ C Change in elastic recoil pressure $(p_{alv} - p_{pl})$

○ D Change in lung volume divided by change in distending pressure $(p_{alv} - p_{pl})$

○ E Lung volume divided by recoil pressure $(p_{alv} - p_{pl})$

respiratory

3.2 **A 65-year-old coal miner with decades of work-related exposure to dust is examined for pulmonary fibrosis. His FEV$_1$ is 75% (normal > 65%) and his arterial oxygen saturation is 92%. His alveolar ventilation is 6000 ml/min at a tidal volume of 600 ml and a breathing rate of 12 breaths/min. Pathological changes in lung compliance and residual volume are also documented in this patient. This patient's residual volume:**

○ A   Cannot be measured directly with a spirometer
○ B   Is part of vital capacity
○ C   Is part of the expiratory reserve volume
○ D   Is the volume at which the lungs tend to recoil outward
○ E   Represents the resting volume of the lungs

3.3 **A 65-year-old coal miner with decades of work-related exposure to dust is examined for pulmonary fibrosis. His FEV$_1$ is 75% (normal > 65%) and his arterial oxygen saturation is 92%. His alveolar ventilation is 6000 ml/min at a tidal volume of 600 ml and a breathing rate of 12 breaths/min. Pathological changes in lung compliance and residual volume are also documented in this patient. What is this patient's anatomical dead space?**

○ A   100 ml
○ B   120 ml
○ C   150 ml
○ D   200 ml
○ E   250 ml

3.4   **A 26-year-old man was seen in the Accident and
Emergency Department following a stab injury to
his left chest in the third intercostal space in the
midaxillary line. He was haemodynamically stable
and his chest X-ray showed a pneumothorax. The
most likely response in this patient upon entry of
air into the chest would be for the:**

O   A   Lung to collapse inward and the chest wall to collapse
         inward

O   B   Lung to collapse inward and the chest wall to spring
         outward

O   C   Lung to expand outward and the chest wall to spring
         inward

O   D   Lung to expand outward and the chest wall to spring
         outward

O   E   Lung volume to be unaffected and chest wall to spring
         outward

3.5   **Under normal conditions the amount of O_2 taken
up is a function of pulmonary blood flow; that
is, normally, O_2 transfer is perfusion-limited.
Which of the following conditions would favour a
diffusion limitation of O_2 transfer from alveolar
to pulmonary capillary blood?**

O   A   Breathing hyperbaric gas mixture
O   B   Chronic obstructive lung disease
O   C   Increased ventilatory rate
O   D   Mild exercise
O   E   Pulmonary oedema

respiratory

3.6 **A 42-year-old woman committed suicide by a self-inflicted gunshot wound through her mouth, which injured her brainstem. She died of immediate respiratory failure as result of this injury. Which of the following statements accurately describes the interaction of respiratory centres in the brainstem and their effect on respiration?**

○ A Sectioning the brainstem above the pons, near the inferior colliculus of the midbrain results in immediate respiratory arrest

○ B The medullary rhythmicity centre is a discrete group of neurones whose rhythmicity is abolished when the brain is transected above and below this area

○ C Transection above the apneustic centre results in prolonged expiration and very short inspiration

○ D Transection of the afferent fibres of the vagus and glossopharyngeal nerves results in prolonged inspiration and shortened expiration

○ E The apneustic and pneumotaxic centre of the pons are essential for maintenance of the basic rhythm of respiration

3.7 **A 36-year-old patient with multiple rib fractures and flail chest was ventilated in the ICU. In this patient if alveolar ventilation is halved (and if CO_2 production remains unchanged), then:**

○ A Alveolar CO_2 pressure ($p_A(CO_2)$) will be halved

○ B Alveolar O_2 pressure ($p_A(O_2)$) will double

○ C Arterial O_2 pressure ($p_a(O_2)$) will double

○ D Arterial CO_2 pressure ($p_a(CO_2)$) will double

○ E Arterial O_2 pressure ($p_a(O_2)$) will not change

respiratory

3.8 A 35-year-old patient in ICU is given 100% O_2 to breathe. Following this, his arterial blood gases are determined and a $p_a(O_2)$ of 125 mmHg is measured. This result is associated with:

○ A Anatomical right-to-left shunting
○ B Diffusion abnormality
○ C Profound hypoventilation
○ D The normal response
○ E Ventilation/perfusion inequality

3.9 A 38-year-old man with low arterial oxygen saturation is evaluated for anatomical and physiological lung dead space. The anatomical dead space in this patient with a tidal volume of 500 ml is 125 ml when determined by plotting nitrogen concentration versus expired volume after a single inspiration of 100% O_2 (Fowler's method). If the patient's lungs are healthy and the $p_a(CO_2)$ is 40 mmHg, the mixed expired CO_2 tension ($p_E(CO_2)$ should be about:

○ A 0 mmHg
○ B 10 mmHg
○ C 20 mmHg
○ D 30 mmHg
○ E 40 mmHg

respiratory

3.10 **A 68-year-old man with progressively increasing shortness of breath and past history of work-related exposure to asbestos comes for evaluation of his lung function. Which of the following variables must be known to calculate inspiratory reserve volume in this patient?**

○ A Tidal volume and expiratory reserve volume

○ B Tidal volume and residual volume

○ C Tidal volume, vital capacity and expiratory reserve volume

○ D Tidal volume, vital capacity and residual volume

○ E Tidal volume and vital capacity

3.11 **You have been asked to comment on arterial blood gas analysis of a patient that shows a pH = 7.56, bicarbonate = 21 mEq/l, $p(O_2)$ = 50 mmHg and $p(CO_2)$ = 25 mmHg. This patient probably:**

○ A Has severe chronic lung disease

○ B Is an emergency room patient with severely depressed respiration as a result of a heroin overdose

○ C Is a subject in a clinical research experiment who has been breathing a gas mixture of 10% oxygen and 90% nitrogen for a few minutes

○ D Is a lowlander who has been vacationing at high altitude for two weeks

○ E Is an adult psychiatric patient who swallowed an overdose of aspirin

3.12 **If you are flying in the cabin of an aeroplane that is pressurised to an equivalent altitude of 10 000 ft (barometric pressure of 523 mmHg), your $p_A(O_2)$ compared with your predicted $p_A(O_2)$ at sea level will:**

○ A Decrease to < 100 mmHg because the fraction of inspired air that is O_2 (F_iO_2) will be < 0.2

○ B Decrease to < 100 mmHg even though the F_iO_2 is still around 0.2

○ C Not change because water vapour pressure is low at high altitude

○ D Not change because $p_a(CO_2)$ will decrease because of hyperventilation

○ E Not change because the cabin is pressurised

3.13 **Following a routine medical check-up a 35-year-old man in the clinic tells you that his arterial oxygen ($p_a(O_2)$) is usually slightly below the alveolar oxygen ($p_A(O_2)$). He wants to know why this is so. You will tell him that this finding:**

○ A Is due to significant diffusion gradients
○ B Is due to reaction time of O_2 with haemoglobin
○ C Is due to unloading of CO_2
○ D Is normal and due to shunted blood
○ E Is the result of a major cardiac right-to-left shunt (ventricular septal defect)

respiratory

3.14 **A 2-year-old boy with repeated chest infections and frequent episodes of intestinal obstruction was diagnosed with cystic fibrosis. Which of the following statements about cystic fibrosis is CORRECT?**

O   A   Cystic fibrosis is caused by a defective Na^+ transporter across airway epithelial cells, resulting in thick airway mucus

O   B   Cystic fibrosis is more common in African-Americans than in Whites

O   C   Sweat of cystic fibrosis patients has elevated Na^+ and low Cl^- content

O   D   The gene that is abnormal in cystic fibrosis encodes a cAMP-regulated Cl^- channel

O   E   The gene that is abnormal in cystic fibrosis is located on the X chromosome

3.15 **You are asked to assess a patient on an intensive care unit who is ventilated at a frequency of 12 per minute and a tidal volume of 0.6 l. His arterial pH is > 7.6. To correct his respiratory alkalosis, you should:**

O   A   Decrease dead space
O   B   Decrease tidal volume
O   C   Increase oxygen fraction
O   D   Increase minute ventilation
O   E   Use positive end-expiratory pressure (PEEP)

3.16 **A 36-year-old man going for a mountaineering trip to the Himalayas was prescribed acetazolamide (a carbonic anhydrase inhibitor) by his doctor for prevention of mountain sickness. Which of the following statements about the action of acetazolamide is correct? Acetazolamide:**

○ A Causes metabolic alkalosis
○ B Directly suppresses the respiratory drive
○ C Directly increases the respiratory drive
○ D Increases bicarbonate concentration in the urine
○ E Increases hydrogen concentration in the urine

3.17 **Oxygen is carried in the blood in two forms. Most is carried combined with haemoglobin but there is a very small amount dissolved in the plasma. How much oxygen is normally carried in the blood?**

○ A 2 ml oxygen/100 ml blood
○ B 5 ml oxygen/100 ml blood
○ C 10 ml oxygen/100 ml blood
○ D 20 ml oxygen/100 ml blood
○ E 30 ml oxygen/100 ml blood

3.18 **There are three ways by which carbon dioxide is transported in the blood. About 70% of the carbon dioxide is transported to the lungs:**

○ A In the form of bicarbonate ions
○ B In the form of carbonic acid
○ C In the form of carbaminohaemoglobin
○ D In chemical combination with albumin
○ E In the dissolved state in the water of the plasma and cells

respiratory

3.19 The control unit of ventilation consists of a processor (the respiratory centre in the brain), which integrates inputs (emotional, chemical and physical stimuli) and controls an effector (the lungs) via motor nerves arising from the spinal cord. Which of the following can produce the most potent effect in stimulating the respiratory centre and so increasing respiration?

    A Decreases in the blood oxygen tension

    B Decreases in the blood hydrogen ion concentration

    C Decreases in carbon dioxide tension in the cerebrospinal fluid

    D Increases in the blood carbon dioxide tension

    E Increases in the blood hydrogen ion concentration

3.20 In an experiment testing a new muscle relaxant it was noticed that this drug only affected the muscles of inspiration. Which of the following are muscles of inspiration?

    A Abdominal muscles and external intercostals

    B Diaphragm and abdominal muscles

    C Diaphragm and external intercostals

    D Diaphragm and internal intercostals

    E Internal and external intercostals

3.21 Infant respiratory distress syndrome or hyaline membrane disease is caused by lack of surfactant, commonly suffered by premature babies born before 28–32 weeks of gestation. A major function of surfactant is to increase:

    A Alveolar surface tension

    B Pulmonary compliance

    C Release of O_2 from haemoglobin in alveolar capillaries

    D The work of breathing

    E The tendency of the lungs to collapse

respiratory

3.22 **A 25-year-old man is under water in the swimming pool and breathing through a snorkel. He has a respiratory rate of 10/min, a tidal volume of 550 ml and an effective anatomical dead space of 250 ml. What is the alveolar ventilation of this man?**

○   A   2500 ml/min
○   B   3000 ml/min
○   C   3500 ml/min
○   D   4000 ml/min
○   E   4500 ml/min

3.23 **A 25-year-old man is under water in the swimming pool and breathing through a snorkel. He has a respiratory rate of 10/min, a tidal volume of 550 ml and an effective anatomical dead space of 250 ml. Which of the following would cause the greatest increase in alveolar ventilation of this man?**

○   A   A twofold increase in respiration rate
○   B   A twofold increase in tidal volume
○   C   A twofold increase in respiration rate and a shorter snorkel
○   D   A twofold increase in tidal volume and a shorter snorkel
○   E   A longer snorkel

3.24 **A deep-sea diver was airlifted to a tertiary hospital with suspected decompression sickness within 30 min of resurfacing. Decompression sickness:**

○   A   Can occur if one breathes 100% O_2
○   B   Can be treated with inhalation of carbon monoxide
○   C   Can be prevented by rapid decompression
○   D   Is characterised by intense euphoria
○   E   Results from nitrogen bubbles in the body fluids

respiratory

3.25 An arterial blood gas sample from a 36-year-old man shows low $p(O_2)$. If the $p(O_2)$ in the blood is low, the most likely cause is:

○ A Anaemic hypoxia

○ B Histotoxic hypoxia

○ C Hypaemic hypoxia

○ D Hypoxic hypoxia

○ E Stagnant hypoxia

3.26 A 22-year-old man was brought to the Accident and Emergency Department unconscious and hypoventilating. He was thought to be using recreational drugs before this episode. Arterial blood gas analysis was performed as the first step in management of this patient. Which of the following data sets is most consistent with hypoventilation as the principal defect?

	pH	$p_a(CO_2)$ (mmHg)	$p_a(O_2)$ (mmHg)
○ A	7.45	25	71
○ B	7.35	50	69
○ C	7.28	55	81
○ D	7.50	32	65
○ E	7.35	39	221

respiratory

3.27 **A 35-year-old woman with flail chest following chest trauma due to road traffic accident was breathing with the aid of a mechanical ventilator in the intensive care unit. She was heavily sedated and paralysed with muscle relaxant. Suddenly there was a power failure at the hospital and the nurse had to get an Ambu bag to hand-ventilate this patient until the power was restored. Which of the following changes in arterial blood would occur in this patient in the brief period between the power cut and the commencement of hand ventilation?**

	Arterial $p(CO_2)$	pH
A	Decrease	Decrease
B	Decrease	Increase
C	Decrease	No change
D	Increase	Decrease
E	Increase	Increase

3.28 **A 58-year-old man had a prolonged coronary artery bypass operation on cardiopulmonary bypass. Following the surgery, he was bleeding and required transfusion of 3 units of packed red cells, 4 units of fresh-frozen plasma and 1 unit of platelets. On the second postoperative day, he was noticed to be tachypnoeic with increasing oxygen requirements and chest X-ray showed appearances consistent with acute (or adult) respiratory distress syndrome. Which of the following variables is most likely to be lower than normal in this patient?**

A   Alveolar–arterial $p(O_2)$ difference
B   Compliance of the lung
C   Oncotic pressure of alveolar fluid
D   Surface tension of alveolar fluid
E   Work of breathing

respiratory

3.29 **A 28-year-old man has been trekking in the Himalayas for past 2 years. He has developed an increase in ventilation rate and a muscle biopsy reveals increased number of mitochondria. Which of the following physiological changes is also expected to be seen in this man?**

O   A   Decreased production of erythropoietin

O   B   Decreased 2,3-diphosphoglycerate (DPG)

O   C   Increased renal excretion of HCO_3^-

O   D   Increased renal excretion of H^+ ions

O   E   Pulmonary vasodilatation

3.30 **A 62-year-old man was admitted with an exacerbation of chronic obstructive pulmonary disease. His arterial blood gases on air showed pH = 7.29, $p(CO_2)$ = 65.3 mmHg, $p(O_2)$ = 62 mmHg and standard bicarbonate = 30.5 mmol/l. This patient had:**

O   A   Metabolic acidosis

O   B   Metabolic alkalosis

O   C   Mixed acidosis

O   D   Respiratory acidosis

O   E   Respiratory alkalosis

respiratory

3.31 A 28-year-old man was admitted with status epilepticus. He was given intravenous diazepam. Arterial blood gases on 15 l/min via a reservoir bag mask showed pH 7.05, $p(CO_2)$ = 61.5 mmHg, $p(O_2)$ = 115 mmHg and standard bicarbonate = 16 mmol/l. His other results were sodium = 140 mmol/l, potassium = 4 mmol/l and chloride = 98 mmol/l. This patient most likely had:

○   A   Metabolic acidosis
○   B   Metabolic alkalosis
○   C   Mixed acidosis
○   D   Respiratory acidosis
○   E   Respiratory alkalosis

3.32 A 45-year-old man with previous peptic ulcer disease was admitted with persistent vomiting. He looked dehydrated. His blood results were sodium = 140 mmol/l, potassium = 2.5 mmol/l, chloride = 86 mmol/l, pH = 7.5, $p(CO_2)$ = 50 mmHg, $p(O_2)$ = 107 mmHg, standard bicarbonate = 40 mmol/l. This patient had:

○   A   Metabolic acidosis
○   B   Metabolic alkalosis
○   C   Mixed acidosis
○   D   Respiratory acidosis
○   E   Respiratory alkalosis

respiratory

3.33 **A 48-year-old man with pleurisy for 5 days was assessed. A small pneumothorax with a moderate-sized pleural effusion was seen on a chest X-ray. His arterial blood gases on air showed pH = 7.44, $p(CO_2)$ = 23 mmHg, $p(O_2)$ = 234.5 mmHg, standard bicarbonate = 16 mmol/l. This patient had:**

- A   Compensated metabolic acidosis
- B   Compensated metabolic alkalosis
- C   Compensated respiratory acidosis
- D   Compensated respiratory alkalosis
- E   Mixed acidosis

3.34 **A 45-year-old man with type 1 diabetes and diabetic nephropathy was recovering on a surgical ward after a total colectomy and ileotomy. He had persistent metabolic acidosis and the surgeons were concerned about his high potassium concentration and that there may have been some ischaemia in the abdomen causing the acidosis. However, the patient appeared well perfused and had normal vital signs. He had normal fluid balance and his results showed sodium = 130 mmol/l, potassium = 6.5 mmol/l, creatinine = 180 µmol/l (2.16 mg/dl), chloride = 109 µmol/l, 0800 h cortisol = 500 nmol/l (18 µg/dl), pH = 7.29, $p(CO_2)$ = 27 mmHg, $p(O_2)$ = 107 mmHg, standard bicarbonate = 12 mmol/l. This patient had:**

- A   Hyperosmolar diabetic coma
- B   Ketoacidosis
- C   Ischaemic bowel
- D   Lactic acidosis
- E   Renal tubular acidosis

3.35 **If the IXth cranial nerves are blocked bilaterally in the neck the subject will no longer respond to:**

○ A Acidity by causing an increased respiratory minute volume

○ B Alkalosis by causing an increased respiratory minute volume

○ C Hypercapnia by causing an increased respiratory minute volume

○ D Hypocapnia by causing an increased respiratory minute volume

○ E Hypoxia by causing an increased respiratory minute volume

3.36 **The oxygen–haemoglobin dissociation curve is usually a sigmoid plot. The curve will shift to the right with:**

○ A Acute alkalosis
○ B Decrease in $p(CO_2)$
○ C Decrease in temperature
○ D Decrease in 2,3-diphosphoglycerate (DPG)
○ E Exercise

3.37 **A 45-year-old woman suddenly vomits with aspiration of the stomach contents while under general anaesthetic for a laparoscopic cholecystectomy. This is most likely to result in:**

○ A A rise in the intrapleural pressure on the affected side
○ B An increase in the physiological dead space
○ C Bronchitis
○ D Chemical pneumonia
○ E Vasodilatation in the alveoli supplied by that bronchus

respiratory

3.38 A 35-year-old asthmatic woman is to undergo elective repair of a paraumbilical hernia. The consultant anaesthetist requested pulmonary function tests in this woman. Which of the following abnormalities is most likely to be seen in this patient?

○   A   Decreased residual volume

○   B   Decreased first-second forced expiratory volume (FEV_1)/ forced vital capacity (FVC) ratio

○   C   Increased FVC

○   D   Increased forced expiratory volume in the first second (FEV_1)

○   E   Reduced diffusing capacity for carbon monoxide (DL_{CO})

3.39 Two hours after an uneventful cholecystectomy, a 50-year-old woman has the following arterial blood gas analysis on room air:

pH   7.30

$p(CO_2)$ 52 mmHg

$p(O_2)$ 78 mmHg

Which of the following is the most likely cause of these findings?

○   A   Alveolar hypoventilation

○   B   Occult haemorrhage

○   C   Primary cardiac failure

○   D   Peritonitis

○   E   Pulmonary embolus

3.40 **A 54-year-old man complains of increasing dyspnoea. He has been a 2-pack-a-day cigarette smoker for past 30 years. X-ray chest shows widening of intercostal spaces with more blackening bilaterally. In this emphysematous patient on pulmonary function testing the following abnormality is most likely to be seen:**

- A Decreased functional residual capacity
- B Decreased residual volume
- C Increased FEV_1/FVC
- D Increased total lung capacity
- E Increased vital capacity

3.41 **The diffusing capacity for carbon monoxide (DLco) is a measure of the ability of gas to transfer from alveoli to RBCs across the alveolar epithelium and the capillary endothelium. The DLco:**

- A Decreases in patients with polycythaemia
- B Increases in pulmonary embolism
- C Is reported as ml/mmHg
- D Is independent of the area of the blood–gas barrier
- E Is affected by the volume of blood in the pulmonary capillaries

3.42 **A 35-year-old patient was brought to the Accident and Emergency Department following head injury with abnormal breathing pattern characterised by periods of waxing and waning tidal volumes separated by periods of apnoea. This patient has:**

- A Ataxic breathing
- B Biot's breathing
- C Cheyne–Stokes breathing
- D Kussmaul breathing
- E Ondine's curse

respiratory

3.43 **In addition to respiratory functions, such as gas exchange and regulation of hydrogen ion concentration, the lungs also perform non-respiratory functions. One of the non-respiratory functions of lungs is ectopic production of:**

○ A Adrenocorticotrophic hormone (ACTH)
○ B Aldosterone
○ C Angiotensin II
○ D Cortisol
○ E Erythropoietin

3.44 **A 48-year-old man who is a known case of chronic obstructive pulmonary disease (COPD) presented in the Accident and Emergency Department with exacerbation of his respiratory ailment. An arterial blood gas analysis in this patient on room air is most likely to show:**

○ A Metabolic acidosis
○ B Metabolic alkalosis
○ C Mixed acidosis
○ D Respiratory acidosis
○ E Respiratory alkalosis

3.45 **Which of the following is most likely to happen to a 22-year-old man competing in a 1500 metres running event at the Olympics?**

○ A The alveolar–capillary $p(O_2)$ gradient is increased
○ B The CO_2 content of blood is decreased
○ C The CO_2 output is decreased
○ D The O_2 content of mixed venous blood is increased
○ E The O_2 consumption is decreased

3.46 The increase in ventilation that occurs immediately following ascent to high altitude:

○ A Decreases over the next 24 hours

○ B Increases still further over the course in the next 1–3 days

○ C Is augmented by the fall in pH of the cerebrospinal fluid (CSF)

○ D Is caused primarily by the reduced work of breathing because of the less dense air

○ E Is caused by the low $p(O_2)$ in mixed venous blood

3.47 Features of mild carbon monoxide poisoning include:

○ A Decreased arterial O_2 concentration

○ B Decreased arterial $p(O_2)$

○ C Decreased haemoglobin–oxygen affinity

○ D Increased alveolar ventilation

○ E Increased chemoreceptor discharge

3.48 In a patient with anaemia and normal lungs:

○ A Arterial $p(O_2)$ is reduced

○ B Arterial–venous O_2 concentration difference is increased

○ C Arterial O_2 saturation is reduced

○ D Cardiac output is reduced

○ E $p(O_2)$ of mixed venous blood is reduced

respiratory

3.49 Hypoxic pulmonary vasoconstriction:

○ A Acts reflexively via the central nervous system

○ B Improves matching of ventilation and blood flow in some lung diseases

○ C Is not important in the perinatal period

○ D Is irreversible

○ E Requires a $p(O_2)$ of less than 40 mmHg in mixed venous blood

3.50 Pulmonary vascular resistance increases:

○ A At high altitude

○ B During space flight

○ C On exercise

○ D On inspiring 100% oxygen

○ E With anaemia

3.51 A 68-year-old man on the fourth postoperative day following abdominoperineal resection developed sudden-onset dyspnoea, tachypnoea and pleuritic chest pain. A diagnosis of pulmonary embolism was made. Which of the following is most likely to increase in this patient?

○ A Arterial CO_2

○ B Arterial O_2

○ C Alveolar oxygen saturation

○ D Lung volume

○ E Ventilation/perfusion ratio

3.52 **A fireman on a rescue mission got trapped in a burning building. He was eventually rescued by his co-workers in a markedly hypoxic state. Respiration in this fireman will be rapidly influenced by hypoxia through its stimulatory effect:**

○ A Directly on the medullary respiratory neurones

○ B Directly on the oxyhaemoglobin dissociation curve

○ C Directly on the pulmonary mechanoreceptors

○ D On the carotid and aortic chemoreceptors

○ E On the central chemoreceptors

3.53 **A 58-year-old male chronic smoker with chronic obstructive airway disease was admitted for elective right hemicolectomy. The anaesthetist requested pulmonary function tests to evaluate the severity of his respiratory dysfunction. Which of the following abnormalities is most likely to be present in this patient?**

○ A Decreased functional residual capacity

○ B Decreased total lung capacity

○ C Increased carbon monoxide diffusing capacity

○ D Increased FEV_1/FVC

○ E Increased residual volume

respiratory

3.54 A 28-year-old polytrauma victim in the intensive care unit developed acute respiratory distress syndrome characterised by inflammation of the lung parenchyma with concomitant systemic release of inflammatory mediators. Which of the following variables is most likely to be lower than normal in this patient?

○ A   Alveolar–arterial pressure difference
○ B   Lung compliance
○ C   Oncotic pressure of alveolar fluid
○ D   Surface tension of alveolar fluid
○ E   Work of breathing

3.55 A 40-year-old man was trapped in a burning flat. Upon rescue he was noticed to be markedly hypoxic. In this person vasoconstriction in response to hypoxia is most likely to be found in arterial beds in which of the following organs?

○ A   Gut
○ B   Heart
○ C   Kidney
○ D   Lungs
○ E   Skeletal muscle

3.56 The lung has two circulations, the pulmonary circulation that perfuses alveoli and the bronchial circulation that provides nutrients and gas exchange for the conducting airways. What percentage of cardiac output is received by bronchial circulation?

○ A   2%
○ B   12%
○ C   20%
○ D   50%
○ E   70%

3.57 A 35-year-old woman was admitted with a large postpneumonic effusion. Nearly 2 litres of purulent fluid was drained from the chest following insertion of an intercostals drain. What is the normal amount of pleural fluid?

A   10 ml
B   100 ml
C   250 ml
D   500 ml
E   1000 ml

3.58 A normal subject inhales and then holds his breath with glottis open such that his intrapleural pressure (p_{pl}) is −10 cmH$_2$O and alveolar pressure (p_A) is 0. He then closes his glottis and makes an expiratory effort until his p_{pl} = 0. At this point, his alveolar pressure would be closest to:

A   +10 cmH$_2$O
B   Unchanged
C   −10 cmH$_2$O
D   +5 cmH$_2$O
E   −5 cmH$_2$O

3.59 Each year, several thousand premature infants are born with respiratory distress syndrome related to non-functional alveolar surfactant. Which of the following is a recognised effect of the presence of surfactant in lungs?

A   Enhanced alveolar stability
B   Enhanced alveolar surface tension
C   Enhanced atelectasis
D   Enhanced opening pressure in collapsed alveoli
E   Enhanced work of breathing

respiratory

3.60 **Various physiological and physical factors can alter lung airway resistance. The airway resistance will be reduced by:**

A Blockade of β_2-adrenergic receptors

B Increase in airway CO_2

C Release of histamine

D Stimulation of parasympathetic cholinergic fibres

E Stimulation of arterial receptors

3.61 **Breathing requires physical work to be performed by the respiratory muscles to overcome the forces that oppose lung inflation and deflation. In a normally breathing individual maximum amount of work of breathing is required to overcome:**

A Elastance

B Frictional resistance

C Inertia

D Muscle relaxants

E Narcotic overdosage

3.62 **The vessels of the pulmonary circulation are very compliant (easily distensible) and so can serve as a reservoir for the left ventricle. How much blood volume can the pulmonary vessels accommodate in an adult man under normal resting conditions?**

A 150 ml

B 250 ml

C 500 ml

D 1000 ml

E 1500 ml

respiratory

3.63 **Various lung intravascular and extravascular pressures influence pulmonary blood flow and its distribution in the lung. What is the normal mean pulmonary arterial pressure?**

○ A 5 mmHg
○ B 10 mmHg
○ C 15 mmHg
○ D 50 mmHg
○ E 90 mmHg

3.64 **Driving pressure is the difference between inflow and outflow pressure. What is the normal mean intravascular driving pressure for the pulmonary circulation?**

○ A 10 mmHg
○ B 30 mmHg
○ C 50 mmHg
○ D 75 mmHg
○ E 100 mmHg

3.65 **Various humoral substances in the circulation or formed by lung endothelial cells are capable of causing pulmonary vascular smooth muscle to either contract or relax to alter pulmonary vascular resistance. Which of the following substances is most likely to cause pulmonary vasodilatation?**

○ A Catecholamines
○ B Endothelin
○ C Histamine
○ D Nitric oxide
○ E $PGF_{2\alpha}$

respiratory

SECTION 4:
FLUIDS, ELECTROLYTES & ACID–BASE PHYSIOLOGY – QUESTIONS

For each question given below choose the ONE BEST option.

4.1 **A 76-year-old woman was infused hypertonic sodium chloride solution as a treatment for profound hyponatraemia. Infusion of hypertonic sodium chloride solution will:**

○ A Decrease both intracellular and extracellular fluid volumes

○ B Increase both intracellular and extracellular fluid volumes

○ C Increase extracellular osmolarity only

○ D Increase intracellular osmolarity only

○ E Increase extracellular volume and decrease intracellular volume

4.2 **A woman drinks 2 litres of water to replenish the fluids lost by sweating during a period of exercise. Compared with the situation before the period of sweating:**

○ A Her intracellular fluid will be hypertonic

○ B Her extracellular fluid will be hypertonic

○ C Her intracellular fluid volume will be greater

○ D Her extracellular fluid volume will be greater

○ E Her intracellular and extracellular fluid volumes will be unchanged

4.3   Calculate the *net* pressure difference across the capillary wall given the following conditions:

Interstitial fluid hydrostatic pressure = −3 mmHg

Plasma colloid osmotic pressure = 28 mmHg

Capillary hydrostatic pressure = 17 mmHg

Interstitial fluid colloid osmotic pressure = 8 mmHg

Filtration coefficient = 1

- A   −2 mmHg
- B   −1 mmHg
- C   0 mmHg
- D   1 mmHg
- E   2 mmHg

4.4   Which of the following conditions is not likely to be associated with extracellular oedema?

- A   Increased plasma colloid osmotic pressure
- B   Lymphatic blockage
- C   Increased capillary permeability
- D   Increased capillary pressure
- E   Increased interstitial fluid colloid osmotic pressure

4.5   Which of the following changes will decrease the rate of diffusion of a substance?

- A   A decrease in the molecular weight of the substance
- B   An increase in the concentration gradient
- C   An increase in temperature
- D   An increase in the molecular weight of the substance
- E   An increase in membrane permeability

fluids

4.6 **The most important physiological function of the lymphatic system is to:**

○ A Transport fluid and proteins away from the interstitium to the blood

○ B Concentrate proteins in the lymph

○ C Remove particulate materials from the interstitium

○ D Transport antigenic materials to lymph nodes

○ E Create negative pressure in the free interstitial fluid

4.7 **Reabsorption of fluid by the renal peritubular capillaries can be increased by:**

○ A Decreased plasma protein concentration

○ B Decreased filtration fraction

○ C Decreased plasma colloid osmotic pressure

○ D Efferent arteriolar constriction

○ E Increased peritubular capillary hydrostatic pressure

4.8 **The clearance rate for a substance that is freely filtered, but neither secreted nor reabsorbed by the kidney is equal to the:**

○ A Filtration fraction

○ B Renal plasma flow

○ C Glomerular filtration rate

○ D Urinary excretion rate of the substance

○ E Total volume of distribution

fluids

4.9 **The following test results were obtained on specimens from a person during a 24-h period:**

Urine flow rate: 2.0 ml/min

Urine inulin: 1.0 mg/ml

Plasma inulin: 0.01 mg/ml

Urine urea: 220 mmol/l

Plasma urea: 5 mmol/l

What is the glomerular filtration rate?

○ A 100 ml/min

○ B 125 ml/min

○ C 150 ml/min

○ D 175 ml/min

○ E 200 ml/min

4.10 **The following test results were obtained on specimens from a person during a 24-h period:**

Urine flow rate: 2.0 ml/min

Urine inulin: 1.0 mg/ml

Plasma inulin: 0.01 mg/ml

Urine urea: 220 mmol/l

Plasma urea: 5 mmol/l

What is the urea clearance?

○ A 4.4 ml/min

○ B 22 ml/min

○ C 44 ml/min

○ D 88 ml/min

○ E 440 ml/min

fluids

4.11 For which of the following substances would you expect the renal clearance to be the *lowest*, under normal conditions?

○ A Urea
○ B Creatinine
○ C Sodium
○ D Glucose
○ E Water

4.12 When a person is dehydrated, hypotonic fluid will be found in the:

○ A Glomerular filtrate
○ B Proximal tubule
○ C Distal end of the ascending loop of Henlé
○ D Late distal convoluted tubule
○ E Collecting duct

4.13 Destruction of the supraoptic nuclei of the brain will produce which of the following changes in urinary volume and concentration? (Assume that fluid intake equals fluid loss.)

○ A Decreased urinary volume and a very dilute urine
○ B Decreased urinary volume and a concentrated urine
○ C Increased urinary volume and a concentrated urine
○ D Increased urinary volume and a very dilute urine
○ E No change in urine volume and no change in urine concentration

fluids

4.14 **A normal individual on a diet high in K⁺ exhibits increased K⁺ excretion. The major cause of this increased renal excretion of K⁺ is:**

○ A Increased secretion of K⁺ by the distal and collecting tubules

○ B Decreased reabsorption of K⁺ by the proximal tubule

○ C Decreased reabsorption of K⁺ by the loop of Henlé

○ D Decreased aldosterone secretion

○ E Increased glomerular filtration rate (GFR)

4.15 **Which of the following arterial blood acid–base data are for a normal individual?**

		$p(CO_2)$ (mmHg)	$[HCO_3^-]$ (mmol/l)	pH
○	A	29	22.0	7.50
○	B	33	32.0	7.61
○	C	35	17.5	7.32
○	D	40	25.0	7.41
○	E	60	37.5	7.42

4.16 **Which of the following arterial blood acid–base data are for an individual with partially compensated metabolic acidosis?**

		$p(CO_2)$ (mmHg)	$[HCO_3^-]$ (mmol/l)	pH
○	A	29	22.0	7.50
○	B	33	32.0	7.61
○	C	35	17.5	7.32
○	D	40	25.0	7.41
○	E	60	37.5	7.42

fluids

4.17 **Which of the following arterial blood acid–base data are for an individual with fully compensated respiratory acidosis?**

		$p(CO_2)$ (mmHg)	$[HCO_3^-]$ (mmol/l)	pH
○	A	29	22.0	7.50
○	B	33	32.0	7.61
○	C	35	17.5	7.32
○	D	40	25.0	7.41
○	E	60	37.5	7.42

4.18 **Which of the following arterial blood acid–base data are for an individual with uncompensated respiratory alkalosis?**

		$p(CO_2)$ (mmHg)	$[HCO_3^-]$ (mmol/l)	pH
○	A	29	22.0	7.50
○	B	33	32.0	7.61
○	C	35	17.5	7.32
○	D	40	25.0	7.41
○	E	60	37.5	7.42

4.19 **Which of the following arterial blood acid–base data are for an individual with combined respiratory and metabolic alkalosis?**

		$p(CO_2)$ (mmHg)	$[HCO_3^-]$ (mmol/l)	pH
○	A	29	22.0	7.50
○	B	33	32.0	7.61
○	C	35	17.5	7.32
○	D	40	25.0	7.41
○	E	60	37.5	7.42

fluids

4.20 Which of the following substances is actively secreted into the renal tubules?

○ A Amino acids
○ B Chloride
○ C Glucose
○ D Potassium
○ E Sodium

4.21 The most important difference between interstitial fluid and plasma is the:

○ A Concentration of sodium
○ B Concentration of chloride
○ C Osmolarity
○ D Potassium concentration
○ E Protein concentration

4.22 According to the Henderson–Hasselbalch equation, the buffering capacity of the system is maximum when the number of free anions compared with undissociated acid is:

○ A Equal
○ B Exactly half
○ C One-third less
○ D Three times more
○ E Two times more

fluids

4.23 **A 26-year-old woman was seen in the Accident and Emergency Department with profound hypokalaemia. In which of the following conditions will hypokalaemia be most consistently found?**

    A Acute respiratory acidosis
    B Addison's disease
    C Chronic renal failure
    D Diabetic ketoacidosis
    E Prolonged vomiting

4.24 **Which of the following best describes the mechanism for movement of sodium ions between the blood and tissue interstitial fluid in the skeletal muscle of a normal individual?**

    A Active transport through endothelial cell membranes
    B Bulk flow at venous ends of capillaries
    C Diffusion through channels between endothelial cells
    D Diffusion through endothelial cell membrane
    E Filtration at arterial ends of capillaries

4.25 **A 28-year-old man arrived in the Accident and Emergency Department with marked dehydration and metabolic acidosis. Which of the following conditions is most likely to cause marked dehydration and metabolic acidosis?**

    A Complete deprivation of water for 24 h
    B Excessive sweating
    C Severe diarrhoea
    D Severe persistent vomiting
    E Syndrome of inappropriate antidiuretic hormone (ADH) secretion

fluids

4.26 **A 35-year-old man arrived in the Accident and Emergency Department with cerebrospinal fluid (CSF) leaking from his nose following a head injury. Which of the following statements regarding CSF is CORRECT?**

A   It has greater buffering capacity than blood

B   It has a protein content of 20 mg/100 ml

C   It has a higher blood glucose level than plasma

D   It is absorbed through choroid plexus

E   It is nearly 50–60 ml in volume

4.27 **A 25-year-old woman arrived in the Accident and Emergency Department complaining of neck pain with temperature. On examination no neck rigidity was found. The Accident and Emergency Department consultant decided to perform cerebrospinal fluid (CSF) examination. Which of the following statements regarding CSF is CORRECT?**

A   It is actively secreted by the choroid plexus

B   It is the major source of the brain's nutrition

C   It has the same pH as arterial blood

D   It is virtually glucose-free

E   It has low osmolality as compared with plasma

fluids

4.28 **A 36-year-old man with a cerebral abscess was prescribed an antibiotic that could easily penetrate the blood–brain barrier. Which of the following statements regarding the blood–brain barrier is CORRECT?**

○ A It is more permeable in adults than in infants

○ B It permits carbon dioxide to pass via facilitated diffusion

○ C It breaks down in areas of brain that are infected

○ D It is more permeable to water-soluble substances than to lipid-soluble substances

○ E It allows 5-hydroxytryptophan (5HT) to cross to a very limited degree

4.29 **Extracellular body fluid as compared with intracellular body fluid:**

○ A Has lower tonicity

○ B Has greater volume

○ C Contains less chloride

○ D Is relatively rich in glucose

○ E Contains more amino acids

4.30 **A 62-year-old man has undergone Whipple's operation for carcinoma of pancreas. Postoperatively, parenteral nutrition is started. Solution of choice for parenteral nutrition is:**

○ A Crystalline amino acids

○ B Darrow's solution

○ C Plasma albumin

○ D Plasma

○ E Whole blood

fluids

4.31 A 45-year-old woman was seen in the Accident and Emergency Department with extreme generalised oedema with marked expansion of the extracellular space within the subcutaneous tissues, visceral organs and body cavities. The woman has:

○ A Anasarca
○ B Angioedema
○ C Apoptosis
○ D Hyperthecosis
○ E Haemochromatosis

4.32 Arterial blood gas analysis report of a 46-year-old woman in the Accident and Emergency Department showed elevated arterial CO_2 content. The woman is most likely to have which of the following conditions?

○ A Chronic renal failure
○ B Diabetic ketoacidosis
○ C Metabolic acidosis
○ D Metabolic alkalosis
○ E Respiratory alkalosis

4.33 In a person weighing 75 kg the volumes of total body water, intracellular fluid and extracellular fluid are respectively:

○ A 40 l, 30 l, 10 l
○ B 45 l, 30 l, 15 l
○ C 45 l, 35 l, 10 l
○ D 50 l, 25 l, 25 l
○ E 50 l, 35 l, 15 l

fluids

4.34 A 25-year-old Asian man arrived in the Accident and Emergency Department with acute small bowel obstruction. A decision was made to perform exploratory laparotomy. During laparotomy ileal stricture was found and an ileal resection and anastomosis performed. Postoperatively he was kept nil by mouth, with intravenous (IV) antibiotics and IV fluids containing saline and 5% dextrose. A serum biochemistry analysis performed on day 3 showed normal serum potassium level, but on day 5 it showed a low serum potassium level. This is most likely to be due to:

- ○ A Aldosterone deficiency
- ○ B Anaesthetic impairment of intestinal peristalsis
- ○ C Nothing per oral regimen
- ○ D Repeated vomiting of gastric contents before operation
- ○ E Surgical injury

4.35 A person is most likely to feel thirsty in the presence of:

- ○ A Decreased level of angiotensin II
- ○ B Hypoglycaemia
- ○ C Increased ECF volume
- ○ D Increased ICF volume
- ○ E Increased level of angiotensin II

4.36 A 78-year-old woman arrived in the Accident and Emergency Department with severe sodium deficiency. She is most likely to have:

- ○ A Bradycardia
- ○ B Low haematocrit
- ○ C Muscular weakness
- ○ D Severe diarrhoea or vomiting
- ○ E Raised blood pressure

fluids

4.37 **A 28-year-old unconscious patient was brought to the Accident and Emergency Department. The senior house officer (SHO) attending him administered intravenous sodium bicarbonate as a part of the emergency therapy. Intravenous sodium bicarbonate was given to treat:**

○ A Hypokalaemia

○ B Metabolic acidosis

○ C Metabolic alkalosis

○ D Respiratory acidosis

○ E Respiratory alkalosis

4.38 **A 35-year-old man following abdominal surgery received an increased quantity of intravenous normal saline. What is most likely to happen in this patient due to this therapeutic misadventure?**

○ A Decrease in urinary excretion of Na$^+$

○ B Increase in extracellular fluid volume

○ C Increase in renin secretion

○ D Increase in circulating angiotensin level

○ E Increase in serum osmolality

4.39 **A 36-year-old woman with smaller-than-normal kidneys on ultrasound and a history of chronic glomerulonephritis has the following laboratory values:**

Arterial blood	Urine
pH = 7.33 $p_a(O_2)$ = 95 mmHg $p_a(CO_2)$ = 32 mmHg HCO_3 = 18 mEq/l	pH=6.0 protein = positive glucose = negative

fluids

This patient most likely has:

○ A Diabetic ketoacidosis

○ B Respiratory acidosis with some renal compensation

○ C Respiratory acidosis without renal compensation

○ D Metabolic acidosis with some respiratory compensation

○ E Metabolic acidosis without respiratory compensation

4.40 **A 36-year-old woman with smaller-than-normal kidneys on ultrasound and a history of chronic glomerulonephritis has the following laboratory values:**

Arterial blood	Urine
pH = 7.33	pH=6.0
$p_a(O_2)$ = 95 mmHg	protein = positive
$p_a(CO_2)$ = 32 mmHg	glucose = negative
HCO_3^- = 18 mEq/l	

The most likely cause of her acid–base imbalance is:

○ A Decreased ability to produce adequate urinary NH_4^+ excretion

○ B Decreased catabolism of sulphur-containing amino acids (eg methionine, cysteine)

○ C Excess β-hydroxybutyric and acetoacetic acids in her blood

○ D Hypoventilation

○ E Hyperventilation

fluids

SECTION 5:
RENAL PHYSIOLOGY – QUESTIONS

For each question given below choose the ONE BEST option.

5.1 **A substance X has renal clearance greater than inulin but less than para-aminohippuric acid. Which of the following statements best describes the renal handling of substance X?**

- ○ A It is freely filtered and partially reabsorbed
- ○ B It is freely filtered and partially secreted
- ○ C It is freely filtered and totally reabsorbed
- ○ D It is freely filtered and totally secreted
- ○ E It is neither filtered nor secreted

5.2 **In humans, the kidneys together receive roughly 20% of cardiac output, amounting to 1 l/min in a 70-kg adult man. Renal blood flow is closely related to renal plasma flow, which is the volume of blood plasma delivered to the kidney per unit time. Which of the following substances can be used to measure renal plasma flow rate?**

- ○ A Creatinine
- ○ B Inulin
- ○ C Para-aminobenzoic acid (PABA)
- ○ D Para-aminohippuric acid (PAH)
- ○ E Potassium

5.3 Transport maximum (or T_m) refers to the point at which increases in concentration do not result in an increase in movement of a substance across a membrane. In renal physiology, the concept of transport maximum is often discussed in the context of glucose and para-aminohippuric acid (PAH). What is the transport maximum for glucose?

○ A 100
○ B 200
○ C 300
○ D 400
○ E 500

5.4 An 8-year-old school boy developed sore throat. He was treated with an antibiotic and the sore throat resolved. However, 2 weeks later, he developed generalised body oedema, hypertension and haematuria. The most likely diagnosis is:

○ A Acute nephritic syndrome
○ B Bladder stones
○ C Drug reaction
○ D Nephrotic syndrome
○ E Urinary tract infection

renal

5.5 Substance Z is freely filtered but is not secreted, metabolised, or stored in the kidney. The plasma concentration of Z is 1000 mg/l and the urine excretion rate is 25 mg/min. Which of the following values is equal to the rate of tubular reabsorption of substance Z (in mg/min) if the inulin clearance is 100 ml/min?

○ A 25
○ B 75
○ C 250
○ D 750
○ E 2500

5.6 A 22-year-old male athlete reports easy fatigability and weakness. Findings on physical examination are unremarkable. Laboratory data are:

Serum	Urine
Na^+ =141 mEq/l	Na^+ = 80 mEq/l
Cl^- = 85 mEq/l	K^+ = 170 mEq/l
K^+ = 2.1 mEq/l	
HCO_3^- = 35 mEq/l	

The most likely diagnosis is:

○ A Aldosterone deficiency
○ B Anxiety reaction with hyperventilation
○ C Diabetes mellitus with ketoacidosis
○ D Ingestion of anabolic steroids
○ E Surreptitious use of diuretics

renal

5.7 **A 35-year-old woman with hypertension and hypokalaemia is suspected of having hyperaldosteronism. In addition to serum aldosterone measurement, initial evaluation of this patient should include measurement of which of the following?**

○ A Plasma adrenocorticotrophic hormone (ACTH)

○ B Plasma cortisol

○ C Plasma prolactin

○ D Plasma renin

○ E Urinary sodium

5.8 **A 36-year-old previously fit and healthy woman reported 'swelling up' that had worsened over the past 4 weeks. Her blood pressure was 160/95 mmHg. Examination showed ascites and marked ankle oedema. Auscultation of the chest revealed bilateral pleural effusions with normal heart sounds. Laboratory studies showed:**

Blood urea nitrogen (BUN) = 30 mg/dl

Creatinine = 2.8 mg/dl

Albumin = 2.0 mg/dl

Alanine transaminase (ALT) = 25 U/l

Bilirubin = 1 mg/dl

Urine analysis shows 3+ albumin and no cells

Which of the following is the most likely cause of the ascites and oedema?

○ A Acute tubular necrosis

○ B Cirrhosis of the liver

○ C Congestive heart failure

○ D Interstitial renal disease

○ E Nephrotic syndrome

renal

5.9 **A 35-year-old man has recently developed hypertension with haematuria. He is suspected to have some form of glomerulonephritis. Which of the following substances will be most appropriate for measuring glomerular filtration rate (GFR) in this patient?**

○ A Creatinine

○ B ^{51}Cr-EDTA

○ C Inulin

○ D Para-aminohippuric acid (PAH)

○ E Urea

5.10 **A 48-year-old woman with a 10-year history of progressive systemic sclerosis (scleroderma) undergoes an emergency laparotomy for a perforated appendix with peritonitis. During the immediate postoperative period, she has a blood pressure of 100/50 mmHg. Over the next 3 days, her serum creatinine level increases, *and* her urinary output decreases to 250 ml/day. On postoperative day 4, she has mild shortness of breath. Her peripheral oxygen saturation on room air is 89%. Laboratory studies show a potassium level of 6.2 mEq/l, blood urea nitrogen (BUN) of 64 mg/dl, and creatinine level of 4.5 mg/dl. Which of the following is the most appropriate next step in the management of this woman?**

○ A Fluid bolus with 2 l of lactated Ringer's solution

○ B Haemodialysis

○ C Intravenous administration of angiotensin-converting enzyme (ACE) inhibitors

○ D Intravenous administration of morphine

○ E Peritoneal dialysis

renal

111

5.11 A 16-year-old girl with gross facial and ankle oedema was diagnosed with nephrotic syndrome. In this patient oedema is most probably due to:

○ A Arterial occlusion

○ B Decreased oncotic pressure

○ C Increased capillary hydrostatic pressure

○ D Lymphatic obstruction

○ E Venous obstruction

5.12 A 15-year-old boy was seen in the Accident and Emergency Department with localised oedema of his lips and tongue. Which of the following conditions will cause localised oedema?

○ A Angio-oedema

○ B Cardiac failure

○ C Cirrhosis

○ D Hypoproteinaemia

○ E Sodium retention

5.13 Glucose is an essential substrate for the metabolism of most cells. The transport of glucose in the renal tubular cells occurs via:

○ A Active transport

○ B Concentration gradient

○ C Facilitated diffusion

○ D Secondary active transport with sodium

○ E Secondary active transport with potassium

renal

5.14 **Which of the following is most likely to be seen if a sample of fluid leaving the proximal tubule in a person with normal kidneys is analysed?**

A It will be hypertonic compared with plasma

B It will have more K^+ than plasma

C It will have more HCO_3^- ions than plasma

D It will have similar pH to that in ureter

E It will have no amino acids

5.15 **To maintain a normal plasma bicarbonate, the kidney must secrete H^+ into the tubular lumen. Which of the following statements regarding secretion of hydrogen ions in renal tubules is CORRECT?**

A The process of H^+ secretion is coupled with regeneration of chloride

B Maximum H^+ secretion occurs in the descending limb of the loop of Henlé

C H^+ secretion occurs by active transport

D H^+ secretion results in secretion of equal moles of HCO_3^- ions

E H^+ secretion increases the pH of urine

5.16 **The normal glomerular filtration rate (GFR) for both kidneys is 125 ml/min per 1.73 m^2 of body surface area. GFR increases by:**

A Afferent arteriolar constriction

B Angiotensin II release

C Efferent arteriolar constriction

D Reducing renal blood flow

E Sympathetic stimulation

renal

5.17 **A 40-year-old diabetic woman has glycosuria. This may occur due to inadequate glucose reabsorption at:**

○ A Collecting duct

○ B Distal convoluted tubule

○ C Glomerulus

○ D Loop of Henlé

○ E Proximal convoluted tubule

5.18 **During routine antenatal check-up of a pregnant patient at 16 weeks gestation it was discovered that she had high blood pressure, proteinuria (400 mg/day), serum albumin of 2.0 g/dl, creatinine 0.8 mg/dl, and peripheral oedema. She had normal blood pressure on her first antenatal check-up. Which of the following diagnoses is most appropriate for this patient?**

○ A Chronic renal failure

○ B Glomerulonephritis

○ C Nephrotic syndrome

○ D Polycystic kidney disease

○ E Pre-eclampsia

renal

5.19 A 28-year-old man decides to donate a kidney to his brother who is in chronic renal failure, after human leukocyte antigen (HLA) typing suggests that he would be a suitable donor. He is admitted to the hospital and his right kidney is removed and transplanted into his brother. Which of the following indices would be expected to be decreased in the donor after full recovery from the operation?

○ A Creatinine clearance
○ B Creatinine production
○ C Plasma creatinine concentration
○ D Plasma sodium concentration
○ E Plasma chloride concentration

5.20 The mesangium is an inner layer of the glomerulus, within the basement membrane surrounding the glomerular capillaries. It has extraglomerular mesangial cells that:

○ A Are major contributors to the extracellular matrix
○ B Form the juxtaglomerular apparatus in combination with the macula densa and juxtaglomerular cells
○ C Phagocytose glomerular basal lamina components
○ D Phagocytose immunoglobulins
○ E Provide structural support for and regulate blood flow of the glomerular capillaries by their contractile activity

renal

5.21   The distal convoluted tubule (DCT) is a portion of nephron between the loop of Henlé and the collecting duct system. DCT:

○   A   Forms part of the juxtaglomerular complex

○   B   Is capable of reabsorbing hydrogen ions by a mechanism that involves carbonic anhydrase

○   C   Is capable of secreting sodium ions in exchange for potassium ions

○   D   Is capable of secreting Ca^{2+} in response to parathyroid hormone

○   E   Reabsorbs approximately 50% of the water in the glomerular filtrate

5.22   A 55-year-old diabetic is on haemodialysis for management of chronic renal failure (equivalent to a reduction in the total number of nephrons). Which of the following abnormalities is most likely to be seen in this patient?

○   A   High specific gravity of the urine

○   B   Hypercalcaemia

○   C   Hypophosphataemia

○   D   Increased erythropoietin release

○   E   Low plasma HCO_3^-

5.23   A 38-year-old man with end-stage renal disease had a successful renal transplant from a living, related donor. In this patient:

○   A   Immunosuppression is not required

○   B   Renal transplant can be judged successful if the glomerular filtration rate is 10 ml/min

○   C   Renal transplant can be expected to restore abnormal calcium and phosphorous metabolism towards normal

○   D   Renal transplant can be expected to cure anaemia even in disease of bone marrow

○   E   Rejection of renal transplant will involve only cellular mechanisms

renal

5.24 **A 45-year-old trauma victim develops acute renal failure secondary to mismatched blood transfusion. His urine volume is 20 ml/day, urine pH = 4.9, urine specific gravity = 1.055, Hb+++. Which of the following physiological abnormalities of acute renal failure will be most life threatening for this patient?**

A Acidosis

B Fluid overload

C Raised blood urea nitrogen (BUN)

D Raised serum creatinine level

E Raised serum urea level

5.25 **A 65-year-old man following prostatectomy complained of incontinence. He is most likely to have:**

A Functional incontinence

B Mixed incontinence

C Overflow incontinence

D Stress incontinence

E Urge incontinence

5.26 **A defect in which part of the renal tubule will affect absorption of amino acids and glucose the most?**

A Collecting duct

B Collecting tubule

C Distal convoluted tubule

D Loop of Henlé

E Proximal convoluted tubule

renal

5.27 **In an experiment the juxtaglomerular cells in the kidney were selectively destroyed. This will result in loss of production of:**

○ A Aldosterone
○ B Angiotensin
○ C Erythropoietin
○ D Renin
○ E Urodilatin

5.28 **Which part of the nephron will have to be selectively destroyed to stop the macula densa from performing its function?**

○ A Afferent arteriole
○ B Distal convoluted tubule
○ C Efferent arteriole
○ D Juxtaglomerular cells
○ E Loop of Henlé

5.29 **A child has ingested an overdose of a drug. Which of the following is most likely to reduce the renal excretion of this drug?**

○ A Alkalinisation of urine
○ B Extensive binding of drug to plasma proteins
○ C Haemodialysis
○ D Induced diuresis
○ E Induction of hepatic microsomal enzymes

renal

5.30 If the medullary thick ascending limb of loop of Henlé is selectively destroyed this will result in:

○ A Reduced absorption of water
○ B Reduced passive transport of sodium
○ C Reduced active transport of sodium
○ D Reduced passive transport of chloride
○ E Reduced production of erythropoietin

5.31 Interference with active reabsorption of sodium by the kidney is most likely to cause:

○ A A rise in blood pressure
○ B A rise in plasma potassium ion level
○ C A rise in interstitial fluid volume
○ D A rise in plasma specific gravity
○ E A rise in the volume of urine passed in a given time

5.32 A patient is brought to casualty with profuse haemorrhage resulting in hypotension and tachycardia. Which part of the kidney is going to compensate?

○ A Collecting ducts
○ B Distal convoluted tubule
○ C Proximal convoluted tubule
○ D Thick limb of loop of Henlé
○ E Thin limb of loop of Henlé

renal

5.33 **A 75-year-old man was seen in the Accident and Emergency Department complaining of loss of control over the bladder function. Which of the following statements about micturition is CORRECT?**

○ A Higher centres in the brainstem primarily serve to enhance the micturition reflex

○ B Patients with damage to the lumbar spinal cord lose their micturition reflex (atonic bladder)

○ C Patients with damage to the sacral spin cord have an intact micturition reflex but lose almost all voluntary control over micturition (automatic bladder)

○ D Sympathetic fibres originating in LI and L2 provide continuous tone to the external sphincter, thereby preventing micturition unless desired

○ E Urination will occur if inhibition of the external sphincter through spinal reflex pathways is stronger than the voluntary constrictor signals to the external sphincter from the brain

5.34 **A 35-year-old woman has been diagnosed with idiopathic hyperfunction of the juxtaglomerular apparatus (Bartter's syndrome). Typical findings in patients with Bartter's syndrome are:**

○ A Decreased sensitivity of blood vessels to angiotensin

○ B Low renin levels

○ C Low angiotensin levels

○ D Low aldosterone levels

○ E Very high blood pressure

renal

5.35 A 35-year-old patient with acute glomerulonephritis has a total plasma $[Ca^{2+}]$ = 2.5 mmol/l and a glomerular filtration rate of 160 l/day. What is the estimated daily filtered load of calcium?

○ A 64 mmol/day

○ B 120 mmol/day

○ C 240 mmol/day

○ D 400 mmol/day

○ E 500 mmol/day

5.36 A 15-year-old girl had a past episode of minimal change glomerulonephritis. On follow-up examination, her urinary protein normalised and now is negative. There is very little protein in her glomerular filtrate because:

○ A All serum proteins are too large to fit through the glomerular pores

○ B Of a combination of pore size and negative charges lining the pores

○ C Of active reabsorption of filtered protein by the glomerular epithelial cells

○ D Of metabolism of filtered proteins by the urinary flora

○ E Positive charges line the pores, which repel serum proteins

5.37 A patient with long-standing renal vascular disease has developed chronic renal insufficiency due to a net functional loss of nephrons. If we assume that production of urea and creatinine is constant and that the patient is in a steady state, a 50% decrease in the normal glomerular filtration rate (GFR) will:

○ A Decrease plasma urea concentration

○ B Greatly increase plasma Na^+

○ C Increase the per cent of filtered Na^+ excreted

○ D Not affect plasma creatinine

○ E Significantly decrease plasma K^+

renal

5.38 **A 48-year-old man was admitted to the Accident and Emergency Department with exacerbation of his chronic obstructive pulmonary disease. An arterial blood gas on room air showed respiratory acidosis. The patient's renal excretion of potassium would be expected to:**

○ A Fall, since the filtered load of potassium to the tubules falls in acidosis

○ B Fall, since tubular secretion of potassium is inversely coupled to acid secretion

○ C Rise, since acid and potassium excretion are coupled

○ D Rise, since acidosis is a stimulus to renin secretion by the juxtaglomerular apparatus

○ E Rise, since acidosis increases the affinity of the aldosterone receptor for aldosterone

5.39 **In a normal kidney, a large increase in glomerular filtration rate (GFR) would be expected to occur following:**

○ A An increase in mean arterial pressure from 90 mmHg to 140 mmHg

○ B Vasoconstriction of glomerular afferent arterioles

○ C Vasoconstriction of vasa recta

○ D Strong, acute sympathetic stimulation to kidney

○ E Substantial increases in renal blood flow

5.40 **During a marathon attempt a runner collapses and is admitted with severe acute dehydration. This patient most likely has:**

○ A Decreased baroreceptor firing rate

○ B Decreased plasma osmolarity

○ C High renal water excretion

○ D Low plasma ADH levels

○ E Low water permeability of collecting duct tubular cells

renal

5.41 Renin, also known as angiotensinogenase, is a circulating enzyme released mainly by juxtaglomerular cells in the juxtaglomerular apparatus of the kidneys. Plasma renin levels are decreased in patients with:

○ A Heart failure
○ B Primary aldosteronism
○ C Renal artery stenosis
○ D Salt restriction
○ E Upright posture

5.42 A 79-year-old patient with congestive heart failure and peripheral oedema is given a diuretic. Which of the following diuretics promotes diuresis by opposing the action of aldosterone?

○ A Carbonic anhydrase inhibitor
○ B Loop diuretic
○ C Mannitol
○ D Thiazide
○ E Potassium-sparing diuretic

5.43 In an experiment the primary site of salt and water reabsorption in the kidney was selectively destroyed. Which of the following is the primary site of salt and water reabsorption in the kidney?

○ A Collecting duct
○ B Glomerulus
○ C Juxtaglomerular apparatus
○ D Proximal tubule
○ E Thick ascending limb of the loop Henlé

renal

5.44 **In an experiment the renal site characterised by low water permeability under normal circumstances was selectively destroyed. Which of the following renal sites is characterised by low water permeability under normal circumstances?**

O A Collecting duct

O B Glomerulus

O C Juxtaglomerular apparatus

O D Proximal tubule

O E Thick ascending limb of the loop of Henlé

5.45 **Approximately 80% of phosphate is absorbed in the proximal convoluted tubule. Phosphate reabsorption in the proximal convoluted tubule:**

O A Is due to active co-transport with calcium ions

O B Is due to active co-transport with chloride ions

O C Is due to passive diffusion down its electrochemical gradient

O D Is inhibited by calcitonin

O E Is inhibited by parathyroid hormone

SECTION 6: GASTROINTESTINAL PHYSIOLOGY – QUESTIONS

For each question given below choose the ONE BEST option.

6.1 **A 40-year-old woman was brought to the Accident and Emergency Department complaining of sudden onset of pain in right hypochondrium accompanied by nausea and vomiting. An abdominal ultrasound scan showed presence of gallstones. Gallstones are composed mainly of:**

○ A Bilirubin
○ B Bile salts
○ C Calcium
○ D Cholesterol
○ E Lecithin

6.2 **You have just eaten a beefburger consisting mainly of complex foodstuffs. The breakdown of complex foodstuffs is accomplished by which of the following chemical reactions?**

○ A Dehydration
○ B Hydrolysis
○ C Neutralisation
○ D Oxidation
○ E Reduction

6.3 **Pasta is an important dietary source of complex starches. Complex starches are mainly digested by enzymes secreted from the:**

A Pancreas

B Large intestine

C Salivary glands

D Small intestine

E Stomach

6.4 **In the stomach, chief cells release pepsinogen. Pepsinogen is activated by:**

A Acid pH and pepsin

B Cholecystokinin

C Chymotrypsin

D Gastrin and pepsin

E Trypsin and acid pH

6.5 **Amino acids are the major form in which proteins and peptides are absorbed in the small intestine. Which process transports amino acids across the luminal surface of the epithelium that lines the small intestine?**

A Co-transport with the chloride ion

B Co-transport with glucose

C Co-transport with the sodium ion

D Primary active transport

E Simple diffusion

gastrointestinal

6.6 **The initial phase of protein digestion occurs in the stomach (the gastric phase) and is carried out by pepsin. However, the stomach does not digest itself because:**

○ A Acid is not secreted between meals

○ B Bicarbonate is secreted between meals

○ C Gastric mucosal cells are not digestible

○ D Gastric mucosal cells transport hydrogen ions out of the gastric mucosa

○ E The acid is completely neutralised by food

6.7 **Fat metabolism is in a constant state of dynamic equilibrium, in which some fats are constantly oxidised to meet energy requirements and some fats are synthesised and stored. Stored fat is usually transported from one part of the body to another in the form of:**

○ A Cholesterol

○ B Free fatty acids

○ C Glycerol

○ D Neutral fat

○ E Triglycerides

6.8 **A balance of essential amino acids is necessary for a high degree of net protein utilisation, which is the mass ratio of amino acids converted to proteins to amino acids supplied. The essential amino acids:**

○ A Are all found in all dietary proteins

○ B Are necessary to provide adequate amounts of ATP

○ C Are necessary for synthesis of cholesterol

○ D Can be formed in the body

○ E Must be present in the diet

gastrointestinal

6.9 Colonoscopy of a 38-year-old woman with long-standing ulcerative colitis revealed multiple foci of high-grade dysplasia. The entire colon of this patient had to be removed to prevent colon carcinoma. Which of the following is most likely to happen in this patient with total colectomy and ileostomy?

○ A Following total colectomy and ileostomy, the volume and water content of ileal discharge decreases over time

○ B Long-term survival is not possible, since the colon is a vital organ

○ C Long-term survival is possible, but parenteral nutrition is required to maintain fluid and electrolyte balance

○ D This patient is at increased risk of anaemia due to malabsorption of iron

○ E This patient is at increased risk of anaemia due to malabsorption of vitamin B_{12}

6.10 A 35-year-old man has a history of recurring attacks of pancreatitis, eruptive xanthomas and increased plasma triglyceride levels (2000 mg/dl) associated with chylomicrons. Deficiency of which of the following is the likely cause of these symptoms?

○ A Apo-B-100 receptor

○ B Apo-B-48

○ C HMG-CoA reductase

○ D Low-density lipoprotein (LDL) receptors

○ E Lipoprotein lipase

gastrointestinal

6.11 A 40-year-old man has complained of diarrhoea for 10 days. On examination there is no fever and the patient tells you that the diarrhoea stops when he stops taking food. The most likely cause of diarrhoea is:

○ A Drug induced
○ B Inflammatory
○ C Motility related
○ D Osmotic
○ E Secretory

6.12 Which of the following is most likely to happen if the ileum of a patient is completely resected?

○ A Deficiency of fat content of the stool
○ B Extracellular fluid volume deficiency
○ C Increased iron absorption
○ D Increased calcium absorption
○ E Vitamin B_{12} deficiency

6.13 Triglycerides play an important role in metabolism as energy sources and transporters of dietary fat. They contain more than twice as much energy (9 kcal/g) as carbohydrates and proteins. Which one of the following has the highest content of triglycerides?

○ A Chylomicron
○ B High-density lipoprotein (HDL)
○ C Intermediate-density lipoprotein (IDL)
○ D Low-density lipoprotein (LDL)
○ E Very-low-density lipoprotein (VLDL)

gastrointestinal

6.14 **Vitamin B_{12} is the most chemically complex of all the vitamins. Vitamin B_{12} absorption depends on:**

○ A Ca^{2+}

○ B Fe^{3+}

○ C HCl

○ D Intrinsic factor

○ E Transferrin

6.15 **Iron-deficiency anaemia is often seen in patients following gastrectomy. The reason for this anaemia is:**

○ A Acid secreted by stomach enhances iron absorption

○ B Iron is absorbed in stomach

○ C Intrinsic factor is necessary for iron absorption

○ D Iron is released from heme inside the gastric mucosal cells

○ E Pepsin sets iron free

6.16 **A 6-year-old boy is diagnosed with an inherited metabolic disorder of carbohydrate metabolism that is characterised by an abnormally increased concentration of hepatic glycogen with normal structure and no detectable increase in serum glucose from gluconeogenesis after oral intake of protein-rich diet. These two observations suggest that the disease is a result of the absence of which of the following enzymes?**

○ A Fructokinase

○ B Glucokinase

○ C Glucose-6-phosphatase

○ D Phosphoglucomutase

○ E UDPG–glycogen transglucosylase

gastrointestinal

6.17 **Defecation is the act or process by which humans eliminate solid or semi-solid waste material from the digestive tract. Defecation:**

○ A Is an involuntary act

○ B Is initiated by stretch receptors in the wall of the small intestine

○ C Is solely controlled by spinal centres

○ D Is facilitated by assuming a standing posture to align and dilate the recto–anal junction

○ E Is facilitated by employing the Valsalva manoeuvre

6.18 **A 48-year-old man has been unable to eat for 7 days because of an obstructing lesion in the oesophagus. Which of the following is the major source of fuel being oxidised by his skeletal muscles?**

○ A Muscle creatine phosphate

○ B Muscle glycogen

○ C Muscle triglycerides

○ D Serum fatty acids

○ E Serum glucose

6.19 **A neonate develops abdominal distension with failure to pass meconium. X-ray films of the abdomen show markedly dilated loops of small bowel and colon. Which of the following is the most likely diagnosis?**

○ A Aganglionosis in the rectum

○ B Atrophy of the colonic mucosa

○ C Hypertrophic pyloric stenosis

○ D Meckel's diverticulum

○ E Multiple polyps in the colon

gastrointestinal

131

6.20 **Gastric acid is, together with several enzymes and the intrinsic factor, one of the main secretions of the stomach. Which of the following statements regarding control of gastric acid secretion from oxyntic cells is CORRECT?**

- A Acetylcholine increases gastric acid secretion
- B Gastrin reduces gastric acid secretion
- C Histamine reduces gastric acid secretion
- D Prostaglandin increases gastric acid secretion
- E Somatostatin increases gastric acid secretion

6.21 **A patient underwent total gastrectomy because of a proximal gastric cancer. Which of the following digestive enzymes will be produced in inadequate amounts after the surgery in this patient?**

- A Amylase
- B Chymotrypsin
- C Trypsin
- D Pepsin
- E Proelastase

6.22 **Over the past 4 months, a 50-year-old man has had increasing difficulty swallowing solids and liquids. He has also had regurgitation of undigested solids and liquids. Clinical examination shows no abnormalities. A barium swallow shows dilatation of the distal oesophagus with loss of peristalsis in the distal two-thirds. Which of the following is the most likely diagnosis in this patient?**

- A Achalasia
- B Diffuse oesophageal spasm
- C Oesophageal cancer
- D Oesophageal candidiasis
- E Oesophageal reflux

gastrointestinal

6.23 The small intestine is where the most chemical digestion takes place. Which of the following is an enzyme secreted by mucosa of small intestine?

- A Cholecystokinin
- B Enterokinase
- C Gastrin
- D Lactase
- E Secretin

6.24 A 40-year-old obese woman comes to you in the surgical outpatient clinic complaining of right upper quadrant abdominal pain, which occurs whenever she takes a fatty meal. Which of the following substances may be involved in the pathophysiology of this woman's complaint?

- A Cholecystokinin
- B Chymotrypsin
- C Gastrin
- D Secretin
- E Somatostatin

6.25 The digestive functions of saliva include moistening food and helping to create a food bolus, so it can be swallowed easily. When saliva is freshly formed at ultimate stimulation its pH is:

- A 2.0
- B 4.4
- C 6.0
- D 7.4
- E 8.0

gastrointestinal

6.26 A 38-year-old woman presented in the Accident and Emergency Department with severe abdominal pain radiating to the back. Her serum amylase was markedly elevated. The most likely diagnosis will be?

○ A Cholecystitis
○ B Ectopic pregnancy
○ C Hepatitis
○ D Pancreatitis
○ E Renal spasm

6.27 A patient with gastric hyperacidity was prescribed a proton pump inhibitor. Which of the following statements regarding gastric acid secretion is CORRECT?

○ A At maximum rates of H^+ secretion, H^+ is pumped against a concentration gradient of $10:1$

○ B Cl^- is transported to the lumen of the gland along a concentration gradient

○ C H^+ is transported across the mucosal membrane, using the H^+/Na^+-ATPase system

○ D The mucosal surface of the stomach is always electrically positive

○ E When acid secretion is stimulated in the stomach, the potential difference between mucosa and serosa falls to -20 mV

gastrointestinal

6.28 **Hepatic bile is modified in the gallbladder. Which of the following modifications in hepatic bile takes place in the gallbladder?**

○ A Chloride is added
○ B Calcium is concentrated
○ C H^+ ions are removed
○ D Sodium is added
○ E Water is added

6.29 **Biliary atresia is a rare condition in newborn infants in whom the common bile duct between the liver and the small intestine is blocked or absent with resultant bile retention in the liver. Which of the following statements regarding bile is CORRECT?**

○ A All the steroids and lipids in the bile undergo an enterohepatic circulation
○ B Bile is stored in the gallbladder during digestion
○ C Bile secretion is stimulated by somatostatin
○ D Bile becomes more acidic in the gallbladder
○ E The total estimated bile output per day is about 200–300 ml

6.30 **A mother has given a feed to her child, but after a few minutes the child defecates. This is probably due to:**

○ A Enterogastric reflex
○ B Enterocolic reflex
○ C Gastrocolic reflex
○ D Gastro-oesophageal reflex
○ E Oesophagoenteric reflex

gastrointestinal

6.31 **A patient suffering from severe diarrhoea characteristically has:**

○ A   A decrease in the sodium content of the body

○ B   A metabolic alkalosis

○ C   An increase in the bicarbonate content of the body

○ D   An increase in the magnesium content of the body

○ E   An increase in the potassium content of the body

6.32 **Jaundice is yellowing of the skin, sclerae and other tissues caused by excess circulating bilirubin. Jaundice is likely to be due to:**

○ A   Common bile duct obstruction if the serum amino transferases are elevated and alkaline phosphatase is low

○ B   Haemolytic disease if plasma albumin is low and globulin high

○ C   Haemolytic disease if prothrombin time is prolonged

○ D   Hepatic disease if plasma albumin is low and serum aminotransferase elevations > 500 units

○ E   Hepatic disease if plasma acid phosphatase level is raised

6.33 **A 40-year-old woman, who is jaundiced, presents to you with reports of laboratory tests that reveal conjugated hyperbilirubinaemia. Urine bilirubin levels are significantly above normal while urine urobilinogen levels are significantly below normal. Which of the following is the most likely cause of her jaundice?**

○ A   Blockage of the common bile duct

○ B   Deficiency of glucuronyl transferase

○ C   Gilbert syndrome

○ D   Haemolytic anaemia

○ E   Primary shunt hyperbilirubinaemia

gastrointestinal

6.34 A 48-year-old man with chronic pancreatitis underwent Whipple's operation (for extensive disease at the head of the pancreas). Which of the following statements about pancreas is CORRECT?

- A The endocrine pancreas comprises 98% of the gland
- B The exocrine pancreas secretes approximately 150–250 ml of pancreatic juice per day
- C The exocrine pancreas is stimulated by the sympathetic nervous system
- D The pH of the pancreatic juice is alkaline
- E The pancreatic juice contains enzymes that complete the digestion of only carbohydrates since other food stuffs are digested earlier

6.35 The columnar epithelial cells of the pancreatic ducts secrete most of the aqueous component of the pancreatic juice. In the aqueous component of the pancreatic juice:

- A Cl^- increases threefold above basal levels during high secretory rates
- B HCO_3^- content is greater in response to secretin
- C HCO_3^- and Cl^- concentrations usually vary directly
- D Na^+ is more than in plasma
- E K^+ is less than in plasma

6.36 Abolition of the cephalic phase of pancreatic secretion:

- A Will mainly affect HCO_3^- secretion
- B Will mainly affect enzymatic secretion
- C Will result in 10% reduction in maximal pancreatic secretion
- D Will result after vagotomy
- E Will result after administration of a sympathetic antagonist

gastrointestinal

137

6.37 Deficiency of maltase in the brush border of small intestine:

○ A Does not prevent hydrolysis of maltose because it can be hydrolysed by pancreatic amylase

○ B Decreases rate of absorption of ingested glucose

○ C Results in lack of absorption of lactose

○ D Results in decreased frequency of stool

○ E Results in increased passage of maltose in stool

6.38 A 46-year-old woman following chemotherapy has been having persistent vomiting. Vomiting:

○ A Is a reflex controlled by a centre in the pons

○ B Is not influenced by higher centres in the brain

○ C Is accompanied by hyperchloraemic metabolic acidosis

○ D Is accompanied by hypochloraemic metabolic alkalosis

○ E Is associated with hyperkalaemia

6.39 A 58-year-old man was brought to the Accident and Emergency Department following a haemorrhagic stroke affecting his brainstem. Which of the following can occur in this patient without brainstem co-ordination?

○ A Chewing

○ B Gastric emptying

○ C Primary oesophageal peristalsis

○ D Swallowing

○ E Vomiting

gastrointestinal

6.40 The motility pattern primarily responsible for the propulsion of chyme along the small intestine is:

○ A Haustrations

○ B Myogenic contractions

○ C Peristaltic waves

○ D Segmentation

○ E The migrating motor complex

6.41 Lab report of liver function tests of a patient with jaundice showed predominantly conjugated hyperbilirubinaemia. Which of the following conditions is most likely to be responsible for conjugated hyperbilirubinaemia?

○ A Acute haemolytic crisis in sickle cell disease

○ B Gilbert syndrome

○ C Haemolysis due to rhesus incompatibility

○ D Obstructive jaundice due to carcinoma of common bile duct

○ E Physiological jaundice of the newborn

6.42 A 45-year-old polytrauma patient developed massive haematemesis due to acute stress ulceration in the stomach. He was treated with a continuous infusion of omeprazole. Which of the following is the site of action of omeprazole?

○ A Active H^+ and Cl^- co-transport

○ B Cl^-/HCO_3^- exchange

○ C H^+/K^+-ATPase

○ D Na^+/K^+ pump

○ E Passive diffusion of H^+

gastrointestinal

6.43 Gastrointestinal (GI) resistance vessels are affected by their unique vascular properties, by the presence of vasodilator metabolites, by autonomic nerves and by a variety of circulating agents. Which of the following circulating factors dilates GI resistance vessels?

○ A Adrenaline
○ B Angiotensin II
○ C Noradrenaline
○ D Vasoactive intestinal peptide
○ E Vasopressin

6.44 Gastric blood flow is influenced by both neural and humoral factors. Which of the following factors reduces gastric blood flow?

○ A Acetylcholine
○ B Gastrin
○ C Histamine
○ D Vagal stimulation
○ E Vasopressin

6.45 The basal metabolic rate (BMR) is defined as the rate of calorie consumption after an overnight fast, in the absence of any muscular activity, with the patient in a restful state. Which of the following factors is most likely to reduce BMR?

○ A Decrease in body temperature
○ B Hyperthyroidism
○ C Increase in ambient temperature
○ D Shivering
○ E Stress

gastrointestinal

SECTION 7: NEUROPHYSIOLOGY – QUESTIONS

For each question given below choose the ONE BEST option.

7.1 **Prefrontal leukotomy is no longer prevalent as a treatment for psychiatric disorders, because of undesirable and permanent side-effects. Which of the following is a recognised side-effect of prefrontal leukotomy?**

- ○ A Anger
- ○ B Confusion
- ○ C Global aphasia
- ○ D Motor aphasia
- ○ E Receptive aphasia

7.2 **Electroencephalogram of an adult patient shows waves with a frequency range of 8–12 Hz. Which of the following waves is most probably seen?**

- ○ A Alpha
- ○ B Beta
- ○ C Delta
- ○ D Gamma
- ○ E Theta

7.3 **A middle-aged patient following a stroke developed dysarthria, nystagmus and a tremor that worsens with directed movement. This patient most probably has:**

○ A Cerebellar disease

○ B Damage to pontine and caudate nuclei

○ C Hyperthyroidism

○ D Parkinsonism

○ E Spinal cord transection

7.4 **During a neurological examination, a patient exhibited extension of his toes when the plantar surface of his foot was stroked. An additional neurological finding might be:**

○ A Atrophy

○ B Fasciculations

○ C Hyporeflexia

○ D Hypotonia

○ E Spasticity

7.5 **Parkinsonism is a known disorder of motor function. The primary area involved in this disease is:**

○ A Basal ganglia

○ B Motor cortex

○ C Neostriatum

○ D Red nucleus

○ E Substantia nigra

7.6 Neurotransmitters are chemicals that are used to relay, amplify and modulate electrical signals between a neurone and another cell. Which of the following is a neurotransmitter of the nigrostriatal pathway?

- A Dopamine
- B Gamma-aminobutyric acid (GABA)
- C Glycine
- D Serotonin
- E Noradrenaline

7.7 A lesion of the lateral geniculate nucleus of the thalamus will affect:

- A Hearing
- B Smell
- C Taste
- D Touch
- E Vision

7.8 A lesion of the suprachiasmatic nucleus of hypothalamus will affect:

- A Autonomic function
- B Regulation of circadian rhythm
- C Regulation of water balance
- D Temperature regulation
- E Sexual maturity

7.9 **Lesion of which of the following parts of the brain is most likely to affect rapid eye movement (REM) sleep?**

- A Basal ganglia
- B Frontal lobe
- C Hypothalamus
- D Pons
- E Sulcus terminalis

7.10 **A patient complaining of loss of fine touch and proprioception sense in the lower part of the body (below T6) will have a lesion of:**

- A Anterior limb of internal capsule
- B Cuneate nucleus
- C Descending corticospinal tract
- D Gracile nucleus
- E Lateral spinothalamic tract

7.11 **A patient complaining of loss of pain and temperature sensation in the left leg is most likely to have a lesion of the:**

- A Left corticospinal tract
- B Left anterior spinothalamic tract
- C Left lateral spinothalamic tract
- D Right anterior spinothalamic tract
- E Right lateral spinothalamic tract

7.12 **A lesion of the posterior column–medial lemniscus system is most likely to affect:**

○ A Fine touch
○ B Hearing
○ C Pain sensation
○ D Temperature sensation
○ E Visual acuity

7.13 **Which of the following substances is most likely to be associated with production of pain after an injury?**

○ A Acetylcholine
○ B Adrenaline
○ C Bradykinin
○ D Gamma-aminobutyric acid (GABA)
○ E Substance P

7.14 **A 60-year-old man suffered a stroke. During the recovery phase it was noticed that he had developed a tremor in his fingers. The tremor was most pronounced when he reached for his coffee cup or pointed to an object. Which component of the motor system is most likely to be involved?**

○ A Basal ganglia
○ B Cerebellum
○ C Cerebral cortex
○ D Frontal eye field
○ E Motor nucleus of the thalamus

7.15 A 22-year-old man complaining of headache, nausea and feeling of being unwell for 2 days was seen in the Accident and Emergency Department. He was intolerant to bright light and sounds. Lumbar puncture performed by the on call consultant showed glucose < 40 mg/dl, protein > 4.5 mg/dl and neutrophil leukocytosis. What is the most likely diagnosis?

- A Cervical tumour
- B Cerebral malaria
- C Encephalitis
- D Intracerebral haemorrhage
- E Meningitis

7.16 A 26-year-old man is seen in the Accident and Emergency Department with a lower motor neurone lesion of long standing. This patient will have:

- A Hyperaesthesia
- B Hyper-reflexia
- C Muscle wasting
- D Positive Babinski's sign
- E Spasticity

7.17 **A 30-year-old man is seen in the Accident and Emergency Department complaining of progressive weakness in his arms and legs over the past 4 days. He has been well except for an upper respiratory tract infection 10 days ago. His temperature is 37.8 °C (100 °F), blood pressure is 130/80 mmHg, pulse is 94 beats/min, and respirations are 42 breaths/min and shallow. There is symmetrical weakness of both sides of the face and of the proximal as well as distal muscles of the upper and lower extremities. Sensations are intact. No deep tendon reflexes can be elicited. The plantar responses are flexor. Which of the following is the most likely diagnosis?**

○ A Acute disseminated encephalomyelitis
○ B Guillain–Barré syndrome
○ C Myasthenia gravis
○ D Poliomyelitis
○ E Polymyositis

7.18 **A 12-year-old child fell on his back from the second storey of a building. On arrival in the Accident and Emergency Department he was assessed by the consultant neurologist who told the parents that the child had developed Brown–Séquard syndrome due to hemisection of the spinal cord at the mid-thoracic level. What clinical signs were elicited by the neurologist to arrive at the diagnosis?**

○ A Contralateral spastic paralysis, contralateral loss of vibration and proprioception (position sense) and contralateral loss of pain and temperature sensation beginning one or two segments below the lesion

○ B Contralateral spastic paralysis, ipsilateral loss of vibration and proprioception (position sense) and contralateral loss of pain and temperature sensation beginning one or two segments below the lesion

○ C Ipsilateral spastic paralysis, ipsilateral loss of vibration and proprioception (position sense) and contralateral loss of pain and temperature sensation beginning one or two segments below the lesion

○ D Ipsilateral spastic paralysis, contralateral loss of vibration and proprioception (position sense) and contralateral loss of pain and temperature sensation beginning one or two segments below the lesion

○ E Ipsilateral spastic paralysis, ipsilateral loss of vibration and proprioception (position sense) and ipsilateral loss of pain and temperature sensation beginning one or two segments below the lesion

7.19 **A soldier received a gunshot wound in his back, which resulted in hemisection of the spinal cord on the right side. On clinical examination this patient will have:**

O A Exaggeration of the knee jerk on the left side

O B Impaired two-point discrimination and vibratory sensibility on the left side of body below the lesion

O C Loss of pain and temperature sensibility on the right side of the body beginning two to three segments below the lesion

O D Loss of conscious proprioception in the limbs on the right side that are supplied by dorsal roots below the lesion

O E Spastic paralysis of muscles on the left side of the body below the lesion

7.20 **Which of the following structures in the body is depolarised by mechanical distortion and is independent of K+ channels?**

O A Neuromuscular junction

O B Organ of Corti

O C Pacinian corpuscle

O D Rods and cones

O E Sinoatrial (SA) node

7.21 **Stretch reflex such as knee jerk tends to be exaggerated:**

O A After cerebellar hemisphere damage

O B Immediately following spinal cord transection above the segment responsible for reflex

O C In extrapyramidal disorders like Parkinsonism

O D In upper motor neurone lesion

O E When the subject allows his arm muscles to relax

7.22 A lesion of the reticular activating system will affect:

○ A Co-ordination of endocrine activity
○ B Level of wakefulness
○ C Regulation of micturition
○ D Regulation of gastrointestinal motility
○ E Release of endocrine secretions

7.23 If the ventromedial nucleus of the hypothalamus is destroyed the affected individual will have:

○ A Loss of appetite
○ B Loss of circadian rhythm
○ C Loss of regulation of antidiuretic hormone secretion
○ D Loss of satiety
○ E Loss of vision

7.24 A 58-year-old man suffered a stroke that mainly affected his thalamus. Which of the following abnormalities is most likely to be seen in this patient after the stroke?

○ A Increased sexual drive
○ B Increased temperature
○ C Hyperaesthesia
○ D Hypotonia
○ E Thirst

7.25 A 62-year-old man has a tremor that is caused by a cerebellar lesion. This tremor is most readily differentiated from that caused by loss of the dopaminergic nigrostriatal tracts in that:

○ A It is decreased during activity

○ B It is present at rest

○ C It only occurs during voluntary movements

○ D Its amplitude remains constant during voluntary movements

○ E Its frequency is very regular

7.26 Pupil size is an important indicator of brainstem function. Which of the following statements about pupil diameter is CORRECT?

○ A Atropine causes pupil constriction

○ B Decrease in parasympathetic activity in fibres innervating the inner eye muscles during darkness results in pupil constriction

○ C General increase in sympathetic tone during emotional excitement results in pupil constriction

○ D Increase in sympathetic activity in fibres innervating the inner eye muscles during darkness results in pupil constriction

○ E Phentolamine causes pupil constriction

7.27 The introduction of cold water into one ear may cause giddiness and nausea. The primary cause of this effect of temperature is:

○ A Convection currents in endolymph

○ B Decreased discharge rate in vestibular afferents

○ C Decreased movement of ampullar cristae

○ D Increased discharge rate in vestibular afferents

○ E Temporary immobilisation of otoliths

neurophysiology

7.28 **You are in a closed room listening to music. Suddenly the pitch of the singer's voice increases. Which of the following physiological responses occurs as the pitch of a sound is increased?**

A A greater number of hair cells become activated

B The amplitude of maximal basilar membrane displacement increases

C The frequency of action potentials in auditory nerve fibres increases

D The location of maximal basilar membrane displacement moves toward the base of the cochlea

E Units in the auditory nerve become responsive to a wider range of sound frequencies

7.29 **A 35-year-old woman has a history of progressive muscle weakness. Which of the following diagnostic signs or procedures would support a diagnosis of myasthenia gravis?**

A A small dose of physostigmine is likely to worsen the symptoms

B A large dose of physostigmine is likely to improve the symptoms

C Response of skeletal muscles to direct electrical stimulation is weakened

D Response of skeletal muscle to nerve stimulation is weakened

E The patient should be given α-bungarotoxin to determine the number of acetylcholine binding sites at the postjunctional membrane

7.30 **Which of the following events typically occurs during rapid eye movement (REM) sleep?**

○ A Enuresis

○ B Night terrors

○ C Sleep spindles

○ D Somnambulism

○ E Penile erections

7.31 **You see a patient with damage to the left cervical sympathetic chain ganglia as a result of a neck tumour. Which of the following physical signs would be expected?**

○ A Increased sweat secretion on the left side of the face

○ B Lateral deviation of the left eye

○ C Pale skin on the left side of the face

○ D Ptosis (hanging of the upper eyelid) on the left side

○ E Pupil dilatation of the left eye

7.32 **A 16-year-old girl has hyperopia. Which of the following statements regarding this patient is CORRECT?**

○ A The eyeball of this patient is too long

○ B The lens of this patient has reduced elasticity

○ C The lens of this patient has unusually large refractive power

○ D This patient's condition can be corrected with convex glasses

○ E This patient is nearsighted

7.33 **Which of the following conditions is associated with a decrease in skeletal muscle tone?**

A   Activation of γ-fibres

B   Anxiety

C   Lower motor neurone lesions

D   Parkinson's disease

E   Upper motor neurone lesions

7.34 **The 'dark current' of retinal photoreceptors is generated by:**

A   Cl⁻ channels

B   Non-selective cation channels

C   Non-selective anion channels

D   The ryanodine receptor

E   The Na^+/K^+ pump

7.35 **Following an acute stroke a patient denies the presence of paralysis of his left upper and lower extremities. The most likely cortical lesion in this patient is localised in the:**

A   Posterior inferior gyrus of left frontal lobe

B   Posterior superior gyrus of left temporal lobe

C   Right precentral gyrus

D   Right postcentral gyrus

E   Right posterior parietal cortex

neurophysiology

7.36 A 35-year-old woman is found to have depressed hearing at all frequencies of sound when tested by air conduction but to have normal bone conduction for all frequencies. What is the most likely cause of deafness in this woman?

A Destruction of the cochlea

B Damage to auditory association area

C Fibrosis causing fixation of the ossicles

D Lesion of the auditory nerve

E Poor hair cell function in cochlea

7.37 Why is a sudden loud sound more likely to damage the cochlea than a loud sound that develops slowly?

A A sudden sound carries more energy

B A sudden sound directly damages the vestibular nerve

C The fluid pressure in the scala tympani decreases as a sound becomes louder

D There is a latent period before the attenuation reflex can occur

E The tympanic membrane becomes flaccid as a sound becomes louder

7.38 During a routine preschool examination a 5-year-old boy is found to have difficulty focusing on distant objects. Which of the following statements regarding far accommodation is CORRECT?

A The ciliary muscles are relaxed

B The focal length of the lens is short

C The lens is rounded

D The pupils are constricted (accommodation response)

E The zonular fibres are relaxed

7.39 **A 56-year-old man presents with headache, nausea, left-sided ocular pain and blurred vision. On examination his cornea appears cloudy and the pupils are fixed in a mid-dilated position. Ocular pressure is 48 mmHg (normally < 20 mmHg). Which of the following statements about intraocular pressure is CORRECT?**

○ A Anti-inflammatory corticosteroids are the drug of choice for this patient

○ B Decreased pupil size reduces flow out of ocular chamber

○ C Glaucoma is not a rare cause of blindness in the UK

○ D Intraocular pressure varies by as much as 50% from day to day

○ E Intraocular pressure is mainly determined by the rate of production of the aqueous humour

7.40 **Monitoring regional cerebral blood flow (rCBF) is a method of measuring the dynamics of the physiological substrate of speech. During periods of silent counting, rCBF increases within the:**

○ A Broca's area

○ B Motor cortex

○ C Medial temporal lobe

○ D Occipital cortex

○ E Supplementary motor area

7.41 **A 25-year-old man, who was backseat passenger on a motorcycle, was brought to the Accident and Emergency Department following a head-on collision with a speeding motor car. On arrival in the Accident and Emergency Department a haematoma was noticed on the nape of his neck. A computed tomography (CT) scan revealed a haematoma pressing on the spinal cord in the region of the lateral portion of the dorsal columns. Which of the following functions is most likely to be affected by this lesion?**

- A   Fine motor control of the ipsilateral fingers
- B   Motor control of the contralateral foot
- C   Proprioception from the ipsilateral leg
- D   Sweating of the ipsilateral face
- E   Vibratory sensations from the ipsilateral arm

7.42 **A patient developed decerebrate rigidity following a head injury. Which of the following lesions is most likely to be associated with decerebrate rigidity in this patient?**

- A   Haemorrhage in lateral ventricle
- B   Intercollicular brainstem transection
- C   Internal capsule haemorrhage
- D   Occipital cortex laceration
- E   Parietal cortex contusion

7.43 **While on a holiday a 26-year-old man fell from the second storey of a hotel. He sustained complete transection of the spinal cord at the level of T6. In the immediate post-injury period he is most likely to have:**

A Areflexia

B Decerebrate rigidity

C Exaggerated spinal reflexes below the level of transaction

D Denervation supersensitivity in spinal cord neurones

E Sprouting of the central terminals of primary afferent fibres

7.44 **A 56-year-old diabetic and hypertensive woman suffered a haemorrhagic stroke affecting the primary somatic sensory cortex. Where is the primary somatic sensory cortex located?**

A Central sulcus

B Occipital lobe

C Precentral gyrus

D Postcentral gyrus

E Sylvian fissure

7.45 **A 58-year-old woman with long-standing atrial fibrillation suffered an embolic stroke that affected her primary motor cortex. Where is the primary motor cortex located?**

A Cerebellar vermis

B Occipital lobe

C Precentral gyrus

D Postcentral gyrus

E Sylvian fissure

SECTION 8: ENDOCRINE PHYSIOLOGY – QUESTIONS

For each question given below choose the ONE BEST option.

8.1 A 35-year-old woman is diagnosed as having diabetes insipidus. In this patient although vasopressin (ADH) significantly contributes to fluid and electrolyte balance, it does not appear to closely regulate blood volume in the long run. Blood volume is maintained at near normal levels in this patient because:

- ○ A Plasma oncotic pressure increases
- ○ B Renal blood flow decreases
- ○ C Sympathetic reflexes decrease glomerular filtration
- ○ D The peripheral renin–angiotensin system is stimulated
- ○ E Water intake is appropriately adjusted

8.2 Glucagon is secreted by the α-cells of the pancreatic islets. Which of the following is most likely to induce glucagon secretion?

- ○ A High serum concentration of glucose
- ○ B Low serum concentration of amino acids
- ○ C Low serum concentration of glucose
- ○ D Secretion of somatostatin by the pancreatic δ-cells
- ○ E Parasympathetic stimulation

8.3 **A 46-year-old hypertensive woman has secondary hyperaldosteronism. Aldosterone release in secondary hyperaldosteronism occurs primarily in response to:**

O A Angiotensin II

O B Atrial natriuretic peptide

O C High volume states (fluid overload)

O D Hypernatraemia

O E Hypokalaemia

8.4 **A 36-year-old head-injury patient developed syndrome of inappropriate antidiuretic hormone secretion (SIADH). This patient manifesting SIADH would be expected to have:**

O A High serum sodium due to the direct stimulatory effect of ADH on distal tubular sodium resorption

O B High serum sodium due to the concentrating effect of ADH-induced water excretion in the collecting tubules

O C Low serum sodium due to the dilutional effect of ADH-induced water retention in the collecting tubules

O D Low serum sodium due to a direct inhibitory effect of ADH on distal tubular sodium resorption

O E No change in serum sodium, since the dilutional effect of ADH-induced water retention is balanced by a direct stimulatory effect of ADH on distal tubular sodium resorption

8.5 **Antidiuretic hormone (ADH) is a peptide hormone liberated from a preprohormone precursor that is synthesised in the hypothalamus as it is transported to the posterior pituitary. ADH secretion is most increased by:**

O A Decreased plasma osmolarity

O B Decreased plasma volume

O C Hypothalamic releasing factor

O D Increased plasma osmolarity

O E Increased plasma volume

8.6 **You are asked to see a diabetic patient in the Accident and Emergency Department who has a blood glucose level of 200 mg/dl but, surprisingly, a dipstick test is negative for urinary glucose. How could this finding be explained?**

O A Dipstick tests are more sensitive for reducing sugars other than glucose

O B Patient has diabetes insipidus

O C Patient is in a state of antidiuresis

O D Patient has defective tubular glucose transporters

O E Patient has significantly reduced glomerular filtration rate

endocrine

8.7 **The glycogen stored in the liver is affected by several hormones. Which of the following shows the correct effects of hormones on liver glycogen content?**

	Catecholamines	Glucocorticoids	Glucagon
A	Decreased	Decreased	Decreased
B	Decreased	Decreased	Decreased
C	Decreased	Increased	Decreased
D	Increased	Decreased	Increased
E	Increased	Increased	Decreased

8.8 **A 38-year-old woman presents with a plasma thyroid-stimulating hormone (TSH) 12.5 mU/l (normal < 5 mU/l) and a T_3 resin uptake of 19% (normal 25–35%). Which of the following clinical symptoms and signs would you expect in this patient?**

- A Anxiety
- B Increased body temperature
- C Palpitations
- D Periorbital swelling and lethargy
- E Tachycardia

8.9 **A 79-year-old male patient with chronic renal failure and a glomerular filtration rate of 25 ml/min (normal 120 ml/min) is admitted to the hospital because of a spontaneous fracture of the left humerus. X-ray shows numerous subperiosteal erosions with low bone density. The most likely cause of this patient's fracture is:**

- A Osteomalacia due to primary hyperparathyroidism
- B Osteomalacia due to secondary hyperparathyroidism
- C Osteoporosis due to old age
- D Osteoporosis due to lack of sex steroids
- E Rickets due to lack of dietary vitamin D

8.10 **A patient presents with a brain tumour that has caused blockage of the hypothalamic–hypophyseal venous portal system. Increased secretion of which of the following hormones is most likely to be expected in this patient?**

○ A Adrenocorticotrophic hormone
○ B Follicle-stimulating hormone
○ C Growth hormone
○ D Prolactin
○ E Thyroid-stimulating hormone

8.11 **A 42-year-old woman has Addison's disease. In Addison's disease, one would expect:**

○ A High blood levels of cortisol
○ B Hypertension
○ C Hypoglycaemia between meals
○ D Hypopigmentation
○ E Increased metabolic rate

8.12 **A 26-year-old woman has Graves' disease. In this woman, one would least likely expect:**

○ A Goitre
○ B Increased metabolic rate
○ C Increased sweating
○ D Increased thyroid-stimulating hormone (TSH) secretion
○ E Weight loss

endocrine

8.13 **Growth hormone and glucagon are both polypeptide hormones. Both growth hormone and glucagon:**

◯ A Decrease blood glucose concentration

◯ B Increase blood glucose concentration

◯ C Increase gluconeogenesis

◯ D Increase glycogenolysis

◯ E Increase lipolysis

8.14 **Liver is the main site of glycogenolysis and gluconeogenesis. Which of the following hormones increases hepatic glycogenolysis and promote gluconeogenesis?**

◯ A Cortisol

◯ B Glucagon

◯ C Growth hormone

◯ D Insulin

◯ E Secretin

8.15 **Hormone-sensitive lipase breaks down triglycerides to release free fatty acids. Which of the following hormones impairs hydrolysis of triglycerides to fatty acids by inhibiting hormone-sensitive lipase?**

◯ A Cortisol

◯ B Glucagon

◯ C Growth hormone

◯ D Hydrocortisone

◯ E Insulin

8.16 **The most common cause for goitre in the world is iodine deficiency; this condition is commonly called endemic goitre. A person with endemic goitre would be expected to have:**

○ A Mental retardation

○ B High plasma levels of thyroid-stimulating hormone (TSH)

○ C High plasma levels of thyroxine

○ D Low production of thyroglobulin

○ E Low plasma levels of TSH

8.17 **Patients with hyperthyroidism have high plasma levels of thyroxine. High plasma levels of thyroxine:**

○ A Cause exophthalmos

○ B Cause somnolence

○ C Deplete fat stores

○ D Increase body weight

○ E Produce hypothermia

8.18 **Vitamin D regulates the calcium and phosphorus levels in the blood by promoting their absorption from food in the intestines and by promoting reabsorption of calcium in the kidneys. The active form of vitamin D is:**

○ A 1,25-Dihydroxycholecalciferol

○ B Calcitonin

○ C Cholecalciferol

○ D Ergosterol

○ E Parathyroid hormone

8.19 A 26-year-old man has elevated parathyroid hormone levels secondary to a solitary parathyroid adenoma. Elevated parathyroid hormone levels lead to:

○ A Decreased activity of osteoclasts

○ B Decreased calcium absorption from the intestines

○ C Decreased renal phosphate excretion

○ D Increased formation of 1,25-dihydroxycholecalciferol

○ E Increased renal excretion of calcium

8.20 Parathyroid hormone is a polypeptide secreted by the parathyroid glands. The secretion of parathyroid hormone is controlled by the concentration of:

○ A Calcium bound to citrate anions

○ B Calcium bound to plasma proteins

○ C Calcium inside of the bone matrix

○ D Extracellular ionised calcium

○ E Intracellular phosphate

8.21 Hormones known classically as posterior pituitary hormones are synthesised by the hypothalamus. They are then stored and secreted by the posterior pituitary into the bloodstream. Which of the following hormones is secreted by the posterior pituitary gland?

○ A Follicle-stimulating hormone

○ B Luteinising hormone

○ C Prolactin

○ D Thyroid-stimulating hormone (TSH)

○ E Vasopressin

endocrine

8.22 **A 4-year-old girl has developed rickets due to vitamin D deficiency. Which of the following might be expected in this patient with rickets due to vitamin D deficiency?**

○ A Decreased plasma parathyroid hormone concentration

○ B Hypercalcaemia

○ C Low plasma concentration of 1,25-dihydroxycholecalciferol

○ D Normal plasma phosphate concentration

○ E Suppressed osteoclastic activity

8.23 **In an untreated adrenalectomised subject, a physician would most likely find:**

○ A Increased blood glucose

○ B Increased daily excretion of 17-hydroxysteroids

○ C Increased daily excretion of 17-ketosteroids

○ D Increased skin pigmentation

○ E Increased volume of extracellular fluid

8.24 **A 56-year-old woman on long-term steroid therapy was brought to the Accident and Emergency Department unconscious and hypotensive. On enquiry from the ambulance crew it was discovered that she had been unwell for last few days and had stopped taking her oral prednisolone. She most likely has:**

○ A Addisonian crisis

○ B Diabetic ketoacidosis

○ C Hypothyroidism

○ D Primary hyperaldosteronism

○ E Sheehan's syndrome

endocrine

8.25 **A 6-year-old boy with short stature and delayed bone age is started on recombinant growth hormone therapy. Which of the following laboratory findings is most likely to be seen after 3 months of therapy?**

    A Decreased serum insulin-like growth factor-1 concentration

    B Decreased serum free fatty acid levels

    C Increased alkaline phosphatase activity

    D Increased acid phosphatase concentration

    E Increased blood urea nitrogen (BUN) concentration

8.26 **A 23-year-old student has severe diarrhoea resulting from an intestinal parasite that he acquired on a trip to the Far East. He loses 4.0 l of intestinal fluid over a 6-hour period, but feels too sick to drink any fluids. His urine output during the 6-hour ordeal is only 0.1 l. Which of the following physiological changes is most likely to be found in this patient at the end of the 6-hour period as compared with the hour before the onset of diarrhoea?**

    A Decreased plasma angiotensin II levels

    B Decreased urine osmolarity

    C Increased extracellular fluid volume

    D Increased glomerular filtration rate

    E Increased plasma aldosterone levels

endocrine

8.27 **A 48-year-old woman has secondary hyperaldosteronism. Which of the following can produce secondary hyperaldosteronism?**

○ A Increased adrenocorticotrophic hormone (ACTH)
○ B Increased angiotensin II
○ C Increased cortisol
○ D Increased renin
○ E Salt excess

8.28 **A women was brought to the Accident and Emergency Department semi-conscious, with a history of post-partum haemorrhage (PPH) 10 years back. She has been on growth hormone replacement therapy as well as thyroxine since then. What is the most likely diagnosis?**

○ A Addison's disease
○ B Cushing's syndrome
○ C Hypothyroidism
○ D Sheehan's syndrome
○ E SIADH

8.29 **The insulin receptor is a transmembrane receptor. The intracellular domain of the insulin receptors has which of the following enzyme activities?**

○ A Adenylyl cyclase
○ B Phosphodiesterase
○ C Phospholipase C
○ D Phosphoprotein phosphatase
○ E Tyrosine kinase

endocrine

8.30 **A 36-year-old woman is diagnosed with a phaeochromocytoma. She is most likely to have increased serum levels of:**

O   A Aldosterone

O   B Cortisol

O   C Noradrenaline

O   D Oxytocin

O   E Vasopressin

8.31 **Growth hormone is a 191-amino-acid, single-chain polypeptide hormone that is synthesised, stored and secreted by the somatotroph cells within the lateral wings of the anterior pituitary gland, which stimulates growth and cell reproduction in humans. Secretion of growth hormone is increased by:**

O   A Cortisol

O   B Exercise

O   C Free fatty acids

O   D Hyperglycaemia

O   E Somatostatin

8.32 **Aldosterone and cortisol are steroid hormones. Steroid hormones act via:**

O   A Altering ion channels

O   B Formation of cAMP

O   C Formation of DAG + IP_3

O   D Gene transcription

O   E Tyrosine kinase activity

8.33 **A 15-year-old girl is seen in the endocrinology clinic because of irritability, restlessness, difficulty concentrating, and deteriorating academic performance over the past 2 months. She has had occasional palpitations and a 1-kg weight loss during this period despite an increased appetite. Menarche was at the age of 12 years, and her menses occur at regular intervals. Examination shows no abnormalities. Serum tri-iodothyronine (T$_3$) and thyroxine (T$_4$) levels are increased. Which of the following is the most likely diagnosis?**

○ A Attention-deficit/hyperactivity disorder
○ B Diabetes mellitus
○ C Hyperthyroidism
○ D Pituitary adenoma
○ E Thyroid cancer

8.34 **A 48-year-old woman was diagnosed as having tertiary hypothyroidism. Which of the following abnormalities is a feature of tertiary hypothyroidism?**

○ A Antithyroid antibodies
○ B Decreased plasma levels of cholesterol and triglycerides
○ C Exaggerated reflexes
○ D High serum T$_3$ levels
○ E Hypothalamic failure

endocrine

8.35 **A 40-year-old woman underwent total thyroidectomy for a follicular carcinoma of the thyroid gland. Which one of the following after-effects would you expect after total thyroidectomy in this patient?**

○ A Elevated total T_4

○ B Elevated free T_4

○ C Elevated T_3

○ D Elevated thyroid-stimulating hormone (TSH)

○ E Elevated calcium level

8.36 **Tumours of the adrenal medulla that are actively producing catecholamines are called phaeochromocytomas. Patients with these tumours experience sudden periodic increases in catecholamine blood levels. During such an episode patients may experience:**

○ A Anxiety

○ B Decreased heart rate

○ C Decreased blood pressure

○ D Decreased blood glucose

○ E Decreased sweat secretion

8.37 **Patients who are hyperparathyroid usually suffer from a tumour (adenoma) of one of the parathyroid glands. Which of the following is most likely to be seen in a patient with hyperparathyroidism?**

○ A Less bone resorption

○ B Less calcium absorption from the small intestine

○ C Less phosphate absorption from the small intestine

○ D Increased calcitriol

○ E Tetany

8.38 **21-Hydroxylase is an enzyme that is involved with the biosynthesis of the steroid hormones, aldosterone and cortisol. A 2-year-old baby girl with deficiency of 21-hydroxylase is most likely to have:**

O A Congenital adrenal hyperplasia
O B Conn's syndrome
O C Cushing's syndrome
O D Klinefelter's syndrome
O E Turner's syndrome

8.39 **Which of the following reactions is stimulated by adrenocorticotrophic hormone (ACTH) to promote the production of cortisol?**

O A 11-Deoxycortisol to cortisol
O B 17-Hydroxyprogesterone to 11-deoxycortisol
O C Cholesterol to pregnenolone
O D Progesterone to 17-hydroxyprogesterone
O E Pregnenolone to progesterone

8.40 **Insulin deficiency results in diabetes mellitus. Which of the following is a recognised metabolic effect of insulin?**

O A Decreased amino acid uptake
O B Decreased esterification of fatty acids
O C Decreased gluconeogenesis
O D Decreased glycogen synthesis
O E Decreased potassium uptake

endocrine

8.41 **You have been asked to review the thyroid function tests report of a patient who shows T_3 value of 3 (< normal), T_4 value of 8 (< normal) and thyroid-stimulating hormone (TSH) value of 200 (high). What is the most likely diagnosis?**

○ A Hyperparathyroidism

○ B Hyperpituitarism

○ C Hyperthyroidism

○ D Hypoparathyroidism

○ E Hypothyroidism

8.42 **Beta-endorphin is a cleavage product of pro-opiomelanocortin (POMC). POMC is the precursor hormone for:**

○ A Adrenocorticotrophic hormone (ACTH)

○ B Cortisol

○ C Growth hormone

○ D Prolactin

○ E Thyroid-stimulating hormone (TSH)

8.43 **Cortisol and adrenal androgens are synthesised from cholesterol. Which of the following substances is an intermediary in the metabolism of cortisol and androgens?**

○ A Aldosterone

○ B Corticosterone

○ C Oestrogen

○ D Pregnenolone

○ E Progesterone

8.44 **A 22-year-old woman has puffy eyes and hoarse voice. Her plasma thyroid-stimulating hormone (TSH) concentration is low but increases markedly when she is given thryrotrophin-releasing hormone (TRH). She probably has:**

○ A Hyperthyroidism due to a thyroid tumour

○ B Hyperthyroidism due to a primary abnormality in the hypothalamus

○ C Hypothyroidism due to a primary abnormality in the hypothalamus

○ D Hypothyroidism due to a primary abnormality in pituitary gland

○ E Hypothyroidism due to a primary abnormality in thyroid gland

8.45 **Follicle-stimulating hormone (FSH) is a glycoprotein hormone synthesised and secreted by gonadotrophs in the anterior pituitary gland. In men FSH:**

○ A Acts as an antagonist of testosterone

○ B Inhibits Sertoli cells

○ C Inhibits sperm maturation

○ D Secretion is completely suppressed by testosterone

○ E Stimulates the synthesis of androgen-binding protein

8.46 **A 34-year-old man with parathyroid adenoma has hypercalcaemia. A high plasma calcium level causes:**

○ A Bone demineralisation

○ B Decreased secretion of calcitonin

○ C Decreased blood coagulability

○ D Increased formation of 1,25-dihydroxycholecalciferol

○ E Short QT interval on ECG

endocrine

8.47 **Cortisol (or hydrocortisone) is the most important human glucocorticoid. It is essential for life and regulates or supports a variety of important cardiovascular, metabolic, immunological and homeostatical functions. Cortisol:**

O A Decreases normal sensitivity of vascular smooth muscle to the vasoconstrictor effects of catecholamines

O B Deficiency results in filling of vascular beds

O C Enables kidney to retain potassium

O D Enables kidney to lose sodium

O E Increases normal sensitivity of vascular smooth muscle to the vasoconstrictor effects of catecholamines

8.48 **Which of the following effects on salivary secretion will be observed as a result of aldosterone release?**

O A Reabsorption of HCO_3^-

O B Reabsorption of Na^+

O C Reabsorption of K_+

O D Secretion of Cl^-

O E Secretion of Na^+

8.49 **Which of the following hormones will an individual be unable to produce if zona glomerulosa cells in the adrenal glands are completely destroyed?**

O A Adrenaline

O B Aldosterone

O C Cortisol

O D Dehydroepiandrosterone

O E Oestrogen

endocrine

8.50 **A 40-year-old woman is diagnosed as having chronic primary adrenal insufficiency due to destruction of the adrenal glands by tuberculosis. Which of the following effects is most likely to be found in this patient?**

○ A Hyperglycaemia

○ B Hypokalaemia

○ C Hyponatraemia

○ D Hypopigmentation

○ E Hypophosphataemia

8.51 **A 22-year-old male type I diabetic was received in the Accident and Emergency Department in ketoacidosis. What is the basic pathophysiology of diabetic ketoacidosis?**

○ A Action of glucagon

○ B Decreased deacylase

○ C Decreased enzyme production by liver

○ D Increased ketone bodies formation

○ E Insulin deficiency

8.52 **The hormonal analysis of a 40-year-old man shows elevation of parathyroid hormone (PTH) in serum. Which of the following statements regarding PTH is most likely to be CORRECT?**

○ A PTH secretion is increased by 1,25-dihydroxycholecalciferol

○ B PTH secretion is increased by a high plasma level of ionised calcium

○ C PTH secretion is increased by increased plasma magnesium level

○ D PTH secretion is increased by increased plasma phosphate level

○ E PTH secretion is increased by PTH-releasing hormone

endocrine

8.53 **Catecholamines are produced in the adrenal medulla. Which of the following effects is most likely to be seen in response to the release of catecholamines from the adrenal medulla?**

O A Decreased blood levels of free fatty acids and ketone bodies

O B Decreased plasma lactic acid level

O C Increased blood level of glucose due to glycogenolysis in liver and muscle cells

O D Increased bronchial constriction

O E Increased muscle and splanchnic blood flow

8.54 **A 65-year-old diabetic patient has poorly controlled diabetes mellitus. Which of the following biochemical changes is associated with inadequately controlled diabetes?**

O A Abnormally rapid fall of blood glucose following a meal

O B Abnormally low concentration of fatty acids in blood

O C Increased protein breakdown

O D High rate of glycogen synthesis in liver

O E Decreased gluconeogenesis

8.55 **Biochemical mechanisms of signal transduction follow the pharmacological subdivisions of the adrenergic receptors. Stimulation of either β_1 or β_2 receptors:**

O A Activates adenylate cyclase

O B Activates guanylate cyclase

O C Activates gene transcription

O D Inhibits adenylate cyclase

O E Inhibits guanylate cyclase

8.56 **Which of the following hormones exhibits a diurnal rhythm in its secretion?**

O A Adrenocorticotrophic hormone (ACTH)

O B Adrenaline

O C Aldosterone

O D Parathyroid hormone

O E Prolactin

8.57 **A 48-year-old woman on long-term steroid therapy for rheumatoid arthritis has now developed Cushing's syndrome. Administration of glucocorticoids in high doses for prolonged periods results in:**

O A Hypotension

O B Increased libido

O C Purple striae on the trunk

O D Rapid weight loss

O E Thickening of skin

8.58 **Aldosterone is the primary mineralocorticoid. Which of the following is the primary stimulus for the release of aldosterone?**

O A Angiotensin II

O B Cortisol

O C High blood volume

O D Hypernatraemia

O E Hypokalaemia

endocrine

8.59 **Although named for their critical role in carbohydrate metabolism, glucocorticoids produce a number of diverse physiological actions. In humans, cortisol is the major glucocorticoid and the terms are used interchangeably. Which of the following effects is most likely to be seen following cortisol release?**

- O A Decreased gluconeogenesis
- O B Decreased mobilisation of fatty acids and glycerol from adipose tissue
- O C Decreased phagocytosis by white blood cells
- O D Decreased stabilisation of lysosomal membranes
- O E Decreased utilisation of amino acids for the formation of protein in the liver

8.60 **A series of photographs taken of a middle aged man over a period of two decades demonstrates gradual coarsening of facial features and progressive protrusion of the brows. Upon enquiry the patient reports having to wear larger shoes and gloves than he did as a young man. Which one of the following pairs of hormones normally regulates the hormone responsible for these changes?**

- O A Thyrotrophin-stimulating hormone (TSH) and adrenocorticotrophic hormone (ACTH)
- O B Luteinising hormone (LH) and human chorionic gonadotrophin (hCG)
- O C Prolactin and FSH
- O D Somatostatin and growth hormone-releasing hormone (GHRH)
- O E Dopamine and noradrenaline

SECTION 9: REPRODUCTIVE PHYSIOLOGY – QUESTIONS

For each question given below choose the ONE BEST option.

9.1 Serum samples from a normal 24-year-old woman with a history of regular 28-day menstrual cycles show a peak in the serum concentration of 17β-oestradiol over the past 12 h. No progesterone is detectable. Which of the following events is expected to occur as result of this hormonal surge?

- A Cessation of menstruation
- B Decreased basal body temperature
- C Onset of menstruation
- D Ovulation
- E Regression of the corpus luteum

9.2 A 19-year-old pregnant woman noted vaginal bleeding. Uterine ultrasound revealed small grape-like cystic structures without evidence of a developing embryo. A diagnosis of complete hydatidiform mole was made at the hospital. Further analysis is most likely to reveal that:

- A The genotype of the mole is triploid
- B The genotype of the mole is 46,XX and is completely paternal in origin
- C Human chorionic gonadotrophin (hCG) levels are markedly decreased
- D Serum levels of α-fetoprotein are elevated
- E Two or more sperm fertilised the ovum

9.3 **Which of the following would be expected if an antibody that neutralises the activity of human chorionic gonadotrophin (hCG) is administered for 7 days starting 4 weeks after conception?**

○ A Death of the embryo and its subsequent expulsion

○ B Decreased secretion of pituitary LH

○ C Increased secretion of oestradiol

○ D Increased secretion of progesterone

○ E Increased secretion of prolactin

9.4 **Endometrial biopsy from a 24-year-old healthy woman with regular menstrual cycle shows the presence of highly coiled arteries with oedema. Which of the following stages of the menstrual cycle correlates with this description?**

○ A Early proliferative

○ B Late proliferative

○ C Menstruation

○ D Ovulation

○ E Secretory

9.5 **A 39-year-old woman with six previous healthy children and uneventful childbirths was brought to the hospital with severe vaginal bleeding following a difficult vaginal delivery at home. On examination her fundal height was 24-week size. What is the most likely cause of her vaginal bleeding?**

○ A Atony of bladder

○ B Atony of uterus

○ C Bleeding disorder

○ D Cervical tear

○ E Vaginal laceration

9.6 **A 32-year-old woman presented in the antenatal clinic with history of habitual abortion. Deficiency of which of the following hormones is associated with habitual abortion?**

○ A LH
○ B FSH
○ C hCG
○ D Oestrogen
○ E Progesterone

9.7 **Oestrogens are a group of steroid compounds, named for their importance in the oestrous cycle and functioning as the primary female sex hormone. In the body these are all produced from:**

○ A 1,25-Dihydroxycholecalciferol
○ B Aldosterone
○ C Androgens
○ D Cortisol
○ E Corticosterone

9.8 **A 28-year-old woman is in her first trimester of pregnancy. Which of the following changes is most likely to occur in her circulatory system during pregnancy?**

○ A Blood volume remains unchanged
○ B Blood flow to the brain increases
○ C Cardiac output increases
○ D Cutaneous vasoconstriction occurs
○ E Mean arterial pressure is maximum in the first trimester

reproductive

9.9 **A 26-year-old woman is 16 weeks pregnant. Which of the following respiratory adjustments is most likely to occur during pregnancy in this woman?**

○ A Alveolar ventilation is increased

○ B $p(CO_2)$ is increased

○ C $p(O_2)$ is decreased

○ D The sensitivity of the hypothalamic respiratory centres to $p(CO_2)$ is reduced

○ E Tidal volume is reduced

9.10 **A 29-year-old woman is 12 weeks pregnant. Which of the following renal function adjustments is most likely to take place during pregnancy in this woman?**

○ A Amino acid loss in the urine is decreased

○ B Glomerular filtration is reduced

○ C Glucose loss in the urine is reduced

○ D Renal plasma flow is increased

○ E Solute loss in the urine is reduced

9.11 **Human placental lactogen (hPL) is a placental hormone. hPL:**

○ A Induces lipid synthesis in the pregnant women

○ B Is a steroid hormone

○ C Is also called human chorionic somatotrophin

○ D Is similar in structure and function to growth hormone

○ E Is secreted by the placental cytotrophoblasts

9.12 **A 28-year-old woman is 4 months pregnant. Which of the following parameters is most likely to be decreased in this woman during pregnancy?**

○ A Cardiac output
○ B Gamma-globulins
○ C Glomerular filtration rate (GFR)
○ D $p(CO_2)$
○ E Tidal volume

9.13 **Progesterone is an absolute requirement for maintenance of pregnancy. Which of the following is the major source of progesterone in a woman who is 8 weeks pregnant?**

○ A Corpus luteum
○ B Fetal liver
○ C Maternal liver
○ D Placental cytotrophoblast
○ E Placental syncytiotrophoblast

9.14 **A 25-year-old, 35 weeks pregnant, previously healthy woman is brought to the Accident and Emergency Department complaining of anorexia, nausea, vomiting, fever and yellowish discoloration of the eyes. She is tender in the right hypochondrium. Her blood pressure is normal and there is no past history of alcoholism or viral infections. Which of the following is the most likely reason for this woman's enlarged liver?**

○ A Acute hepatitis
○ B Acute fatty liver
○ C Autoimmune hepatitis
○ D HELLP syndrome
○ E Macronodular cirrhosis

reproductive

9.15 **The secretion of testosterone by interstitial (Leydig) cells in the testes is stimulated by the secretion of which of the following cell types?**

○ A Pituitary acidophils

○ B Pituitary basophils

○ C Primary spermatocytes

○ D Sertoli cells

○ E Spermatogonia

9.16 **Which of the following hormones stimulates respiration and causes the arterial $p(CO_2)$ to fall during pregnancy?**

○ A Cortisol

○ B Glucose

○ C Insulin

○ D Oestrogen

○ E Progesterone

9.17 **Which of the following hormones causes increased circulating level of coagulation factors II, VII, IX and X?**

○ A Follicle-stimulating hormone (FSH)

○ B Human chorionic gonadotrophin (hCG)

○ C Human placental lactogen (hPL)

○ D Oestrogen

○ E Progesterone

9.18 **Which of the following effects is most likely to be seen following bilateral oophorectomy in a woman of reproductive age?**

○ A   Increase uterine growth
○ B   Increase hepatic production of binding proteins
○ C   Reduced bone resorption
○ D   Reduced fat deposition
○ E   Salt and water retention

9.19 **Which of the following hormones is a glycoprotein?**

○ A   Androstenedione
○ B   Human placental lactogen
○ C   Luteinising hormone (LH)
○ D   Oestrogen
○ E   Progesterone

9.20 **If the follicle stimulating hormone (FSH)-producing cells in the anterior pituitary gland were selectively destroyed this would lead to:**

○ A   Decreased level of testosterone
○ B   Decreased level of LH
○ C   Decreased sperm count
○ D   Increased level of testosterone
○ E   Sertoli cells proliferation

reproductive

9.21 **A 16-year-old boy is diagnosed with hypogonadism due to a deficiency of gonadotrophin-releasing hormone (GnRH). Hypogonadism caused by a deficiency of GnRH is termed:**

O   A   Asherman's syndrome

O   B   Kallman's syndrome

O   C   Mendelson's syndrome

O   D   Swyer's syndrome

O   E   Turner's syndrome

9.22 **The Sertoli cell (a kind of sustentacular cell) is a 'nurse' cell of the testes that is part of a seminiferous tubule. Injury to Sertoli cells will affect the production of:**

O   A   FSH

O   B   Inhibin

O   C   LH

O   D   Oestrogen

O   E   Testosterone

9.23 **Androgen-binding protein is a glycoprotein (β-globulin) produced by the Sertoli cells in the seminiferous tubules of the testis that:**

O   A   Binds specifically to testosterone only

O   B   Makes testosterone more lipophilic

O   C   Inhibits spermatogenesis

O   D   Is regulated by oestrogen

O   E   Is regulated by FSH

9.24 **Which of the following is most likely to be seen in a 21-year-old man following removal of testes?**

○ A Increased bone synthesis
○ B Increased calcium retention
○ C Increased deepening of voice
○ D Increased gonadotrophin-releasing hormone secretion
○ E Increased nitrogen retention

9.25 **Which of the following is a feature of seminal fluid produced by seminal vesicles?**

○ A Absence of amino acids
○ B Acidic in nature
○ C Large amounts of ascorbic acid
○ D Large amounts of thromboxane
○ E Rich in lactate

9.26 **Which of the following components of the semen will be deficient if the ampulla of the vas deferens was somehow or other removed from the male reproductive tract without affecting the rest of it?**

○ A Ascorbic acid
○ B Bicarbonate ions
○ C Fructose
○ D Phosphorylcholine
○ E Sperm

reproductive

9.27 **A 23-year-old woman has a progressive increase in serum human chorionic gonadotrophin (hCG) concentrations over an 8-week period. A hydatidiform mole is removed, but the hCG concentration continues to increase. The most likely diagnosis is:**

○ A Adrenal adenoma

○ B A second non-invasive mole

○ C Choriocarcinoma

○ D Ectopic pregnancy

○ E Pituitary insufficiency

9.28 **Activation of spermatozoa is an essential step for successful fertilisation. Activation of spermatozoa:**

○ A Is a calcium-dependent event

○ B Is a glucose-dependent event

○ C Occurs before ejaculation takes place

○ D Requires magnesium for successful completion

○ E Takes place in the epididymis

9.29 **Lactation does not occur during pregnancy because the action of prolactin is blocked by increased concentrations of which of the following hormones?**

○ A Growth hormone

○ B Human chorionic somatomammotrophin

○ C Insulin

○ D Progesterone

○ E Thyroxine

9.30 **Which of the following hormones produces contraction of the smooth muscle cells underlying the milk-producing alveolar cells?**

○ A FSH
○ B Oestrogen
○ C Oxytocin
○ D Progesterone
○ E Prolactin

9.31 **Which of the following hormones prevents menstrual cycle during the early post-partum period?**

○ A FSH
○ B Oestrogen
○ C Oxytocin
○ D Progesterone
○ E Prolactin

9.32 **A 32-year-old woman is in labour. Which of the following substances is the most important factor for initiation of labour in this woman?**

○ A Maternal ACTH
○ B Maternal cortisol
○ C Maternal oxytocin
○ D Maternal prolactin
○ E Maternal prostaglandin

reproductive

9.33 Which of the following is a recognised effect of oestrogen on parturition?

○ A Decreased gap-junction formation in myometrium
○ B Enhancement of effects of progesterone
○ C Inhibition of prostaglandin output
○ D Inhibition of myometrial contractility
○ E Stimulation of the number of oxytocin receptors in the decidua and myometrium

9.34 Which of the following is a feature of the antral phase of ovarian cycle in a woman of reproductive age?

○ A Degeneration of corpus luteum
○ B Formation of corpus luteum
○ C Formation of Graafian follicles
○ D High levels of progesterone
○ E Luteinisation of the granulosa cells

9.35 A 34-year-old woman has developed progressive hirsutism over the face and body for the past 2 years. She takes no medications. Her blood pressure is 116/80 mmHg. Examination shows a slightly abnormal amount of hair growth over the upper lip, chin, chest, and abdomen. There is no truncal obesity or purple striae. She has also developed oligomenorrhoea. Pelvic examination suggested enlarged ovaries. Which of the following is the most likely diagnosis?

○ A Adrenal adenoma
○ B Congenital adrenal hyperplasia
○ C Cushing's syndrome
○ D Hypothyroidism
○ E Polycystic ovarian syndrome

9.36 **Free testosterone is transported into the cytoplasm of target tissue cells, where it can bind to the androgen receptor or can be converted to dihydrotestosterone. Conversion of testosterone to dihydrotestosterone is brought about by:**

○ A 3β-Hydroxysteroid dehydrogenase

○ B 5α-Reductase

○ C 17β-Hydroxylase

○ D 17,20-Desmolase

○ E 20,22-Desmolase

9.37 **Testosterone is the male sex hormone. Testosterone is synthesised in the testes from:**

○ A Cholesterol

○ B Glycine

○ C Oestrogen

○ D Taurine

○ E Tyrosine

9.38 **Testosterone is the biologically important product of the Leydig cell. In plasma:**

○ A 2% testosterone circulates as free testosterone

○ B 22% testosterone circulates as free testosterone

○ C 98% testosterone circulates as free testosterone

○ D Testosterone is completely bound to proteins

○ E Testosterone is not normally found

reproductive

9.39 **Which of the following components of semen will be absent following radical prostatectomy?**

A Ascorbic acid

B Alkaline phosphatase

C Citric acid

D Fructose

E Phosphorylcholine

9.40 **Following menopause, secretion of which of the following hormones increases?**

A FSH

B Oxytocin

C Oestrogen

D Prolactin

E hCG

9.41 **A 45-year-old woman comes to you with a 3-month history of episodes (of about 5 min) in which she becomes overwhelmingly hot and sweats so much that her clothes become wet. Menses are regular, but the intermenstrual interval has decreased by 5 days over the past 6 months. Her temperature is 37°C (98.6°F), blood pressure is 110/70 mmHg, and pulse is 74 beats/min. Examination shows no other abnormalities. Which of the following is the most likely explanation for these findings?**

A Carcinoid tumour

B Excessive caffeine ingestion

C Generalised anxiety disorder

D Hot flush

E Hyperthyroidism

9.42 **A normal healthy woman became pregnant. On her first antenatal visit she had haemoglobin concentration of 12 g/dl. After 24 weeks of gestation she had haemoglobin of 10 g/dl with normal blood picture. The most likely cause is:**

○ A Folate-deficiency anaemia

○ B Iron-deficiency anaemia

○ C Thalassaemia

○ D Vitamin B_{12} deficiency

○ E Physiological response

9.43 **Menstrual bleeding serves as a sign that a woman has not become pregnant. Menstrual bleeding is a consequence of:**

○ A Progesterone withdrawal

○ B Proliferative phase of endometrium

○ C Prostaglandin withdrawal

○ D Secretory phase of endometrium

○ E Thickening of endometrium

9.44 **Which of the following substances is transported by facilitated diffusion across the placental barrier?**

○ A Amino acids

○ B Conjugated steroids

○ C Glucose

○ D Nucleotides

○ E Water-soluble vitamins

reproductive

9.45 Infertility in the man can be:

○ A Explained by failure of the sperms in a sample of semen to remain motile for more than 24 h

○ B Explained by finding that 10% of the sperms in a sample are definitely abnormal

○ C Explained by finding a sperm count that is 50% below average

○ D Explained by failure of testis to descend

○ E Treated effectively in some cases with large doses of vitamin E

9.46 What is the normal sperm count per ejaculate?

○ A 10–20 million

○ B 25–50 million

○ C 70–80 million

○ D 100–110 million

○ E 200–500 million

9.47 In the normal healthy 25-year-old woman menstruation:

○ A Always occurs every 4 weeks except during or immediately after pregnancy

○ B Is a period of secretion by the endometrium of the uterus

○ C Occurs 1–2 days after ovulation

○ D Occurs after the demise of corpus luteum in the ovary

○ E Occurs several hours after the formation of a corpus luteum in the ovary

reproductive

9.48 **A patient at 3–4 weeks of gestation develops marked pruritus. Among the diagnostic possibilities is:**

- ○ A Cholestasis of pregnancy
- ○ B Diabetes insipidus
- ○ C Hyperthyroidism
- ○ D Pancreatitis
- ○ E Pancreatic cancer

9.49 **Capacitation of sperms takes place in the uterus. Capacitation allows:**

- ○ A Decreased energy metabolism
- ○ B Enhanced motility
- ○ C Inhibition of acrosome reaction
- ○ D Release of FSH
- ○ E Release of LH

9.50 **A 28-year-old woman is 5 months pregnant with her second child. Pregnancy and delivery of her first child were unremarkable. Which of the following combinations poses a significant risk of haemolytic anaemia for her second child?**

	Mother	First child	Second child
○ A	Rh-negative	Rh-negative	Rh-positive
○ B	Rh-negative	Rh-positive	Rh-positive
○ C	Rh-positive	Rh-positive	Rh-negative
○ D	Rh-positive	Rh-negative	Rh-positive
○ E	Rh-positive	Rh-positive	Rh-positive

reproductive

ANSWERS

SECTION 1:
GENERAL PHYSIOLOGY –
ANSWERS

1.1

Answer: C　Gap junctions

A gap junction is a junction between certain animal cell types that allows different molecules and ions to pass freely between cells. The junction connects the cytoplasm of cells. One gap junction is composed of two connexons (or hemichannels), which connect across the intercellular space. They are analogous to the plasmodesmata that join plant cells. In vertebrates, gap-junction hemichannels are primarily homo- or hetero-hexamers of connexin proteins. Invertebrate gap junctions comprise proteins from the hypothetical innexin family. However, the recently characterised pannexin family, functionally similar but genetically distinct from connexins and expressed in both vertebrates and invertebrates, probably encompasses the innexins. Gap junctions formed from two identical hemichannels are called homotypic, while those with differing hemichannels are heterotypic. In turn, hemichannels of uniform connexin composition are called homomeric, while those with differing connexins are heteromeric. Channel composition is thought to influence the function of gap-junction channels but it is not yet known how.

Gap junctions:

- allow for direct electrical transmission between cells

- allow for chemical transmission between cells, through the transmission of small second messengers, such as IP_3 and Ca^{2+}

- allow any molecule smaller than 1 kDa to pass through.

1.2

Answer: D Lysosomes

Lysosomes are organelles that contain digestive enzymes (acid hydrolases) to digest macromolecules. They are found in both animal and plant cells but they are rare in plant cells. They are built in the Golgi apparatus. The name comes from the Greek words 'lysis', which means dissolution or destruction and 'soma', which means body. They are frequently nicknamed 'suicide-bags' by cell biologists due to their role in autolysis. Lysosomes were discovered by the Belgian cytologist Christian de Duve in the 1949. The lysosomes are used for the digestion of macromolecules from phagocytosis (ingestion of cells), from the cell's own recycling process (where old components such as worn out mitochondria are continuously destroyed and replaced by new ones and receptor proteins are recycled) and for autophagic cell death, a form of programmed self-destruction or autolysis, of the cell, which means that the cell is digesting itself. Other functions include digesting foreign bacteria that invade a cell and helping repair damage to the plasma membrane by serving as a membrane patch, sealing the wound. Lysosomes also do much of the cellular digestion required to digest tails of tadpoles and to remove the web from the fingers of a 3–6-month-old fetus. This process of programmed cell death is called apoptosis.

1.3

Answer: B Synthesis of proteins

The rough endoplasmic reticulum (ER) contains protein-manufacturing ribosomes (the ribosomes on its surface are responsible for its being named 'rough') and transports proteins destined for membranes and secretion. Rough ER is connected to the nuclear envelope as well as linked to the cis cisternae of the Golgi complex by vesicles that shuttle between the two compartments. The rough ER works in concert with the Golgi apparatus to target new proteins to their proper destinations.

1.4

Answer: A   Acts like haemoglobin and binds with O_2

Myoglobin is a single-chain globular protein of 153 amino acids, containing a haem (iron-containing porphyrin) prosthetic group in the centre around which the remaining apoprotein folds. With a molecular weight of 16 kDa, it is the primary oxygen-carrying pigment of muscle tissues. Unlike the blood-borne haemoglobin, to which it is structurally related, this protein does not exhibit co-operative binding of oxygen, since positive co-operativity is a property reserved for multimeric proteins. Instead, the binding of oxygen by myoglobin is unaffected by the oxygen pressure in the surrounding tissue. Myoglobin is often cited as having an 'instant binding tenacity' to oxygen given its hyperbolic oxygen dissociation curve. In 1958, John Kendrew and associates successfully determined the structure of myoglobin by high-resolution X-ray crystallography. For this discovery, John Kendrew shared the 1962 Nobel Prize in chemistry with Max Perutz.

1.5

Answer: A   It is monosynaptic

A stretch reflex is a muscle contraction in response to stretching within that muscle. It is a monosynaptic reflex that provides automatic regulation of skeletal muscle length. Muscle spindles are sense organs sensitive to stretch of the muscle in which they lie. The patellar (knee-jerk) reflex is an example. Another example is the group 1a fibres in the calf muscle, which synapse with motor neurones supplying muscle fibres in the same muscle. A sudden stretch, such as tapping the Achilles' tendon, causes a reflex contraction in the muscle as the spindles sense the stretch and send an action potential to the motor neurones, which then cause the muscle to contract; this particular reflex causes a contraction in the soleus–gastrocnemius group of muscles. This reflex can be enhanced by the Jendrassik manoeuvre. Jendrassik's manoeuvre (Erno Jendrassik, Hungarian physician, 1858–1921) is a medical manoeuvre wherein the patient flexes both sets of fingers into a hook-like form and interlocks those sets of fingers together. The tendon below the patient's knee is then hit with a reflex hammer. The elicited response is compared with the reflex

general

result of the same action when the manoeuvre is not in use. Often a larger reflex response will be observed when the patient is occupied with the manoeuvre, as the manoeuvre may prevent the patient from consciously inhibiting or influencing his or her response to the hammer. This manoeuvre is particularly useful in that, even if the patient is aware that the interlocking of fingers is just a distraction to elicit a larger reflex response, it still functions properly.

1.6

Answer: B   Mitochondrion

A mitochondrion (plural mitochondria) is a membrane-enclosed organelle, found in most eukaryotic cells. Mitochondria are sometimes described as 'cellular power plants', because they convert food molecules into energy in the form of ATP via the process of oxidative phosphorylation. A typical eukaryotic cell contains about 2000 mitochondria, which occupy roughly one-fifth of its total volume. Mitochondria contain DNA that is independent of the DNA located in the cell nucleus. They have the ability to regenerate and replicate spontaneously.

1.7

Answer: E   Red blood cells

An electron transport chain (also called electron transport system or electron transfer chain) is a series of membrane-associated electron carriers mediating biochemical reactions that produce ATP, which is the energy currency of life. Only two sources of energy are available to living organisms: oxidation–reduction (redox) reactions and sunlight (photosynthesis). Organisms that use redox reactions to produce ATP are called chemotrophs. Organisms that use sunlight are called phototrophs. Both chemotrophs and phototrophs utilise electron transport chains to convert energy into ATP. The overall purpose of the electron transport chain is to create ATP using energy contained in high-energy electrons.

This is achieved through a three-step process:

- Gradually sap energy from a high-energy electron in a series of individual steps.

- Use that energy to forcibly unbalance the proton concentration across the membrane.

- Use the proton concentration's drive to rebalance itself as a means of producing ATP.

Electron transport chains are present in the mitochondria. Energy sources such as glucose are initially metabolised in the cytoplasm. The products are imported into mitochondria. Mitochondria continue the process of catabolism using metabolic pathways including the Krebs cycle, fatty acid oxidation and amino acid oxidation.

The end-result of these pathways is the production of two energy-rich electron donors, NADH and $FADH_2$. Electrons from these donors are passed through an electron transport chain to oxygen, which is reduced to water. This is a multi-step redox process that occurs on the mitochondrial inner membrane. The enzymes that catalyse these reactions have the remarkable ability to simultaneously create a proton gradient across the membrane, producing a thermodynamically unlikely high-energy state with the potential to do work. Although electron transport occurs with great efficiency, a small percentage of electrons are prematurely leaked to oxygen, resulting in the formation of the toxic free radical, superoxide.

Four membrane-bound complexes have been identified in mitochondria. Each is an extremely complex transmembrane structure that is embedded in the inner membrane. Three of them are proton pumps. The structures are electrically connected by lipid-soluble electron carriers and water-soluble electron carriers. The overall electron transport chain is:

NADH → Complex I → Q → Complex III → Cytochrome c → Complex IV → O_2

↑

Complex II

Much of our knowledge of mitochondrial function results from the study of toxic compounds. Specific inhibitors were used to distinguish the electron transport system from the phosphorylation system and helped to define the sequence of redox carriers along the respiratory chain. If the chain is blocked then all the intermediates on the substrate side of the block become more reduced, while all those on the oxygen side become more oxidised. It is easy to see what has happened, because the oxidised and reduced carriers often differ in their spectral properties. If a variety of different inhibitors are available then many of the respiratory carriers can be placed in the correct order. Atractyloside transport inhibitor blocks the adenine nucleotide porter by binding to the outward-facing conformation (contrast with bongkrekic acid). It has no effect on submitochondrial particles, which re-seal spontaneously after sonication with the membranes inside-out. This ATP/ADP transport inhibitor resembles oligomycin when used with intact mitochondria. Of all the options given in this question, red blood cells are the only cell type that do not have mitochondria and hence will not be affected by electron transport chain inhibitor, atractyloside.

1.8

Answer: D   Sodium ions flow inward

A local membrane depolarisation caused by an excitatory stimulus causes some voltage-gated sodium channels in the neurone cell-surface membrane to open and therefore sodium ions diffuse in through the channels along their electrochemical gradient. Being positively charged, they begin a reversal in the potential difference across the membrane from negative-inside to positive-inside. Initially, the inward movement of sodium ions is also favoured by the negative-inside membrane potential. Overall, the ions are under the influence of the *driving force,* the difference between the membrane potential and the equilibrium potential of sodium.

1.9

Answer: A   Use anaerobic metabolism

Skeletal muscle fibres can be divided into two basic types, type I (slow-twitch fibres) and type II (fast-twitch fibres). Type I muscle fibres (slow-oxidative fibres) use primarily cellular respiration and, as a result, have relatively high endurance. To support their high-oxidative metabolism, these muscle fibres typically have lots of mitochondria and myoglobin and so appear red or what is typically termed 'dark' meat in poultry. Type I muscle fibres are typically found in muscles of animals that require endurance, such as chicken leg muscles or the wing muscles of migrating birds (eg, geese). Type II muscle fibres use primarily anaerobic metabolism and have relatively low endurance. These muscle fibres are typically used during tasks requiring short bursts of strength, such as sprints or weightlifting. Type II muscle fibres cannot sustain contractions for significant lengths of time and are typically found in the 'white' meat (eg, the breast) of chicken.

There are two subclasses of type II muscle fibres, type IIa (fast-oxidative) and IIb (fast-glycolytic). The Type IIa fast-oxidative fibres actually also appear red, due to their high content of myoglobin and mitochondria. Type IIb (fast-glycolytic) tire the fastest and are the prevalent type in sedentary individuals. These fibres appear white histologically, due to their low oxidative demand, manifested by the lack of myoglobulin and mitochondria (relative to the type I and type IIa fibres). Some research suggests that these subtypes can switch with training to some degree. The biochemical difference between the three types of muscle fibres is in their myosin heavy chains.

1.10

Answer: D   Monocyte

A monocyte is a leukocyte, part of the human body's immune system that protects against blood-borne pathogens and moves quickly (approx. 8–12 hours) to sites of infection in the tissues. Monocytes are usually identified in stained smears by their large bilobed nucleus. They are produced by the bone marrow from haemopoietic stem cell precursors called monoblasts. Monocytes circulate in the bloodstream for about one to three days and then typically move into tissues throughout the body. They consist of between 3 and 8% of the leukocytes in the blood. In the tissues, monocytes mature into different types of macrophages at different anatomical locations. Monocytes are responsible for phagocytosis (ingestion) of foreign substances in the body. Monocytes can perform phagocytosis using intermediary (opsonising) proteins such as antibodies or complement that coat the pathogen, as well as by binding to the microbe directly via pattern-recognition receptors that recognise pathogens. Monocytes are also capable of killing infected host cells via antibody, termed antibody-mediated cellular cytotoxicity. Vacuolisation may be present in a cell that has phagocytosed foreign matter.

Monocytes that migrate from the bloodstream to other tissues are called macrophages. Macrophages are responsible for protecting tissues from foreign substances, but are also suspected to be the predominant cells involved in triggering atherosclerosis. They are cells that possess a large smooth nucleus, a large area of cytoplasm and many internal vesicles for processing foreign material.

A *monocyte count* is part of a complete blood count and is expressed either as a ratio of monocytes to the total number of white blood cells counted or by absolute numbers. Both may be useful in determining or refuting a possible diagnosis. Monocytosis is the state of excess monocytes in the peripheral blood. It may be indicative of various disease states. Examples of processes that can increase a monocyte count include:

- chronic inflammation
- stress response
- hyperadrenocorticism
- immune-mediated disease
- pyogranulomatous disease
- necrosis
- red cell regeneration.

1.11

Answer: A   Erythropoietin

Erythropoietin, or EPO, is a glycoprotein hormone that is a cytokine for erythrocyte (red blood cells) precursors in the bone marrow. Also called haematopoietin or haemopoietin, it is produced by the kidney and is the hormone regulating red blood cell production. Erythropoietin is available as a therapeutic agent produced by recombinant DNA technology in mammalian cell culture. It is used in treating anaemia resulting from chronic renal failure or from cancer chemotherapy. Its use is also believed to be common as a doping agent in endurance sports such as bicycle racing, triathlons and marathon running.

1.12

Answer: D   IgG

IgG is a monomeric immunoglobulin, built of two heavy chains γ and two light chains. Each molecule has two antigen-binding sites. This is the most abundant immunoglobulin and is approximately equally distributed in blood and in tissue liquids, constituting 75% of serum immunoglobulins in humans. This is the only isotype that can pass through the placenta, thereby providing protection to the newborn in its first weeks of life before its own immune system has developed. It can bind to many kinds of pathogens, for example viruses, bacteria and fungi, and protects the body against them by complement activation (classic pathway), opsonisation or phagocytosis and neutralisation of their toxins. There are four subclasses: IgG1 (66%), IgG2 (23%), IgG3 (7%) and IgG4 (4%):

- IgG1, IgG3 and IgG4 cross the placenta easily
- IgG3 is the most effective complement activator, followed by IgG1 and then IgG2
- IgG4 does not activate complement
- IgG1 and IgG3 bind with high affinity to Fc receptors on phagocytic cells
- IgG4 has intermediate affinity and IgG2 affinity is extremely low.

1.13

Answer: A   A positive

According to the ABO blood typing system there are four different kinds of blood types: A, B, AB or O.

- Blood group A - If you belong to the blood group A, you have A antigens on the surface of your red blood cells and B antibodies in your blood plasma.

- Blood group B - If you belong to the blood group B, you have B antigens on the surface of your red blood cells and A antibodies in your blood plasma.

- Blood group AB - If you belong to the blood group AB, you have both A and B antigens on the surface of your red blood cells and no A or B antibodies at all in your blood plasma.

- Blood group O - If you belong to the blood group O, you have neither A nor B antigens on the surface of your red blood cells but you have both A and B antibodies in your blood plasma.

Many people also have a so-called Rh factor on the red blood cell's surface. This is also an antigen and those who have it are called Rh+. Those who have not are called Rh−. A person with Rh− blood does not have Rh antibodies naturally in the blood plasma (as one can have A or B antibodies, for instance) but they can develop Rh antibodies in the blood plasma if they receive blood from a person with Rh+ blood, whose Rh antigens can trigger the production of Rh antibodies. A person with Rh+ blood can receive blood from a person with Rh− blood without any problems. So, in this vignette the patient's blood group is A positive as he has antigen A, antibody B and Rh antigens.

1.14

Answer: C   It is the largest immunoglobin molecule

IgM forms polymers where multiple immunoglobulins are covalently linked together with disulphide bonds, normally as a pentamer or occasionally as a hexamer. It has a large molecular mass of approximately 900 kDa (in its pentamer form). The J chain is attached to most pentamers, while hexamers do not possess the J chain due to space constraints in the complex. Because each monomer has two antigen binding sites, an IgM has 10 of them; however, it cannot bind 10 antigens at the same time because they hinder each other. Because it is a large molecule, it cannot diffuse well and is found in the interstitium only in very low quantities. IgM is primarily found in serum; however, because of the J chain, it is also important as a secretory immunoglobulin.

Due to its polymeric nature, IgM possesses high avidity and is particularly effective at complement activation. It is sometimes called a 'natural antibody', but it is likely that the antibodies arise due to sensitisation in the very young to antigens that are naturally occurring in nature. For example anti-A and anti-B IgM antibodies can be formed in early life as a result of exposure to anti-A- and anti-B-like substances that are present on bacteria or perhaps also on plant materials. In germ-line cells, the gene segment encoding the μ constant region of the heavy chain is positioned first among other constant-region gene segments. For this reason, IgM is the first immunoglobulin expressed by mature B cells.

IgM is also by far the physically largest antibody in the circulation. IgM antibodies are mainly responsible for the clumping (agglutination) of red blood cells if the recipient of a blood transfusion receives blood that is not compatible with his/her blood type. IgM antibodies appear early in the course of an infection and usually do not reappear after further exposure. IgM antibodies do not pass across the human placenta. These two biological properties of IgM make it useful in the diagnosis of infectious diseases. Demonstrating IgM antibodies in a patient's serum indicates recent infection or, in serum from a neonate, indicates intrauterine infection such as congenital rubella.

general

1.15

Answer: E   Vascular endothelium

Factor VIII (FVIII) is an essential clotting factor. The lack of normal FVIII causes haemophilia A, an inherited bleeding disorder. The gene for Factor VIII is located on the X chromosome (Xq28). FVIII is a glycoprotein pro-cofactor. Factor VIII is synthesised predominantly in the vascular endothelium and is not affected by liver disease. In fact, levels usually are elevated in such instances. It is also synthesised and released into the bloodstream by the liver. In the circulating blood, it is mainly bound to von Willebrand factor (vWF, also known as factor VIII-related antigen) to form a stable complex. Upon activation by thrombin or factor Xa, it dissociates from the complex to interact with factor IXa in the coagulation cascade. It is a co-factor to factor IXa in the activation of factor X, which, in turn, with its co-factor factor Va, activates more thrombin. Thrombin cleaves fibrinogen into fibrin, which polymerises and crosslinks (using factor XIII) into a blood clot. No longer protected by vWF, activated FVIII is proteolytically inactivated in the process (most prominently by activated protein C and factor IXa) and quickly cleared from the bloodstream. FVIII concentrated from donated blood plasma or alternatively recombinant FVIII can be given to haemophiliacs to restore haemostasis. So, FVIII is also known as antihaemophilic factor. The transfer of a plasma by-product into the bloodstream of a patient with haemophilia often led to the transmission of diseases such as HIV and hepatitis before purification methods were improved. In the early 1990s, pharmaceutical companies began to produce recombinant synthesised factor products, which now prevent nearly all forms of disease transmission during replacement therapy.

1.16

Answer: A   Autosomal dominant

von Willebrand's disease (vWD) is the most common hereditary coagulation abnormality described in humans, although it can also be acquired as a result of other medical conditions. It arises from a qualitative or quantitative deficiency of von Willebrand factor (vWF), a multimeric protein that is required for platelet adhesion. It is known to affect humans and, in veterinary medicine, dogs. There are three types of hereditary vWD, but other factors such as ABO blood group may also play a part in the cause of the condition. The various types of vWD present with varying degrees of bleeding tendency. Severe internal or joint bleeding is rare (only in type 3 vWD); bruising, nosebleeds, heavy menstrual periods (in women) and blood loss during childbirth (rare) may occur. Death may occur

The *vWF* gene is located on chromosome 12 (12p13.2). It has 52 exons spanning 178 kbp. Types 1 and 2 are inherited as autosomal dominant traits and type 3 is inherited as autosomal recessive. Occasionally type 2 also inherits recessively. In humans, the incidence of vWD is roughly about 1 in 100 individuals. Because most forms are rather mild, they are detected more often in women, whose bleeding tendency shows during menstruation. The actual abnormality (which does not necessarily lead to disease) occurs in 0.9–3% of the population. It may be more severe or apparent in people with blood group O. Acquired vWD can occur in patients with autoantibodies. In this case the function of vWF is not inhibited but the vWF–antibody complex is rapidly cleared from the circulation. A form of vWD occurs in patients with aortic valve stenosis, leading to gastrointestinal bleeding (Heyde's syndrome). This form of acquired vWD may be more prevalent than is presently thought. Acquired vWF has also been described in the following disorders: Wilms' tumour, hypothyroidism and mesenchymal dysplasias.

Patients with vWD normally require no regular treatment, although they are always at increased risk for bleeding. Prophylactic treatment is sometimes given for patients with vWD who are scheduled for surgery. They can be treated with human-derived medium purity factor VIII concentrates. Mild cases of vWD can be trialled on desmopressin (1-desamino-8-D-arginine vasopressin, DDAVP) (antihaemophilic factor, more commonly known as humate-P), which works by raising the patient's own plasma levels of vWF by inducing release of vWF stored in the Weibel–Palade bodies in the endothelial cells.

general

1.17

Answer: C   Iron is more efficiently absorbed in the ferrous state (Fe^4) than in the ferric state (Fe^{3+})

The absorption of non-haem iron in any food is strongly affected by the composition of the meals. Iron is more efficiently absorbed in the ferrous state (Fe^{2+}) than in the ferric state (Fe^{3+}) and commercial iron preparations often contain vitamin C to prevent oxidation of Fe^{2+} to Fe^{3+}. Still, only 3–6% of the ingested daily iron is actually absorbed in the upper gastrointestinal tract. Seventy per cent of the total body iron is used for haemoglobin and myoglobin; the remainder is stored as readily exchangeable ferritin and some is stored in less easily mobilised haemosiderin. When old red blood cells are destroyed by the tissue macrophage system, haem is separated from globin and degraded to biliverdin. Iron in the plasma is bound to the iron-transporting protein transferrin. Transferrin level (total iron-binding capacity) and saturation are clinically important indicators of iron-deficiency anaemia.

1.18

Answer: C   Patients with haemophilia A usually have a normal bleeding time

Prolonged bleeding time is characteristic of platelet disorders, eg, thrombocytopaenia. Patients with haemophilia A or B (ie absence of factor VIII or IX, respectively) have a prolonged partial thromboplastin time (PTT), but do not have a prolonged bleeding time. Ca^{2+} is a necessary co-factor for blood coagulation, and chelation of Ca^{2+} ions by citrate inhibits coagulation. Von Willebrand factor is part of the factor VIII complex and also promotes platelet adherence to the vascular subendothelium. Patients who lack this factor (von Willebrand's disease) have both a prolonged PTT and a prolonged bleeding time. Disseminated intravascular coagulation results in depletion of coagulation factors and accumulation of fibrin split products.

1.19

Answer: B   Decrease the rate of rhythmicity of the sinoatrial (SA) node by inducing hyperpolarisation

The toxic effects of nerve gas derive from its ability to inhibit the enzyme cholinesterase. The inhibition of this naturally occurring degradative enzyme engenders a massive accumulation of acetylcholine evoking an overstimulation of the acetylcholine receptors throughout the body. In the heart, specifically, acetylcholine released by the vagal nerve stimulates muscarinic receptors in the cells of the sinoatrial (SA) node. This results in the opening of potassium channels and hyperpolarisation of the SA node. It therefore takes longer for sodium leakage to cause the membrane potentials of these cells to reach the threshold required for an action potential. The rate of rhythmicity is so decreased. A similar hyperpolarisation of the fibres at the atrioventricular (AV) junction decreases conduction velocity of atrial impulses to the ventricle. The force of ventricular contractions is not affected by the vagus nerve.

1.20

Answer: C   Hyperpolarisation to about -70mV

Increasing the membrane's conductance to chloride will result in chloride influx and the membrane potential approaching the value dictated by the chloride equilibrium potential (calculated from the Nernst equation), which is about -70 mV for neurones. A value of -30 mV is near the Nernst potential for Cl^- ions in smooth muscle cells, but not in neurones; $+30$ mV is near the Nernst potential for Na^+ ions. The membrane potential would remain unchanged only if the cell resting membrane potential is already at the Nernst potential of the ion channels that were opened. Action potentials occur if the cell membrane is depolarised above threshold.

1.21

Answer: A   The cell will depolarise if its membrane potential is positive with respect to the equilibrium potential for chloride ions

Although electrogenic pumps may contribute to the membrane potential of certain cells, the major determinants of membrane potential are the external and internal concentrations of permeant ions and their relative permeabilities in the membrane. Decreasing the conductance causes the membrane potential to move away from the equilibrium potential for that ion. So, a decrease in the conductance of a membrane to chloride ions causes the cells to depolarise – that is, become more positive – if the membrane potential is positive with respect to the chloride equilibrium potential. Conversely, increasing the conductance for an ion causes the membrane potential to approach the equilibrium potential for that ion. External and internal ion chloride concentrations are needed to calculate the Nernst potential for this ion, but a simple comparison of these two values does not allow predictions about the change in membrane potential.

1.22

Answer: E   Reflex inhibition of motor neurones

The stimulation of receptors in the Golgi tendon organs leads to the inverse stretch reflex. This reflex is responsible for the relaxation that is observed when a muscle is subjected to a strong stretch. Impulses from the organs travel in type Ib fibres to the spinal cord, where they activate inhibitory interneurones. These in turn suppress the activity of motor neurones and therefore lead to relaxation of the extrafusal muscle fibres attached to the tendons. The state of contraction of intrafusal fibres, the gamma-efferent discharge rate and the activity in group II afferent fibres control the stretch reflex, which, distinct from the inverse stretch reflex, is mediated by the Golgi tendon organs.

1.23

Answer: B The opening of multiple ion channels in the muscle membrane caused by spontaneous release of a small amount of neurotransmitter

Acetylcholine, the transmitter at the muscle endplate, may be released spontaneously in small packets or quanta, without the presynaptic terminal being depolarised by an action potential. These quanta are believed to represent the contents of single vesicles containing about 10 000 molecules of acetylcholine. Release of acetylcholine activates many ion channels in the muscle to produce a miniature endplate potential. Current through single ion channels can only be observed with special methods (patch clamping), but not with microelectrodes used to measure membrane potentials. While ion channels do open spontaneously even in the absence of neurotransmitter, the amplitude of these currents is much smaller than the amplitude of miniature endplate potentials occurring during spontaneous release of vesicles from the nerve terminal. The opening of multiple ion channels in the postsynaptic membrane in response to a single presynaptic action potential would produce a large endplate potential of much greater amplitude than miniature endplate potentials possess.

1.24

Answer: A A combination of gradual inactivation outward I_K along with the presence of an inward 'funny' current (I_f) due to opening of channels permeable to both Na^+ and K^+ ions

One of the principal distinguishing features of nodal cell action potentials is the gradual diastolic depolarisation, the so-called pacemaker potential. When the pacemaker potential reaches threshold, an action potential is generated and propagated along conducting pathways to other cardiac fibres (the basis of autorhythmicity of cardiac pacemaker cells). During the diastolic period the outward I_k (or delayed rectifier current mainly responsible for polarisation) is slowly deactivated. At the same time there is activation of poorly selective channels (permeable to both Na^+ and K^+), which gives rise to a slow 'funny' inward current due mainly to

Na^+. Fast Na^+ channels are responsible for action potentials in nerve cells and skeletal muscle fibres. An increase in delayed rectifier K^+ current would counteract any cell membrane depolarisation. Changes in anion permeability do not contribute significantly to the pacemaker potential, but may play a role in the repolarisation phase of the ventricular action potential. The ratio of intracellular to extracellular ion concentration shows no measurable change during action potentials. Due to the small membrane capacitance, movement of a very small number of ions across the cell membrane is sufficient to create the membrane potential.

1.25

Answer: E   The breakdown of glycogen to lactic acid

Energy can be derived from either aerobic or anaerobic sources. Although aerobic oxidative processes can provide a significant amount of energy, these processes are too slow to provide all of the energy required. Although stores of ATP and creatine phosphate are present in muscle, they provide sufficient energy for only very brief periods of exercise (a few seconds). Deaminated proteins may undergo gluconeogenesis, in which they are converted to glucose or glycogen, but this pathway is not normally used for strenuous exercise. The breakdown of glycogen to lactic acid provides sufficient energy rapidly enough to support brief periods of strenuous exercise (many seconds to a few minutes). The depletion of glycogen and production of lactic acid contribute to an energy debt, which is repaid via oxidative metabolism in the period after exercise.

1.26

Answer: C   Increased heat production by skeletal muscle

Malignant hyperthermia is due to a genetic variation of the skeletal muscle ryanodine receptors (sarcoplasmic Ca^{2+} release channels). Halothane and several other drugs may trigger excessive Ca^{2+} release, leading to muscle contractures, increased muscle metabolism and an enormous increase in heat production. This condition is fatal if not treated promptly with a ryanodine receptor antagonist such as dantrolene. An increased hypothalamic temperature set point occurs during febrile episodes of infectious diseases. Such change of set point is due to increased blood levels of interleukin-1. Convectional heat loss (eg, lack of appropriate clothing during winter) would result in cooling of the body temperature. Increased sweat production is a consequence, but not the cause, of malignant hyperthermia.

1.27

Answer: B   MCHC = haemoglobin concentration/haematocrit

Mean corpuscular haemoglobin concentration (MCHC) is calculated simply by dividing the haemoglobin concentration (8 g/dl) by the haematocrit (0.3). Normal range is 31–36 g/dl and this patient has a hypochromic anaemia (MCHC = 8/0.3 = 26.7 g/dl). Dividing the haemoglobin concentration × 10 by erythrocyte number yields mean corpuscular haemoglobin (MCH). Normal range is 25.4–34.6 pg/cell and this patient has significantly reduced cellular haemoglobin content (MCH = 8 × 10/4 = 20 pg/cell). Mean corpuscular volume (MCV) is calculated by dividing haematocrit × 1000 by erythrocyte number (4 × 10^6/μl). Normal range is 80–100 fl and this patient has a microcytic anaemia (MCV = 0.3 × 1000/4 = 75 fl). Microcytic, hypochromic anaemia is characteristic for iron-deficiency.

1.28

Answer: E   Promotes lipolysis

Adrenaline, a catecholamine, has numerous effects on metabolism, mostly mediated by β-receptors. It has a direct lipolytic effect on fat cells because it activates the hormone-sensitive lipase, releasing free fatty acids into the circulation. Adrenaline has a potent effect on liver cells causing glycogenolysis, releasing large quantities of glucose within minutes into the bloodstream. It inhibits glycogen synthesis. This action is mediated by β-receptors linked to adenylate cyclase. By the same mechanism, adrenaline also inhibits glycogen synthesis in skeletal muscle cells and promotes muscle glycogenolysis. However, the freed glucose is directly utilised by the muscle and not released into the bloodstream. Under some conditions stimulation of sympathetic nerves can increase insulin and glucagon secretion; however, it is doubtful that these effects are of physiological

general

significance. The main factor controlling both insulin and glucagon secretion is the blood glucose level. Increased blood glucose levels increase insulin secretion and suppress glucagon secretion, while low blood glucose levels increase glucagon secretion and inhibit insulin secretion.

1.29

Answer: B   PGE$_2$ sensitises nociceptive nerve endings, causing pain

Local inflammatory processes are often painful. This is due to sensitisation of nociceptive nerve endings by PGE$_2$. Non-steroidal anti-inflammatory drugs (NSAIDs) inhibit prostaglandin synthesis and help to alleviate the pain. Thromboxane A$_2$ and prostacyclin (PGI$_2$) are both derived from PGH$_2$, but have opposite effects on platelets and blood vessels. Thromboxane A$_2$, released from platelets, promotes vasoconstriction and platelet aggregation while PGI$_2$, released from endothelial cells, is a potent vasodilator and inhibits platelet aggregation. Most prostaglandins have a large range of actions and they may contract or relax smooth muscle cells depending on tissue source and species. In humans PGF$_{2\alpha}$ constricts bronchial smooth muscle and PGE$_2$ relaxes it. An increase in prostaglandin production by fetal membranes is believed to be a major factor for onset of uterine contractions and labour in humans.

1.30

Answer: B   Due to hydrolysis of fibrin by plasmin

Plasmin lyses fibrin and fibrinogen and is the active component of the fibrinolytic system. Plasminogen is a protein made in the liver. Cleavage of a single arginine–valine bond converts plasminogen to active plasmin. Streptokinase has no direct effect on fibrin. Its action is due to formation of plasmin from its inactive precursor plasminogen. Neither plasmin nor streptokinase inhibits sfibrinolysis. ε-Aminocaproic acid inhibits fibrinolysis by inhibiting the conversion of plasminogen to plasmin. Streptokinase does not act on tissue plasminogen activator (TPA). Streptokinase, urokinase and recombinant human TPA all activate plasminogen and are used clinically in early treatment of myocardial infarction.

1.31

Answer: C   γ-Interferon

Despite tremendous progress in understanding the role of cytokines in normal and pathological processes, the therapeutic and research potential of these substances has only just begun to be explored. Interferons, by definition, elicit a non-specific antiviral activity by inducing specific RNA synthesis and protein expression in neighbouring cells. Common interferon inducers are viruses, double-stranded RNA and micro-organisms. INF-γ is produced mainly by CD4+ and CD8+ T cells and to a lesser extent by B cells and natural killer cells. INF-γ has antiviral and antiparasitic activity and is synergistic with INF-α and INF-β, but its main biological activity appears to be immunomodulatory. Among its many functions are activation of macrophages and enhanced expression of MHC-II proteins (DP, DQ and DR) or macrophages. The other two common human interferons are INF-α and INF-β, derived from leukocytes and fibroblasts, respectively. INF-α is currently in clinical use against hairy cell leukaemia, Kaposi's sarcoma and venereal warts (condyloma acuminata). In addition to the common inducers, INF-β production by fibroblasts is also elicited by TNF and IL-1. In contrast to INF-α, INF-β is strictly species-specific. INF-β appears to be useful for treatment of squamous sarcomas, viral encephalitis and possibly multiple sclerosis. Macrophages produce IL-1 and TNF. The effects of IL-1 and TNF are widespread and include activation of T cells, B cells, fever induction and many others.

1.32

Answer: A   Dietary iron is more readily absorbed when ferritin stores of the intestinal epithelium are low

Only a small amount (5–15%) of dietary iron is absorbed by the body. Much of the iron entering the intestinal mucosa is not transferred to the plasma, but remains trapped as ferritin inside the epithelial cells and is lost when the cells are shed. Patients with chronic iron-deficiency anaemia have low ferritin stores and therefore a larger rate of intestinal iron absorption because of this mucosal regulatory mechanism. Intrinsic factor is produced by parietal cells of the stomach. Its presence is crucial for intestinal absorption of vitamin

general

B_{12}, but not iron. Its absence causes a macrocytic megaloblastic anaemia. Iron is virtually exclusively absorbed in the duodenum and proximal jejunum and not the terminal ileum. Only iron kept soluble, either as haemoglobin or myoglobin or bound to low-weight organic molecules is absorbed by intestinal epithelial cells. Ferrous iron (Fe^{2+}) is better absorbed than ferric iron (Fe^{3+}) and commercial iron preparations often contain an antioxidant like vitamin C to keep iron in the ferrous state.

1.33

Answer: B   K+ channels

The resting membrane potential of excitable cells is largely due to the selective permeability of the cell membrane to potassium ions. The Na+/K+ pump generates the ion gradient across the cell membrane (ie, high intracellular K+, high extracellular Na+), but it is the back diffusion of K+ ions through K+ channels that are open at rest, which charges the cell membrane. If the cell membrane were a perfect K+ electrode, the membrane potential would equal the equilibrium potential for K+ as predicted by the Nernst equation. In reality, the resting membrane potential is more positive because of small contributions by Na+ channels, Cl− channels and non-selective cation channels.

1.34

Answer: E   Normal MCV

Mean corpuscular volume is calculated from haematocrit and RBC count: mean corpuscular volume (MCV) [fl] haematocrit × 1000/RBC [$10^6/\mu l$] = 0.27 1000/3 = 90 fl, which is within the normal range. Mean corpuscular haemoglobin concentration is calculated from blood haemoglobin and RBC count MCHC [g/dl] − haemoglobin [g/dl]/haematocrit = 11/0.27 = 41 g/dl and is higher than normal. Red blood cell diameter cannot be calculated from the data given, but is probably less than normal in this patient (*see also* answer to 1.27).

1.35

Answer: D   Spherocytosis

Spherocytes are small, round red blood cells with a decreased cell membrane surface area. They usually have a normal mean corpuscular volume but a smaller than normal diameter since they are rounded. This makes them more vulnerable to plasma or salt solutions with decreased osmotic pressure. Spherocytes are seen in haemolytic anaemias and hereditary spherocytosis, an autosomal dominant disorder involving a molecular abnormality of the cytoskeleton (spectrin deficiency). The decreased cell surface area makes the red blood cells less flexible while traversing the spleen's microcirculation, resulting in anaemia and sometimes jaundice. Iron-deficiency anaemia is characterised by smaller-than-normal cells with decreased mean corpuscular volume and since membrane flexibility is not affected these cells have normal or near normal osmotic fragility. Sickle cells and target cells as seen in thalassaemia and chronic liver disease have a decreased osmotic fragility (ie, are less vulnerable to changes in osmolarity).

1.36

Answer: D   The adult red blood cell to have an ovoid shape rather than the usual biconcave disc shape

Vitamin B_{12} and folic acid are essential for the synthesis of DNA. Lack of either vitamin leads to decreased DNA and so failure of nuclear maturation and division. The erythroblastic cells of the bone marrow become larger than normal and are called *megaloblasts*. The adult red blood cell has a flimsy membrane and is often large with an ovoid shape rather than the usual biconcave disc shape. Therefore, vitamin B_{12} or folic acid deficiency causes *maturation failure* in the process of erythropoiesis.

1.37

Answer: B   Hypochromic anaenia

Iron is a primary nutritive factor necessary for formation of haemoglobin. Iron is present in the diet in only very small quantities and even then is rather poorly absorbed from the gastrointestinal tract; therefore, many people fail to form sufficient quantities of haemoglobin to fill the red blood cells as they are being produced. This causes *hypochromic anaemia,* in which the number of cells may be normal but the amount of haemoglobin in each cell is far below normal.

1.38

Answer: D   Liver disease

Most of the coagulation factors are formed in the liver. Therefore, hepatitis, cirrhosis and other diseases of the liver can depress the normal coagulation system, causing a person to bleed excessively. Another cause of decreased coagulation factor production by the liver is vitamin K deficiency. Vitamin K is necessary for formation of prothrombin, factor VII, factor IX and factor X.

1.39

Answer: C   Polycythaemia anaemia

Pernicious anaemia refers to a type of autoimmune anaemia. Antibodies are directed against intrinsic factor or parietal cells, which produce intrinsic factor. Intrinsic factor is required for vitamin B_{12} absorption, so impaired absorption of vitamin B_{12} can result. Blood testing typically shows a macrocytic, normochromic anaemia and low levels of serum vitamin B_{12}. A Schilling test can then be used to distinguish between pernicious anaemia, vitamin B_{12} malabsorption and vitamin B_{12} deficiency. Approximately 90% of individuals with pernicious anaemia have antibodies for parietal cells; however, only 50% of individuals with these antibodies have the disease. Pernicious anaemia is more common among women (1.6 : 1) with a peak occurrence at the age of 60. It has a hereditary component and it is notably more common in people of Northern European ancestry.

Symptoms may include weakness, an abnormally rapid heart beat (tachycardia), shortness of breath, chest pains, an upset stomach including diarrhoea, difficulty walking, numbness and tingling in the extremities, lack of colour (pallor) in the lips, gum and tongue and/or depression. Pernicious anaemia may cause inflammation of the tongue (glossitis). It is also associated with premature greying, blue eyes, vitiligo and blood group A. It is also associated with unpredictable periods of fatigue and an inability to concentrate. Irreversible central nervous system damage may have occurred before treatment. Scissors gait can appear as a late sign of unchecked anaemia. Some sufferers also report mouth ulcers, joint pain and tinnitus as associated with the onset of pernicious anaemia.

Treatment is with vitamin B_{12} (hydroxycobalamin or cyanocobalamin) injected intramuscularly. Body stores (in the liver) are refilled with half a dozen injections in the first couple of weeks and then maintenance with monthly to quarterly injections throughout the life of the patient. Vitamin B_{12} has traditionally been given parenterally to ensure absorption. However, oral replacement is now an accepted route, as it has become increasingly appreciated that sufficient quantities of B_{12} are absorbed when large doses are given. This absorption does not rely on the presence of intrinsic factor or an intact ileum. Generally, 1–2 mg daily is required as a large dose. By contrast, the typical Western diet contains 5–7 µg of vitamin B_{12}.

1.40

Answer: E   It functions as a soluble signal messenger

Platelet-activating factor, also known as PAF or paf-acether, is a potent phospholipid activator and mediator of many leukocyte functions, including platelet aggregation, inflammation and anaphylaxis. It was discovered by French immunologist Jacques Benveniste in 1970. It is produced in response to specific stimuli by a variety of cell types, including neutrophils, basophils, platelets and endothelial cells. Several molecular species of platelet-activating factor have been identified that vary in the length of the O-alkyl side chain. It is an important mediator of bronchoconstriction. Its alkyl group is connected by an ether linkage at the C1 carbon to a 16-carbon chain. The acyl group at the C2 carbon is an acetate unit whose short length increases the solubility of PAF, allowing it to function as a

general

general

soluble signal messenger. It causes platelets to aggregate and blood vessels to dilate. It can cause life-threatening inflammation of the airways to induce asthma-like symptoms. Toxins such as fragments of destroyed bacteria induce the synthesis of PAF, which causes a drop in blood pressure and reduced volume of blood pumped by the heart, which leads to shock and maybe death.

1.41

Answer: A Anaphylotoxin

The complement system is a biochemical cascade of the immune system that helps clear pathogens from an organism. It is derived from many small plasma proteins that work together to form the primary end result of cytolysis by disrupting the target cell's plasma membrane. The actions of the complement system affect both innate immunity and acquired immunity. Activation of this system leads to cytolysis, chemotaxis, opsonisation, immune clearance and inflammation, as well as the marking of pathogens for phagocytosis. The complement system consists of more than 35 soluble and cell-bound proteins, 12 of which are directly involved in the complement pathways. The proteins account for 5% of the serum globulin fraction. Most of these proteins circulate as zymogens, which are inactive until proteolytic cleavage. The complement proteins are synthesised mainly by hepatocytes; however, significant amounts are also produced by monocytes, macrophages and epithelial cells in the gastrointestinal and genitourinary tracts.

The three pathways all generate homologous variants of the protease C3 convertase. The classical complement pathway typically requires antibodies for activation (specific immune response), while the alternate pathway can be activated by C3 hydrolysis or antigens without the presence of antibodies (non-specific immune response). C3 convertase cleaves and activates component C3, creating C3a and C3b and causing a cascade of further cleavage and activation events. C3b binds to the surface of pathogens, leading to greater internalisation by phagocytic cells by opsonisation. C5a is an important chemotactic protein, helping recruit inflammatory cells. Both C3a and C5a have anaphylatoxin activity (mast cell degranulation, increased vascular permeability, smooth muscle contraction). C5b initiates the membrane attack pathway, which results in the membrane attack complex (MAC), consisting of C5b, C6, C7, C8 and polymeric C9. MAC is the cytolytic end-product of the complement cascade; it forms a transmembrane channel, which causes osmotic lysis of the target cell. Kupffer cells help clear complement-coated pathogens. Antibodies, in particular the IgG1 class, can also 'fix' complement.

1.42

Answer: D Spectin

Spectrin is a cytoskeletal protein that lines the intracellular side of the plasma membrane of many cell types, including erythrocytes, in pentagonal or hexagonal arrangements, forming a scaffolding and playing an important role in maintenance of plasma membrane integrity and cytoskeletal structure. The hexagonal arrangements are formed by tetramers of spectrin associating with short actin filaments at either end of the tetramer. These short actin filaments act as junctional complexes allowing the formation of the hexagonal mesh.

1.43

Answer: A Albumin

Serum albumin, often referred to simply as albumin, is the most abundant and the lightest plasma protein in terms of weight in humans. Albumin is essential for maintaining the osmotic pressure needed for proper distribution of body fluids between intravascular compartments and body tissues. Albumin is negatively charged. The glomerular basement membrane is also negatively charged; this prevents the filtration of albumin in the urine. In nephrotic syndrome, this property is lost and there is more albumin loss in the urine. Nephrotic syndrome patients are given albumin to replace the lost albumin. Albumin:

- maintains osmotic pressure

- transports thyroid hormones

- transports other hormones, particularly fat-soluble ones

general

- transports fatty acids ('free' fatty acids) to the liver

- transports unconjugated bilirubin

- transports many drugs

- competitively binds calcium ions (Ca^{2+})

- buffers pH.

1.44

Answer: C   B +ve

According to the ABO blood typing system there are four different kinds of blood types: A, B, AB or O.

- Blood group A - if you belong to the blood group A, you have A antigens on the surface of your red blood cells and B antibodies in your blood plasma.

- Blood group B - if you belong to the blood group B, you have B antigens on the surface of your red blood cells and A antibodies in your blood plasma.

- Blood group AB - if you belong to the blood group AB, you have both A and B antigens on the surface of your red blood cells and no A or B antibodies at all in your blood plasma.

- Blood group O - if you belong to the blood group O, you have neither A nor B antigens on the surface of your red blood cells but you have both A and B antibodies in your blood plasma.

Many people also have a so-called Rh factor on the red blood cell's surface. This is also an antigen and those who have it are called Rh+. Those who have not are called Rh−. A person with Rh− blood does not have Rh antibodies naturally in the blood plasma (as one can have A or B antibodies, for instance) but they can develop Rh antibodies in the blood plasma if they receive blood from a person with Rh+ blood, whose Rh antigens can trigger the production of Rh antibodies. A person with Rh+ blood can receive blood from a person with Rh− blood without any problems. So, in this vignette

general

the patient's blood group is B positive as he has antigen B, antibody A and Rh antigens (see also answer to 1.13).

1.45

Answer: D Iron deficiency anaemia

Iron-deficiency anaemia is the most common type of anaemia and the most common cause of microcytic anaemia. Iron-deficiency anaemia occurs when the dietary intake or absorption of iron is insufficient and haemoglobin, which contains iron, cannot be formed. The principal cause of iron-deficiency anaemia in premenopausal women is blood lost during menses. Iron-deficiency anaemia is the final stage of iron deficiency. When the body has sufficient iron to meet its needs (functional iron), the remainder is stored for later use in the bone marrow, liver and spleen. Iron-deficiency ranges from iron depletion, which yields little physiological damage, to iron-deficiency anaemia, which can affect the function of numerous organ systems. Iron depletion causes the amount of stored iron to be reduced, but has no effect on the functional iron. However, a person with no stored iron has no reserves to use if the body requires more iron: in essence, the amount of iron absorbed by the body is not adequate for growth and development or to replace the amount lost. Iron-deficiency anaemia is characterised by pallor, fatigue and weakness. Because it tends to develop slowly, adaptation occurs and the disease often goes unrecognised for some time. In severe cases, dyspnoea can occur. Unusual obsessive food cravings, known as pica, may develop. Hair loss and light-headedness can also be associated with iron-deficiency anaemia.

Anaemia will be diagnosed on the basis of suggestive symptoms or found on the basis of routine testing, which includes a full blood count (FBC). A sufficiently low haemoglobin or haematocrit value is diagnostic of anaemia and further studies will be undertaken to determine its cause. One of the first abnormal values to be noted on a FBC will be a high red blood cell distribution width, reflecting a varied population of red blood cells. A low MCV, MCH or MCHC and the appearance of the RBCs on visual examination of a peripheral blood smear will narrow the diagnosis to a *microcytic anaemia*.

general

The diagnosis of iron-deficiency anaemia will be suggested by appropriate history (eg, anaemia in a menstruating woman) and by such diagnostic tests as a low serum ferritin, a low serum iron level, an elevated serum transferrin and a high total iron binding capacity. A definitive diagnosis requires a demonstration of depleted body iron stores by performing a bone marrow aspiration, with the marrow stained for iron. Because this is invasive and painful, while a clinical trial of iron supplementation is inexpensive and non-traumatic, patients are often treated without a definitive diagnosis. The diagnosis of iron-deficiency anaemia requires further investigation as to its cause. It can be a sign of other disease, such as colon cancer (as is the case in this vignette), which will cause the loss of blood in the stool. In addition to dietary insufficiency, malabsorption, chronic blood loss, diversion of iron to fetal erythropoiesis during pregnancy, intravascular haemolysis and haemoglobinuria or other forms of chronic blood loss should all be considered.

If the cause is dietary iron deficiency, iron supplements, usually with iron (II) sulphate or iron amino acid chelate, can correct the anaemia. Chelated iron, while not as widely known as iron sulphate, is ten to 15 times more bioavailable per mg and has none of the side-effects of iron sulphate's sulphur content. Iron supplements must be kept out of the reach of children, as iron-containing supplements are a frequent cause of poisoning in the paediatric age group. If malabsorption is present, it may be necessary to administer iron parenterally (eg, as iron dextran). Parenteral iron other than in chelated form, however, is generally poorly tolerated. Follow-up evaluation with a FBC is essential to demonstrate whether the treatment has been effective.

1.46

Answer: B   Erythroid burst-forming units (BFU-E)

Erythroid burst-forming units (BFU-E) differentiate into erythroid colony-forming units (CFU-E) on stimulation by erythropoietin and then further differentiate into erythroblasts when stimulated by other factors.

1.47

Answer: C   Presence of haemoglobin S

Haemoglobin S is an abnormal type of haemoglobin, caused by abnormal composition of the beta chains. When haemoglobin S is exposed to low concentrations of oxygen, it precipitates into long crystals inside the red blood cell, causing the cell to be shaped like a sickle rather than a biconcave disc. The red blood cells become very fragile so that they rupture during passage through the microcirculation, especially in the spleen. The lifespan of the cells is so short that serious anaemia results and the condition is called sickle-cell anaemia. The condition deprives the downstream tissues of oxygen and causes ischaemia and infarction. The disease is chronic and lifelong. Individuals are most often well, but their lives are punctuated by periodic painful attacks. In addition to periodic pain, there may be damage of internal organs, such as stroke. Lifespan is often shortened with sufferers living to an average of 40 years. Sickle-cell anaemia occurs more commonly in people (or their descendants) from parts of the world, such as sub-Saharan Africa, where malaria is or was common.

1.48

Answer: A   Citrate

The citrate ion combines with calcium in the blood to form an un-ionised calcium compound. The lack of ionic calcium prevents coagulation. It is the anticoagulant of choice for blood storage. Following a single transfusion, the citrate ion is removed from the blood within a few minutes by the liver without any dire consequences. Oxalate anticoagulants work in a similar manner, but oxalate is toxic to the body.

1.49

Answer: B   Causes postsynaptic depolarisation

When acetylcholine is released into the synaptic trough it attaches to acetylcholine-gated ion channels on the postsynaptic membrane, causing them to open. The net effect of opening the channels is to allow large numbers of sodium ions to pour inside the fibre. This creates a local potential inside the fibre that initiates an action potential at the muscle membrane.

1.50

Answer: D Troponin

The mechanism of smooth muscle contraction is somewhat different from that of skeletal muscle. In the place of troponin, the smooth muscle contains another regulatory protein, called calmodulin. When calmodulin reacts with calcium ions, it initiates contraction by activating myosin crossbridges.

1.51

Answer: D An increased permeability of the postsynaptic membrane to small cations

Acetylcholine (ACh) diffuses across the synaptic cleft and binds to ACh receptors on the postsynaptic membrane of the skeletal muscle cell. This region is called the motor endplate. The postsynaptic membrane of the neuromuscular junction has many junctional folds. The ACh receptors are localised at the apex of the junctional folds and in close proximity to the active zones. Binding of ACh to the receptor causes directly gated channels in the endplate region to open. When opened, they are permeable to small cations, which under normal circumstances are mainly sodium and potassium. Flux of small cations through these channels leads to a depolarisation of the endplate region towards an equilibrium potential of approximately 0 mV. This potential is called an endplate potential.

1.52

Answer: E Inhibits release of vesicles at all types of synapses

Because entry of calcium from the extracellular medium is required for vesicle mobilisation and fusion with the presynaptic membrane, altering the extracellular calcium concentration affects the number of vesicles released by each nerve action potential. Increasing extracellular calcium concentration increases the number of vesicles released. Conversely, decreasing extracellular calcium concentration decreases the number of vesicles released and, if extracellular calcium is too low, can impair neuromuscular transmission.

1.53

Answer: E   Normally has a concentration between 1.5–4.0 g/l in blood plasma

Fibrinogen (also called factor I) is a 340 kDa glycoprotein synthesised in the liver hepatocytes and megakaryocytes, which normally has a concentration between 1.5–4.0 g/l (normally measured using the Clauss method) in blood plasma. The principal protein of vertebrate blood clotting, fibrinogen, is a hexamer in the form of a symmetrical dimer containing two sets of three different chains (alpha, beta and gamma), linked to each other by disulphide bonds. On the alpha and beta chains, there is a small peptide sequence (called a fibrinopeptide). It is these small peptides that prevent fibrinogen spontaneously forming polymers with itself. The N-terminal sections of these three chains are evolutionarily related and contain the cysteines that participate in the crosslinking of the chains. However, there is no similarity between the C-terminal part of the alpha chain and that of the beta and gamma chains. The C-terminal part of the beta and gamma chains forms a domain of about 270 amino acid residues.

Fibrinogen has a double function: yielding monomers that polymerise into fibrin and acting as a co-factor in platelet aggregation by binding to their GpIIb/IIIa surface membrane proteins. Following the activation of prothrombin to thrombin (factor IIa), thrombin cleaves fibrinopeptide A off the alpha chain and reveals a site in the E domain that can bind to the carboxy terminal end of the gamma chain. Beta chain cleavage occurs more slowly and contributes to the fibril and fibre associations of fibrinogen. These processes convert fibrinogen to fibrin. The active molecules of fibrin stack up on each other, usually incorporating (by trapping) aggregates of platelets and molecules of thrombin. The soluble fibrin molecules are later crosslinked (by factor XIII) with covalent bonds, to form a stable haemostatic plug, so effectively stopping bleeding.

general

Low levels of fibrinogen can indicate a systemic activation of the clotting system, with consumption of clotting factors faster than synthesis. This excessive clotting factor consumption condition is known as 'disseminated intravascular coagulation' or 'DIC'. DIC can be difficult to diagnose, but a strong clue is low fibrinogen levels in the setting of prolonged clotting times (PT or PTT), in the context of acute critical illness such as sepsis or trauma.

1.54

Answer: A   Bilirubin

Bilirubin is a yellow breakdown product of normal haem catabolism. Its levels are elevated in certain diseases and it is responsible for the yellow colour of bruises and the brown colour of faeces. Haemolysis of erythrocytes (red blood cells) releases haemoglobin. This is broken down to haem, as the globin parts are turned into amino acids. The haem is then turned into unconjugated bilirubin in the macrophages of the spleen and bone marrow. It is then bound to albumin and sent to the liver. In the liver it is conjugated with glucuronic acid, making it water-soluble. Much of it goes into the bile and so out into the small intestine. Some of the conjugated bilirubin remains in the large intestine and is oxidised to urobilin and then stercobilin, which gives faeces its colour. Some is reabsorbed and excreted in the urine as urobilinogen. If the liver's function is impaired or biliary drainage blocked, some of the conjugated bilirubin appears in the urine, turning it dark. The reference range for total bilirubin is 2–14 μmol/l or 0.3–1.9 mg/dl.

1.55

Answer: B   Red blood cell count of men is more than that of women

The diameter of a typical human erythrocyte disc is 6–8 μm, much smaller than most other human cells. A typical erythrocyte contains about 270 million haemoglobin molecules, with each carrying four haem groups. Adult humans have roughly $2-3 \times 10^{13}$ red blood cells at any given time (women have about 4 million to 5 million erythrocytes per cubic millilitre of blood and men about 5 million to 6 million;

people living at high altitudes with low oxygen tension will have more). Red blood cells are much more common than the other blood particles: there are about 4000–11 000 white blood cells and about 150 000–400 000 platelets in a cubic millimetre of human blood. The red blood cells store collectively about 3.5 g of iron, more than five times the iron stored by all the other tissues combined.

The process by which red blood cells are produced is called erythropoiesis. Erythrocytes are continuously being produced in the red bone marrow of large bones, at a rate of about 2 million per second. (In the embryo, the liver is the main site of red blood cell production.) The production can be stimulated by the hormone erythropoietin, synthesised by the kidney. Just before and after leaving the bone marrow, they are known as reticulocytes, which comprise about 1% of circulating red blood cells. Erythrocytes develop from stem cells through reticulocytes to mature erythrocytes in about 7 days and live a total of about 120 days. The ageing cells swell up to a sphere-like shape and are engulfed by phagocytes, destroyed and their materials are released into the blood. The main sites of destruction are the liver and the spleen. The haem constituent of haemoglobin is eventually excreted as bilirubin. The blood types of humans are due to variations in surface glycoprotein of erythrocytes.

1.56

Answer: D   Specific cellular mechanism → cytotoxic T cells

The immune system protects organisms from infection with layered defences of increasing specificity. Most simply, physical barriers (first line of defence) prevent pathogens such as bacteria and viruses from entering the body. If a pathogen breaches these barriers, the innate immune system provides an immediate, but non-specific response. Innate immune systems are found in all plants and animals. In humans the innate immune system is comprised of the complement cascade and the innate leukocytes, which include the phagocytes (macrophages, neutrophils and dendritic cells), mast cells, eosinophils, basophils and natural killer cells. These cells identify and eliminate pathogens, either by attacking larger pathogens through contact or by engulfing and then killing micro-organisms. However, if pathogens successfully evade the innate response, vertebrates possess a third layer of protection, the adaptive immune

general

system. Components of the specific adaptive immune system are B and T lymphocytes, cytotoxic T cells, helper T cells and killer T cells. Here, the immune system adapts its response during an infection to improve its recognition of the pathogen. This improved response is then retained after the pathogen has been eliminated, in the form of an immunological memory and allows the adaptive immune system to mount faster and stronger attacks each time this pathogen is encountered.

1.57

Answer: D   Thrombin converts fibrinogen to fibrin

The coagulation of blood is a complex process during which blood forms solid clots. It is an important part of haemostasis (the cessation of blood loss from a damaged vessel) whereby a damaged blood vessel wall is covered by a fibrin clot to stop haemorrhage and aid repair of the damaged vessel. Disorders in coagulation can lead to increased haemorrhage and/or thrombosis and embolism.

The coagulation cascade of secondary haemostasis has two pathways, the contact activation pathway (formerly known as the intrinsic pathway) and the tissue factor pathway (formerly known as the extrinsic pathway) that lead to fibrin formation. It was previously thought that the coagulation cascade consisted of two pathways of equal importance joined to a common pathway. It is now known that the primary pathway for the initiation of blood coagulation is the tissue factor pathway. The pathways are a series of reactions, in which a zymogen (inactive enzyme precursor) of a serine protease and its glycoprotein co-factor are activated to become active components that then catalyse the next reaction in the cascade, ultimately resulting in crosslinked fibrin. Coagulation factors are generally indicated by Roman numerals, with a lower case *a* appended to indicate an active form. The coagulation factors are generally serine proteases (enzymes). There are some exceptions. For example, factor VIII and factor V are glycoproteins and factor XIII is a transglutaminase. Serine proteases act by cleaving other proteins at specific sites. The coagulation factors circulate as inactive zymogens.

The coagulation cascade can be summarised as follows:

- **Tissue Factor Pathway**: the main role of the tissue factor pathway is to generate a 'thrombin burst', thrombin being the single most important constituent of the coagulation cascade in terms of its feedback activation roles. Factor VIIa circulates in a higher amount than any other activated coagulation factor. Following damage to the blood vessel, endothelium tissue factor (TF) is released, forming a complex with factor VIIa (TF–FVIIa), which activates factor IX and factor X. Factor VII itself is activated by thrombin, factor XIa, plasmin, factor XII and factor Xa. The activation of factor Xa by TF–FVIIa is almost immediately inhibited by tissue factor pathway inhibitor (TFPI). Factor Xa and its co-factor, factor Va, form the prothrombinase complex, which activates prothrombin to thrombin. Thrombin then activates other components of the coagulation cascade, including factor V and factor VII (which activates factor XI which in turn activates factor IX) and activates and releases factor VIII from being bound to vWF. Factor VIIIa is the co-factor of factor IXa and together they form the 'tenase' complex, which activates factor X, and so the cycle continues.

- **Contact Activation Pathway**: there is formation of the primary complex on collagen by high-molecular-weight kininogen (HMWK), prekallikrein and factor XII (Hageman factor). Prekallikrein is converted to kallikrein and factor XII becomes factor XIIa. Factor XIIa converts factor XI into factor XIa. Factor XIa activates factor IX, which with its co-factor, factor VIIIa, forms the tenase complex which activates factor X to factor Xa. The minor role that the contact activation pathway has in initiating clot formation can be illustrated by the fact that patients with severe deficiencies of factor XII, HMWK and prekallikrein do not have a bleeding disorder.

- Thrombin has a large array of functions. Its primary role is the conversion of fibrinogen to fibrin, the building block of a haemostatic plug. In addition, it activates factors VIII and V and their inhibitor protein C (in the presence of thrombomodulin) and it activates factor XIII, which forms covalent bonds that crosslink the fibrin polymers that form from activated monomers.

Following activation by the contact factor or tissue factor pathways the coagulation cascade is maintained in a prothrombotic state by the continued activation of factor VIII and factor IX to form the tenase complex, until it is down regulated by the anticoagulant pathways. Various substances are required for the proper functioning of the coagulation cascade:

- Calcium and phospholipid (a platelet membrane constituent) are required for the tenase and prothrombinase complexes to function. Calcium mediates the binding of the complexes via the terminal gamma-carboxy residues on factor Xa and factor IXa to the phospholipid surfaces expressed by platelets. Calcium is also required at other points in the coagulation cascade.

- Vitamin K is an essential factor to a hepatic gamma-glutamyl carboxylase that adds a carboxyl group to glutamic acid residues on factors II, VII, IX and X, as well as protein S, protein C and protein Z. Deficiency of vitamin K (eg in malabsorption), use of inhibiting anticoagulants (warfarin, acenocoumarol and phenprocoumon) or disease (cirrhosis, hepatocellular carcinoma) impairs the function of the enzyme and leads to the formation of PIVKA (proteins formed in vitamin K absence). This causes partial or no gamma-carboxylation and affects the coagulation factors' ability to bind to expressed phospholipid.

1.58

Answer: E Immunoglobin D

Rh disease (also known as **Rh (D) disease, Rhesus disease, RhD haemolytic disease of the newborn, Rhesus D haemolytic disease of the newborn** or **RhD HDN**) is one of the causes of haemolytic disease of the newborn (also known as HDN). The disease ranges from mild to severe. When the disease is mild the fetus may have mild anaemia with reticulocytosis. When the disease is moderate or severe the fetus can have a more marked anaemia and erythroblastosis fetalis. When the disease is very severe it can cause morbus haemolyticus neonatorum, hydrops fetalis or stillbirth.

During any pregnancy a small amount of the baby's blood can enter the mother's circulation. If the mother is Rh negative and the baby is Rh positive, the mother produces antibodies (including IgG) against the Rhesus D antigens on her baby's red blood cells. During this and subsequent pregnancies the IgG is able to pass through the placenta into the fetus and if the level of it is sufficient it will cause a Rhesus D positive fetus to develop Rh disease. The mechanism is maternal anti-D IgG passing through the placenta to the fetus, causing destruction of fetal red blood cells. Generally Rhesus disease becomes worse with each additional Rhesus-incompatible pregnancy.

The incidence of Rh disease in a population depends on the proportion that are Rhesus negative. Many non-White peoples have a very low proportion who are Rhesus negative, so the incidence of Rh disease is very low in these populations. In White populations about 1 in 10 of all pregnancies are of a Rhesus negative woman with a Rhesus positive baby. It is very rare for the first Rhesus positive baby of a Rhesus negative woman to be affected by Rh disease. The first pregnancy with a Rhesus positive baby is significant for a Rhesus negative woman because she can be sensitised to the Rh positive antigen. In White populations about 13% of Rhesus negative mothers are sensitised by their first pregnancy with a Rhesus positive baby. If it were not for modern prevention and treatment, about 5% of the second Rhesus positive infants of Rhesus negative women, would result in stillbirths or extremely sick babies and many babies who managed to survive would be severely ill. Even higher disease rates would occur in the 3rd and subsequent Rhesus positive infants of Rhesus negative woman. By using anti-RhD immunoglobulin (Rho(D)

general

immune globulin) the incidence is massively reduced. Rh disease sensitisation is about ten times more likely to occur if the fetus is ABO compatible with the mother than if the mother and fetus are ABO incompatible.

The main and most frequent sensitising event is childbirth (about 86% of sensitised cases), but fetal blood may pass into the maternal circulation earlier during the pregnancy (about 14% of sensitised cases). Sensitising events during pregnancy include miscarriage, therapeutic abortion, amniocentesis, ectopic pregnancy, abdominal trauma and external cephalic version.

1.59

Answer: D   Plasma cells

Plasma cells (also called **plasma B cells** or **plasmocytes**) are cells of the immune system that secrete large amounts of antibodies. They differentiate from B cells upon stimulation by $CD4^+$ lymphocytes. The B cell acts as an antigen-presenting cell (APC), consuming an offending pathogen. That pathogen gets taken up by the B cell by phagocytosis and broken down within phagosomes after fusion with lysosomes, releasing proteolytic enzymes onto the pathogen. Once the enzymes break down the pathogen, pieces of the pathogen (which are now known as antigenic peptides) are loaded onto major histocompatibility complex II (MHC II) molecules and presented on its extracellular surface. Once on the extracellular surface, the $CD4^+$ T-helper lymphocyte will bind to the MHC II/antigen molecule and cause activation of the B cell, which includes differentiation into a plasma cell and subsequent generation of antibody against the consumed pathogen.

After dividing for around 5 days, mature B cells differentiate into either plasma B cells or memory B cells. Most plasma B cells travel to the spleen or bone marrow to secrete antibodies (approximately 10 000 per second). During the initial stages of an immune response the lifespan of plasma cells is very short, typically only a few days to weeks. However, following the process of affinity maturation, plasma cells can survive for months to years and continue to secrete high levels of antibodies. Memory B cells tend to be longer-lived and can therefore respond quickly upon second exposure to an antigen.

The class of antibody that a plasma cell produces depends on signals, called cytokines, from other immune system cells, such as macrophages and T helper cells. This process is called isotype-switching. For example, plasma cells are likely to secrete IgG3 antibodies if they matured in the presence of the cytokine interferon-gamma. Since B cell maturation also involves somatic hypermutation, these antibodies have a very high affinity for their antigen.

Plasma cells are large lymphocytes with a considerable nucleus-to-cytoplasm ratio and a characteristic appearance on light microscopy. They have basophilic cytoplasm and an eccentric nucleus with heterochromatin in a characteristic cartwheel arrangement. Their cytoplasm also contains a pale zone that on electron microscopy contains an extensive Golgi apparatus and centrioles. Abundant rough endoplasmic reticulum combined with a well-developed Golgi apparatus makes plasma cells well-suited for secreting immunoglobulins. Cancer of plasma cells is termed multiple myeloma. This condition is frequently identified because malignant plasma cells continue producing an antibody, which can be detected as a paraprotein. Common variable immunodeficiency is thought to be due to a problem in the differentiation from lymphocytes to plasma cells. The result is a low serum antibody level and risk of infections.

1.60

Answer: C   A high reticulocyte count

Anaemia refers to a deficiency of red blood cells (RBCs) and/or haemoglobin. This results in a reduced ability of blood to transfer oxygen to the tissues, despite normal $p(O_2)$ in arterial blood, causing hypoxia; since all human cells depend on oxygen for survival, varying degrees of anaemia can have a wide range of clinical consequences. Haemoglobin (the oxygen-carrying protein in the red blood cells) has to be present to ensure adequate oxygenation of all body tissues and organs.

The three main classes of anaemia include excessive blood loss (acutely such as a haemorrhage or chronically through low-volume loss), excessive blood cell destruction (haemolysis) or deficient red blood cell production (ineffective haemopoiesis). In menstruating women, dietary iron deficiency is a common cause of deficient red blood cell production. Anaemia is the most common disorder of the blood. There are several kinds of anaemia, produced by a variety of underlying causes. Anaemia can be classified in a variety of ways, based on the morphology of RBCs, underlying aetiological mechanisms and discernible clinical spectra, to mention a few.

There are two major approaches to classifying anaemias: the 'kinetic' approach, which involves evaluating production, destruction and loss and the 'morphological' approach, which groups anaemia by red blood cell size. The morphological approach uses a quickly available and cheap laboratory test as its starting point (the MCV). On the other hand, focusing early on the question of production may allow the clinician more rapidly to expose cases where multiple causes of anaemia co-exist. Anaemia goes undetected in many people and symptoms can be vague. Most commonly, people with anaemia report a feeling of weakness or fatigue, general malaise and sometimes a poor concentration. People with more severe anaemia often report dyspnoea on exertion. Very severe anaemia prompts the body to compensate by increasing cardiac output, leading to palpitations and sweatiness and to heart failure. Pallor (pale skin, mucosal linings and nailbeds) is often a useful diagnostic sign in moderate or severe anaemia, but it is not always apparent. Other useful signs are cheilosis and koilonychia. A reticulocyte count is a quantitative measure of the bone marrow's capacity to produce new red blood cells. Following haemorrhage, the reticulocyte count is increased, reflecting increased erythropoiesis.

1.61

Answer: C   Physiological polycythaemia

Polycythaemia is a condition in which there is a net increase in the total number of red blood cells in the body. The overproduction of red blood cells may be due to a primary process in the bone marrow (a so-called myeloproliferative syndrome) or it may be a reaction to chronically low oxygen levels or, rarely, a malignancy. Primary polycythaemia, often called polycythaemia vera, polycythaemia rubra vera or erythraemia, occurs when excess red blood cells are produced as a result of an abnormality of the bone marrow. Often, excess white blood cells and platelets are also produced.

Secondary polycythaemia is caused by either natural or artificial increases in the production of erythropoietin that result in an increased production of erythrocytes. In secondary polycythaemia, there may be 6–8 million and occasionally 9 million erythrocytes per cubic millimetre of blood. A type of secondary polycythaemia in which the production of erythropoietin increases appropriately is called physiological polycythaemia. Physiological polycythaemia occurs in individuals living at high altitudes, where oxygen availability is less than at sea level. Many athletes train at higher altitudes to take advantage of this effect – a legal form of blood doping. Actual polycythemia sufferers have been known to use their condition as an athletic advantage for greater stamina.

1.62

Answer: C   Host rejection of cells infected with bacteria will be impaired

Natural killer (NK) cells are a form of cytotoxic lymphocyte that constitute a major component of the innate immune system. NK cells play a major role in the host rejection of both tumours and virally infected cells. They were named 'natural killer' because of the initial notion that they do not require activation to kill cells that are 'missing self' recognition ('missing-self' recognition is a term used to describe cells with low levels of MHC (major histocompatibility complex) class I cell surface marker molecules – a situation that could arise due to viral infection or in tumours under strong selection pressure of killer T cells). Given their strong cytolytic activity and the potential for auto-reactivity, natural killer cell activity is tightly regulated. Natural killer cells must receive an activating signal, which can come in a variety of forms, the most important of which are listed below:

- Cytokines – the cytokines interferon α/β play a crucial role in NK-cell activation. As these are stress molecules, released by cells upon viral infection, they serve to signal to the NK cell the presence of viral pathogens. The ubiquitous activator interleukin-2 as well as interferon γ have also been demonstrated to have the capability of activating NK cells.

- FcR receptor – NK cells, along with macrophages and several other cell types, express the FcR molecule, an activating receptor that binds the Fc portion of antibodies. This allows NK cells to target cells against which a humoral response has been mobilised and lyse cells through antibody-dependent cell cytotoxicity.

- Activating and inhibitory receptors – aside from the FcR receptor, NK cells express a variety of receptors that serve to either activate or suppress cytolytic activity. These bind to various ligands on target cells, both endogenous and exogenous, and have an important role in regulating the NK-cell response.

1.63

Answer: E   Vitamin-K-dependent cloting factors deficiency

Vitamin K is involved in the carboxylation of certain glutamate residues in proteins to form gamma-carboxyglutamate residues (abbreviated GLA residues). GLA residues are usually involved in binding calcium. The GLA residues are essential for the biological activity of all known GLA proteins. To date, 14 human GLA proteins have been discovered and they play key roles in the regulation of three physiological processes:

- blood coagulation (prothrombin [factor II], factors VII, IX, X, protein C, protein S and protein Z)

- bone metabolism (osteocalcin, also called bone GLA protein and matrix GLA protein)

- vascular biology.

Obstructive jaundice is associated with vitamin K deficiency. As a result of the acquired vitamin K deficiency, GLA residues are not or incompletely formed and hence the GLA proteins are inactive. Lack of control of the three processes mentioned above may lead to the following: risk of massive, uncontrolled internal bleeding, cartilage calcification and severe malformation of developing bone or deposition of insoluble calcium salts in the arterial vessel walls.

1.64

Answer: C   Epstein–Barr virus

Burkitt's lymphoma is a type of non-Hodgkin's lymphoma and is most common in equatorial Africa and is co-existent with the presence of malaria. Malaria infection causes reduced immune surveillance of Epstein–Barr virus (EBV), immortalised B cells, so allowing their proliferation. This proliferation increases the chance of a mutation to occur. Repeated mutations can lead to the B cells escaping the body's cell-cycle control, so allowing the cells to proliferate unchecked, resulting in the formation of Burkitt's lymphoma. Burkitt's lymphoma commonly affects the jaw bone, forming a huge tumour mass. It responds quickly to chemotherapy treatment, namely cyclophosphamide, but recurrence is common.

The Epstein–Barr virus, also called human herpesvirus 4 (HHV-4), is a virus of the herpes family (which includes herpes simplex virus and cytomegalovirus) and is one of the most common viruses in humans. Most people become infected with EBV, which is often asymptomatic but commonly causes infectious mononucleosis. It is named after Michael Epstein and Yvonne Barr, who together with Bert Achong discovered the virus in 1964.

1.65

Answer: A   High platelet count

Polycythaemia vera (PV) must be considered in patients with suggestive symptoms, particularly Budd–Chiari syndrome, but is often first suspected because of an abnormal full blood count (eg, haematocrit [Hct] > 54% in men or > 49% in women). Neutrophils and platelets may be increased and morphologically abnormal. Because PV is a panmyelosis, its diagnosis is clear in patients with elevations of all three peripheral blood components, splenomegaly and no cause for a secondary erythrocytosis. However, these findings are not uniformly present. With myelofibrosis, anaemia and thrombocytopenia may develop, with massive splenomegaly. Additional findings include peripheral white blood cell (WBC) and RBC precursors, marked anisocytosis and poikilocytosis and microcytes, elliptocytes and teardrop-shaped cells. Bone marrow examination is generally performed, showing panmyelosis, large

general

and clumped megakaryocytes and sometimes reticulin fibres. Cytogenetic analysis of bone marrow occasionally demonstrates an abnormal clone specific for a myeloproliferative syndrome.

Because the Hct is the ratio of RBCs per unit volume of whole blood, an elevated Hct may be caused by decreased plasma volume (relative or spurious erythrocytosis, also called stress polycythaemia or Gaisböck's syndrome). Measurement of RBC mass has been suggested to be an early test and helps differentiate PV from an elevated Hct due to hypovolaemia. Also, in PV, plasma volume may increase, particularly if splenomegaly is present, making the Hct falsely normal despite erythrocytosis. So, a diagnosis of true erythrocytosis requires demonstration of an increased RBC mass. When measured with radioactive chromium (^{51}Cr)-labelled RBCs, RBC mass > 36 ml/kg in men (normal, 28.3±2.8 ml/kg) and > 32 ml/kg in women (normal, 25.4±2.6 ml/kg) is considered abnormal. Unfortunately, many laboratories do not perform blood volume studies.

1.66

Answer: C   Complexes with factor VIIa to catalyse the conversion of factor X

Tissue factor (TF), also called thromboplastin, factor III or CD142, is a protein present in subendothelial tissue, platelets and leukocytes necessary for the initiation of thrombin formation from the zymogen prothrombin. Thrombin formation ultimately leads to the coagulation of blood. The protein structure of TF consists of three domains:

- A domain that is located outside the cell; this domain binds factor VIIa. The binding of VIIa to TF occurs via protein–protein interactions by both molecules. Factor VIIa is a protein that consists of several domains. One of these domains, the carboxylated GLA domain, binds in the presence of calcium to negatively charged phospholipids. Binding of factor VIIa to negatively charged phospholipids greatly enhances the protein–protein binding of factor VIIa to TF.

- A domain that crosses the hydrophobic membrane.

- A domain of 21 amino acids length inside the cell that is involved in the signaling function of TF.

TF is the cell-surface receptor for the serine protease factor VIIa. The best known function of tissue factor is its role in blood coagulation. The complex of TF with factor VIIa catalyses the conversion of the inactive protease factor X into the active protease factor Xa. Together with factor VII, tissue factor forms the tissue factor or extrinsic pathway of coagulation. This is opposed to the intrinsic (amplification) pathway that involves both activated factor IX and factor VIII. Both pathways lead to the activation of factor X (the common pathway), which combines with activated factor V in the presence of calcium and phospholipid to produce thrombin (thromboplastin activity). TF is related to a protein family known as the 'cytokine receptor class II family'. The members of this receptor family are activated by cytokines. Cytokines are small proteins that can influence the behaviour of white blood cells. Binding of VIIa to TF has also been found to start signaling processes inside the cell. The signaling function of TF/VIIa plays a role in the formation of new blood vessels (angiogenesis) and in the inhibition of the process of cell suicide (apoptosis).

TF is expressed by cells that are normally not exposed to flowing blood, such as subendothelial cells (eg, smooth muscle cells) and cells surrounding blood vessels (eg, fibroblasts). This can change when the blood vessel is damaged by, for example, physical injury or rupture of atherosclerotic plaques. Exposure of TF-expressing cells during injury allows the complex formation of TF with factor VIIa, accelerating activity of factor VIIa about one thousand fold. The inner surface of the blood vessel consists of endothelial cells. Endothelial cells do not express TF except when they are exposed to inflammatory molecules. Another cell type that expresses TF on the cell surface in inflammatory conditions is the monocyte.

1.67

Answer: C   Is able to bind to activated platelets

Factor V is a protein of the coagulation system, rarely referred to as proaccelerin or labile factor. In contrast to most other coagulation factors, it is not enzymatically active but functions as a co-factor. Deficiency leads to predisposition for haemorrhage, while some mutations (most notably) predispose to thrombosis. The gene for factor V is located on the first chromosome (1q23). It is genomically related to the family of multicopper oxidases and is homologous to coagulation factor VIII. The gene spans 70 kb, consists of 25 exons and the resulting protein has a relative molecular mass of approximately 330 000. Factor V circulates in plasma as a single-chain molecule with a plasma half-life of about 12 hours. Half-lives up to 36 hours have been reported, though.

Factor V is able to bind to activated platelets and is activated by thrombin. On activation, factor V is spliced in two chains (heavy and light chain with molecular masses of 110 000 and 73 000, respectively), which are non-convalently bound to each other by calcium. Factor V is active as a co-factor of the thrombinase complex. The activated factor X (FXa) enzyme requires Ca^{2+} and activated factor V to convert prothrombin to thrombin on the cell surface membrane. This is considered part of the common pathway in the coagulation cascade. Factor Va is degraded by activated protein C, one of the principal physiological inhibitors of coagulation. Protein C itself is activated by thrombin, and concentration and action of protein C are therefore important determinants in the negative feedback loop through which thrombin limits its own activation.

Various hereditary disorders of factor V are known. Deficiency is associated with a rare mild form of haemophilia (termed parahaemophilia or Owren parahaemophilia), the incidence of which is about 1:1 000 000. It inherits in an autosomal recessive fashion. Other mutations of factor V are associated with venous thrombosis. They are the most common hereditary causes for thrombophilia (a tendency to form blood clots). The most common one of these, factor V Leiden, is due to the replacement of an arginine residue with glutamine at amino acid position 506 (R506Q). All prothrombotic factor V mutations (factor V Leiden, factor V Cambridge, factor V Hong Kong) make it resistant to cleavage by activated protein C ('APC resistance'). It therefore remains active and increases the rate of thrombin generation.

1.68

Answer: B   Initiates the process of coagulation in conjunction with tissue factor

Factor VII (old name proconvertin) is one of the central proteins in the coagulation cascade. It is an enzyme of the serine protease class. The main role of factor VII (FVII) is to initiate the process of coagulation in conjunction with tissue factor (TF). Tissue factor is found on the outside of blood vessels – normally not exposed to the bloodstream. Upon vessel injury, tissue factor is exposed to the blood and circulating factor VII. Once bound to TF, FVII is activated to FVIIa by different proteases, among which are thrombin (factor IIa), activated factor X and the FVIIa–TF complex itself. The most important substrates for FVIIa–TF are factor X and factor IX.

The action of the factor is impeded by tissue factor pathway inhibitor, which is released almost immediately after initiation of coagulation. Factor VII is vitamin-K-dependent; it is produced in the liver. Use of warfarin or similar anticoagulants impairs its function. The gene for factor VII is located on chromosome 13 (13q34). Deficiency is rare (congenital proconvertin deficiency) and inherits recessively.

Recombinant human factor VIIa (NovoSeven®, eptacog alfa [activated]) has been introduced for use in uncontrollable bleeding in haemophilia patients who have developed inhibitors against replacement coagulation factor. It is being increasingly used in uncontrollable haemorrhage. The rationale for its use in haemorrhage is that it will only induce coagulation in those sites where TF is also present.

1.69

Answer: A   Is a major physiological anticoagulant

Protein C is a major physiological anticoagulant. It is a vitamin-K-dependent serine protease enzyme that is activated by thrombin into activated protein C. The activated form (with protein S as a co-factor) degrades factor Va and factor VIIIa. It should not be confused with C peptide, C-reactive protein or protein kinase C.

The protein C pathway's key enzyme, activated protein C, provides physiological antithrombotic activity and exhibits both anti-inflammatory and anti-apoptotic activities. Its actions are related to development of thrombosis and ischaemic stroke. The protein C pathway of the coagulation of the blood also influences lipids and lipoproteins.

Protein C deficiency is a rare genetic disorder that predisposes to venous thrombosis and habitual abortion. If homozygous, this presents with a form of disseminated intravascular coagulation in newborns, termed purpura fulminans; it is treated by replacing the defective protein C. Activated protein C resistance is the inability of protein C to cleave factors V and/or VIII. This may be hereditary or acquired. The best known and most common hereditary form is factor V Leiden. Acquired forms occur in the presence of elevated factor VIII concentrations. Warfarin necrosis is acquired protein C deficiency due to treatment with the vitamin K inhibitor anticoagulant warfarin. In initial stages of action, inhibition of protein C may be stronger than inhibition of the vitamin-K-dependent coagulation factors (II, VII, IX and X), leading to paradoxical activation of coagulation and necrosis of skin areas. The *PROC* gene is located on the second chromosome (2q13–q14).

1.70

Answer: D   Acts by hydrolysing one arginine–isoleucine bond in factor X to form factor Xa

Factor IX (or Christmas factor or Christmas-Eve factor) is one of the serine proteases of the coagulation system; it belongs to peptidase family S1. Deficiency of this protein causes haemophilia B. Factor IX is inactive unless activated by factor XIa (of the contact pathway) or factor VIIa (of the tissue factor pathway). When activated into factor IXa, it acts by hydrolysing one arginine–isoleucine bond in factor X to form factor Xa. It requires calcium, membrane phospholipids and factor VIII as co-factors to do so. The gene for factor IX is located on the X chromosome (Xq27.1–q27.2). Deficiency of factor IX causes Christmas disease (haemophilia B). Over 100 mutations of factor IX have been described; some cause no symptoms, but many lead to a significant bleeding disorder.

1.71

Answer: E   Deficiency causes haemophilia C

Factor XI or plasma thromboplastin antecedent is one of the enzymes of the coagulation cascade. Like many other coagulation factors, it is a serine protease. Factor XI (FXI) is produced by the liver and circulates as a homodimer in its inactive form. The plasma half-life of FXI is approximately 52 hours. The zymogen factor is activated into factor XIa by factor XIIa (FXIIa), thrombin and it is also autocatalytic. FXI is a member of the 'contact pathway' due to activation by FXIIa (with includes high-molecular-weight kininogen, prekallikrein, factor XII, factor XI and factor IX). Factor XIa activates factor IX by selectively cleaving arginine–alanine and arginine–valine peptide bonds. Factor IXa, in turn, activates factor X.

Inhibitors of factor XIa include protein-Z-dependent protease inhibitor (ZPI, a member of the serine protease inhibitor/serpin class of proteins), which is independent of protein Z (its action on factor X, however, is protein Z-dependent, hence its name). Although synthesised as a single polypeptide chain, FXI circulates as a homodimer. Every chain has a relative molecular mass of approximately 80 000. Typical plasma concentrations of FXI are 5 mg/l, corresponding to a plasma concentration (of FXI dimers) of approximately 30 nM. The *FXI* gene is 23 kb in length, has 15 exons and is found on chromosome 4q32–35.

Deficiency of factor XI causes the rare haemophilia C; this mainly occurs in Ashkenazi jews and is believed to affect approximately 8% of that population, of both sexes. The condition has been described in other populations at around 1% of cases. It is an autosomal recessive disorder. There is little spontaneous bleeding, but surgical procedures may cause excessive blood loss and prophylaxis is required. Low levels of factor XI also occur in many other disease states, including Noonan syndrome. High levels of factor XI have been implicated in thrombosis, although it is uncertain what determines these levels and how serious the procoagulant state is.

1.72

Answer: B   Is mainly synthesised by the vascular endothelium

Factor VIII (FVIII) is an essential clotting factor. The lack of normal FVIII causes haemophilia A, an inherited bleeding disorder. The gene for factor VIII is located on the X chromosome (Xq28). FVIII is a glycoprotein pro-cofactor. Factor VIII is synthesised predominantly in the vascular endothelium and is not affected by liver disease. In fact, levels usually are elevated in such instances. In the circulating blood, it is mainly bound to von Willebrand factor (vWF, also known as factor VIII-related antigen) to form a stable complex. Upon activation by thrombin or factor Xa, it dissociates from the complex to interact with factor IXa of the coagulation cascade. It is a co-factor to factor IXa in the activation of factor X, which, in turn, with its co-factor factor Va, activates more thrombin. Thrombin cleaves fibrinogen into fibrin, which polymerises and crosslinks (using factor XIII) into a blood clot. No longer protected by vWF, activated FVIII is proteolytically inactivated in the process (most prominently by activated protein C and factor IXa) and quickly cleared from the bloodstream. FVIII concentrated from donated blood plasma (Aafact), or alternatively recombinant FVIII, can be given to haemophiliacs to restore haemostasis. So, FVIII is also known as antihaemophilic factor.

1.73

Answer: C   Direct conversion of plasminogen to plasmin

Streptokinase is an extracellular metallo-enzyme produced by β-haemolytic *Streptococcus* and is used as an effective and cheap clot-dissolving medication in some cases of myocardial infarction (heart attack) and pulmonary embolism.

It belongs to a group of medications known as fibrinolytics and works by activating plasminogen through cleavage to produce plasmin. The half-life of streptokinase is 6 hours. Plasmin is produced in the blood to break down the major constituent of blood clots, fibrin, therefore dissolving clots once they have fulfilled their purpose in stopping bleeding. Extra production of plasmin caused by streptokinase breaks down unwanted blood clots, for example, in the lungs (pulmonary embolism).

It is given intravenously as soon as possible after the onset of a heart attack (acute phase of myocardial infarction) to dissolve clots in the coronary arteries. This reduces the amount of damage to the heart muscle. Streptokinase is a bacterial product, so the body will build up an immunity to it. It is recommended that this medication should not be used again after 4 days from the first administration, as it may not be as effective and can also cause an allergic reaction. For this reason, it is usually given only for a person's first heart attack.

1.74

Answer: B It can be found in areas containing mucus

Immunoglobulin A (IgA) is the main immunoglobulin in mucous secretions, including tears, saliva and colostrum as well as respiratory, intestinal, prostatic and vaginal secretions. It is also found in small amounts in blood. Because it is resistant to degradation by enzymes, secretory IgA provides protection against microbes proliferating in body secretions, especially those of the digestive and respiratory tracts. It does not activate complement and opsonises only weakly. Its heavy chains are of the type α. It exists in two forms, IgA1 (90%) and IgA2 (10%) that differ in their structure. IgA1 is composed like other proteins; however, in IgA2 the heavy and light chains are not linked with disulphide but with non-covalent bonds. IgA1 is found in serum and made by bone marrow B cells; however, IgA2 is made by B cells located in the mucosae and has been found to secrete into colostrum, maternal milk, tears and saliva.

IgA is found in secretion in a specific form called secretory IgA, a dimer of two IgA monomers linked by two additional chains. One of these is the J chain (from 'join'), which is a polypeptide of molecular mass 1.5 kDa, rich with cysteine and structurally completely different from other immunoglobulin chains. This chain is formed in the antibody-secreting cells. The dimeric form of IgA in the outer secretions also has a polypeptide of the same molecular mass (1.5 kDa) called the secretory chain and is produced by epithelial cells. It is also possible to find trimeric and even tetrameric IgA. Decreased or absent IgA, termed selective IgA deficiency, can be a clinically significant immunodeficiency.

1.75

Answer: A It binds to allergens and triggers histamine release from mast cells

Immunoglobulin E (IgE) is an antibody subclass (known as 'isotypes'), found only in mammals. Although IgE is typically the least abundant isotype – blood serum IgE levels in a normal ('non-atopic') individual are ~150 ng/ml, compared with 10 mg/ml for the IgGs (the isotypes responsible for most of the classical adaptive immune response) – it is capable of triggering the most powerful immune reactions. Most of our knowledge of IgE has come from research into the mechanism of a form of allergy known as type 1 hypersensitivity.

IgE, which can specifically recognise an 'allergen' (typically this is a protein, such as dust mite DerP1, cat FelD1, grass or ragweed pollen, etc) has a unique long-lived interaction with its high-affinity receptor, Fc epsilon RI, so that basophils and mast cells, capable of mediating inflammatory reactions, become 'primed', ready to release chemicals like histamine, leukotrienes and certain interleukins, which cause many of the symptoms associated with allergy, such as airway constriction in asthma, local inflammation in eczema, increased mucus secretion in allergic rhinitis and increased vascular permeability, ostensibly to allow other immune cells to gain access to tissues, but which can lead to a potentially fatal drop in blood pressure as in anaphylaxis.

1.76

Answer: D   Platelets

In a normal individual, coagulation is initiated within 20 s after an injury occurs to the blood vessel, damaging the endothelial cells. Platelets immediately form a haemostatic plug at the site of injury. This is called primary haemostasis. Secondary haemostasis then follows – plasma components called coagulation factors respond (in a complex cascade) to form fibrin strands, which strengthen the platelet plug. Primary haemostasis is initiated when platelets adhere, using a specific platelet collagen receptor, glycoprotein Ia/IIa, to collagen fibres in the vascular endothelium. This adhesion is mediated by von Willebrand factor (vWF), which forms links between the platelet glycoprotein Ib/IX/V and collagen fibrils. The platelets are then activated and release the contents of their granules into the plasma, in turn activating other platelets and white blood cells. The platelets undergo a change in their shape, which exposes a phospholipid surface for those coagulation factors that require it. Fibrinogen links adjacent platelets by forming links via the glycoprotein IIb/IIIa. In addition, thrombin activates platelets.

1.77

Answer: C   It functions as a co-factor to protein C

Protein S is a vitamin-K-dependent plasma glycoprotein synthesised in the liver. In the circulation, it exists in two forms: a free form and a complex form bound to complement protein C4b. The best characterised function of protein S is its role in the anticoagulation pathway, it functions as a co-factor to protein C in the inactivation of factors Va and VIIIa. Only the free form has co-factor activity.

Protein S can bind to negatively charged phospholipids via the carboxylated GLA domain. This property allows protein S to function in the removal of cells that are undergoing apoptosis. Apoptosis is a form of cell death that is used by the body to remove unwanted or damaged cells from tissues. Cells that are apoptotic (ie, in the process of apoptosis) no longer actively manage the distribution of phospholipids in their outer membrane and hence begin to display negatively charged phospholipids, such as phosphatidyl serine, on the cell surface. In healthy cells, an ATP (adenosine triphosphate)-dependant enzyme removes these from the outer leaflet of the cell membrane. These negatively charged phospholipids are recognised by phagocytes such as macrophages. Protein S can bind to the negatively charged phospholipids and function as a bridging molecule between the apoptotic cell and the phagocyte. This bridging property of protein S enhances the phagocytosis of the apoptotic cell, allowing it to be removed 'cleanly' without any symptoms of tissue damage such as inflammation occurring. Protein S deficiency is a rare blood disorder that can lead to an increased risk of thrombosis.

1.78

Answer: D   It is necessary for the activation of factor XI by factor XIIa

High-molecular-weight kininogen (HMWK), also known as the Williams–Fitzgerald–Flaujeac factor or the Fitzgerald factor or the HMWK–kallikrein factor, is a protein from the blood coagulation system as well as the kinin–kallikrein system. It is a protein that adsorbs to the surface of biomaterials that come in contact with blood in vivo. This protein circulates throughout the blood and quickly adsorbs to the material surfaces. HMWK is one of the early participants of the intrinsic pathway of coagulation, together with factor XII (Hageman factor) and prekallikrein. It is 626 amino acids long and weighs 88–120 kDa (dependent on glycosylation). The kininogen is not enzymatically active and only functions as a co-factor for the activation of kallikrein and Hageman factor. It is also necessary for the activation of factor XI by factor XIIa. The histidine-rich region (amino acids 420 to 510) participates most strongly in coagulation. In addition to its role in blood coagulation, HMWK (like low-molecular-weight kininogen) is a strong inhibitor of cysteine proteinases. Responsible for this activity are three related domains on its heavy chain. HMWK is also a precursor of bradykinin; this vasodilator substance is released through positive feedback by kallikrein.

1.79

Answer: D   Heparin

Antithrombin III is a small molecule that inactivates several enzymes of the coagulation system. It is a glycoprotein produced by the liver. Antithrombin III is a serpin (serine protease inhibitor) that inactivates a number of enzymes from the coagulation system, namely the activated forms of factor X, factor IX, factor II (thrombin), factor VII, factor XI and factor XII. The rate of its reaction with these molecules (ie, its effectiveness) is greatly enhanced by heparin. Antithrombin III deficiency is a rare hereditary disorder that generally comes to light when a patient suffers recurrent venous thrombosis and pulmonary embolism.

1.80

Answer: E   Factor XIII

The coagulation factors are generally serine proteases (enzymes). There are some exceptions. For example, factor VIII and factor V are glycoproteins and factor XIII is a transglutaminase. Factor XIII or fibrin-stabilising factor crosslinks fibrin. When thrombin has converted fibrinogen to fibrin, the latter forms a proteinaceous network in which every E-unit is crosslinked to only one D-unit.

Factor XIII is activated by thrombin into factor XIIIa; its activation into factor XIIIa requires calcium as a co-factor. FXIII is known also as Laki–Lorand factor, after the scientists who first proposed its existence in 1948.

1.81

Answer: A   They activate other immune cells

T helper cells (also known as effector T cells or T cells) are a subgroup of lymphocytes that play an important role in establishing and maximizing the capabilities of the immune system. These cells are unusual in that they have no cytotoxic or phagocytic activity; they cannot kill infected host (also known as somatic) cells or pathogens and without other immune cells they would usually be considered useless against an infection. T helper cells are involved in activating and directing other immune cells and are particularly important in the immune system. They are essential in determining B cell antibody class switching, in the activation and growth of cytotoxic T cells and in maximizing bactericidal activity of phagocytes such as macrophages. It is this diversity in function and their role in influencing other cells that gives T helper cells their name.

Mature T helper cells are believed to always express the surface protein CD4. T cells expressing CD4 are also known as CD4+ T cells. CD4+ T cells are generally treated as having a pre-defined role as helper T helper cells within the immune system, although there are known rare exceptions. For example, there are subgroups of suppressor T cells, natural killer T cells and cytotoxic T cells that are known to express CD4 (although cytotoxic examples have been observed in extremely low numbers in specific disease states, they are usually considered non-existent). All of the latter CD4+ T cell groups are not considered T helper cells. The importance of T helper cells can be seen from HIV, a virus that infects cells that are CD4+ (including T helper cells). Towards the end of an HIV infection the number of functional CD4+ T cells falls, which leads to the symptomatic stage of infection known as the acquired immune deficiency syndrome (AIDS).

general

1.82

Answer: D Skin

Dendritic cells are immune cells and form part of the mammalian immune system. Their main function is to process antigen material and present it on their surface to other cells of the immune system. Dendritic cells are present in small quantities in tissues that are in contact with the external environment, mainly the skin (where they are often called Langerhans cells) and the inner lining of the nose, lungs, stomach and intestines. They can also be found at an immature state in the blood. Once activated, they migrate to the lymphoid tissues where they interact with T cells and B cells to initiate and shape the immune response. At certain development stages they grow branched projections, the dendrites, that give the cell its name. However, these do not have any special relation with neurones, which also possess similar appendages. Immature dendritic cells are also called veiled cells, in which case they possess large cytoplasmic 'veils' rather than dendrites. There are four types of dendritic cells: lymphoid dendritic cells, myeloid dendritic cells, plasmacytoid dendritic cells and follicular dendritic cells. Lymphoid and myeloid dendritic cells evolve from lymphoid or myeloid precursors respectively and so are of haemopoietic origin. The origin of follicular dendritic cell is not yet known, but they share the appearance and function of the other two types. In all these cases, as well as in neurone dendrites, the similar morphology results in a very large contact surface to their surroundings compared with overall cell volume. Follicular dendritic cells are probably not of haemopoietic origin, but simply look similar to true dendritic cells.

1.83

Answer: E They have cytotoxic activity

Cytotoxic T cells (also known as T_C) belong to a subgroup of T lymphocytes that are capable of inducing the death of infected, somatic or tumour cells; they kill cells that are infected with viruses (or other pathogens) or are otherwise damaged or dysfunctional. Most cytotoxic T cells express T-cell receptors that can recognise a specific antigenic peptide bound to class I MHC molecules on an antigen-presenting cell and a glycoprotein called CD8, which is attracted to non-variable portions of the class I MHC molecule. The affinity between CD8 and the MHC molecule keeps the T_C cell and the target cell bound closely together during antigen-specific activation. CD8$^+$ T cells are recognised as T_C cells once they become activated and are generally classified as having a pre-defined cytotoxic role within the immune system. During hepatitis B virus (HBV) infection, cytotoxic T cells play an important pathogenetic role. They contribute to nearly all of the liver injury associated with HBV infection and, by killing infected cells and by producing antiviral cytokines capable of purging HBV from viable hepatocytes, cytotoxic T cells also eliminate the virus.

1.84

Answer: A   Heparin therapy

The partial thromboplastin time (PTT) or activated partial thromboplastin time (aPTT) is a performance indicator measuring the efficacy of both the intrinsic and the common coagulation pathways. Apart from detecting abnormalities in blood clotting, it is also used to monitor the treatment effects with heparin, a major anticoagulant. Values below 25 s and over 39 s (depending on local normal ranges) are generally abnormal. Shortening of the PTT has little clinical relevance. Prolonged aPTT may indicate:

- use of heparin (or contamination of the sample)

- antiphospholipid antibody (especially lupus anticoagulant, which paradoxically increases propensity to thrombosis)

- coagulation factor deficiency (eg, haemophilia).

To distinguish the above causes, *mixing studies* are performed, in which the patient's plasma is mixed (initially at a 50 : 50 dilution) with normal plasma. If the abnormality does not disappear, the sample is said to contain an 'inhibitor' (either heparin, antiphospholipid antibodies or coagulation factor specific inhibitors), while if it does correct, a factor deficiency is more likely. Deficiencies of factors VIII, IX, XI and XII and rarely von Willebrand factor (if causing a low factor VIII level) may lead to a prolonged aPTT correcting on mixing studies.

general

1.85

Answer: D   Liver disease

The prothrombin time (PT) and its derived measures of prothrombin ratio (PR) and international normalised ratio (INR) are measures of the extrinsic pathway of coagulation. They are used to determine the clotting tendency of blood, in the measure of warfarin dosage, liver damage and vitamin K status. The reference range for prothrombin time is usually around 12–15 s; the normal range for the INR is 0.8–1.2. PT measures factors II, V, VII, X and fibrinogen. It is used in conjunction with the activated partial thromboplastin time (aPTT), which measures the intrinsic pathway.

1.86

Answer: B   It is a thrombotic disorder

Heparin-induced thrombocytopaenia (HIT) with or without thrombosis (HITT) is thrombocytopaenia (low platelet counts) due to the administration of heparin. While it is mainly associated with unfractionated heparin (UFH), it can also occur with exposure to low-molecular-weight heparin (LMWH), but at significantly lower rates. Despite the low platelet count, it is a thrombotic disorder, with very high rates of thrombosis, in the arteries with or without venous complications.

HIT typically develops 4–14 days after the administration of heparin. UFH is used in cardiovascular surgery, as prevention or treatment for deep venous thrombosis and pulmonary embolism and in various other clinical scenarios. LMWH is increasingly used in outpatient prophylaxis regimes.

There are two forms of HIT. Type II HIT is the main adverse effect of heparin use. Patients with type I HIT have a transient decrease in platelet count without any further symptoms. This recovers even if heparin is continued to be administered. Platelet counts rarely fall below 100. Type I HIT occurs in 10–20% of all patients on heparin. It is not due to an immune reaction and antibodies are not found upon investigation. Type II HIT is due to an autoimmune reaction with antibodies formed against platelet factor 4 (PF4), neutrophil-activating peptide 2 and interleukin-8, which form complexes with heparin. The most common is the heparin–PF4 complex. It appears that heparin binding to PF4 causes a conformational change in the protein, rendering it antigenic. The antibodies found are most commonly of the IgG class with or without IgM and IgA class antibodies. IgM and IgA are rarely found without IgG antibodies. Type II HIT develops in about 3% of all patients on UFH and in 0.1% of patients on LMWH and causes thrombosis in 30–40% of these patients. The other patients are able to compensate for the activation of haemostasis that leads to thrombosis. Clot formation is mainly arterial and rich in platelets ('white clot syndrome'), in contrast with fibrin-rich clots (which are red due to trapped red blood cells). Most thrombotic events are in the lower limbs; skin lesions and necrosis may also occur at the site of the heparin infusion.

The most important enzyme in type II HIT is thrombin, the generation of which is increased following platelet activation. Platelet activation follows the binding of heparin to PF4 and the cross linking of receptors on the platelet surface.

Genetic risk factors for thrombosis, such as factor V Leiden, prothrombin gene mutation, methylenetetrahydrofolate reductase polymorphism and platelet-receptor polymorphisms, do not increase the risk of developing HIT-associated thrombosis. Risk for HIT is higher in women than in men and HIT occurs more commonly in surgical than in non-surgical settings. Treatment is by prompt withdrawal of heparin and replacement with a suitable alternative anticoagulant. Protamine sulphate, the normal antidote for heparin, is not effective, as the antibodies react with platelets independent of heparin. To block the thrombotic state, lepirudin (Refludan®), fondaparinux, bivalirudin, argatroban, danaparoid or other direct thrombin inhibitors are used. LMWH is contraindicated in HIT.

1.87

Answer: D   It has a smaller risk of heparin-induced thrombocytopenia

Low-molecular-weight heparin (LMWH) is a class of medication used as an anticoagulant in diseases that feature thrombosis, as well as for prophylaxis in situations that lead to a high risk of thrombosis. Heparin is a naturally occurring polysaccharide that inhibits coagulation, the process whereby thrombosis occurs. Natural heparin consists of molecular chains of varying lengths or molecular weights; chains of molecular weight from 5000 to over 40 kDa, make up polydisperse pharmaceutical grade heparin. Heparin derived from natural sources, mainly porcine intestine or bovine lung, can be administered therapeutically to prevent thrombosis. However, the effects of natural, or unfractionated, heparin can be difficult to predict. After a standard dose of unfractionated heparin, coagulation parameters must be monitored very closely to prevent over- or under-anticoagulation.

Low-molecular-weight heparins, in contrast, consist of only short chains of polysaccharide. LMWHs are defined as heparin salts having an average molecular mass of less than 8 kDa and for which at least 60% of all chains have a molecular mass less than 8 kDa. These are obtained by various methods of fractionation or depolymerisation of polymeric heparin. They have a potency of greater than 70 units/mg of antifactor Xa activity and a ratio of antifactor Xa activity to antithrombin activity of >1.5. LMWH differs from unfractionated heparin in the following respects:

- average molecular mass of LMWH is about 3 kDa, whereas for heparin it is about 20 kDa

- once-daily dosing, rather than a continuous infusion of unfractionated heparin

- no need for monitoring of the aPTT coagulation parameter

- possibly a smaller risk of bleeding

- smaller risk of osteoporosis in long-term use

- smaller risk of heparin-induced thrombocytopenia, a feared side-effect of heparin.

1.88

Answer: E   Thrombocytopaenia

Bleeding time is affected by platelet function, certain vascular disorders and von Willebrand disease, but not by other coagulation factors, so in haemophilia it is normal. Diseases that cause prolonged bleeding time include thrombocytopaenia and disseminated intravascular coagulation (DIC). Aspirin and other cyclo-oxygenase inhibitors can prolong bleeding time significantly. While warfarin and heparin have their major effects on coagulation factors, an increased bleeding time is sometimes seen with use of these medications as well. People with von Willebrand's disease usually experience increased bleeding time, as von Willebrand factor is a platelet agglutination protein, but this is not considered an effective diagnostic test for this condition. Normal values fall between 2 and 9 min depending on the method used.

1.89

Answer: B   Deep venous thrombosis

D-dimer is a blood test performed to diagnose thrombosis. Since its introduction in the 1990s, it has become an important test performed in patients suspected of thrombotic disorders. While a negative result practically rules out thrombosis, a positive result can indicate thrombosis but also has other potential causes. Its main use, therefore, is to exclude thromboembolic disease where the probability is low. D-dimer testing is of clinical use when there is a suspicion of deep venous thrombosis (DVT) or pulmonary embolism (PE). In patients suspected of disseminated intravascular coagulation (DIC), D-dimers may aid in the diagnosis. Most sampling kits have 0–300 ng/ml as normal range. Values exceeding 250, 300 or 500 ng/ml (different for various kits) are considered positive. Fibrin degradation products (FDPs) are formed whenever fibrin is broken down by enzymes (eg, plasmin). Determining FDPs is not considered useful, as this does not indicate whether the fibrin is part of a blood clot or being generated as part of inflammation.

D-dimers are unique in that they are the breakdown products of a fibrin mesh that has been stabilised by factor XIII. This factor crosslinks the E-element to two D-elements. This is the final step in the generation of a thrombus. Plasmin is a fibrinolytic enzyme that organises clots and breaks down the fibrin mesh. It cannot, however, break down the bonds between one E and two D units. The protein fragment so left over is a D-dimer. D-dimer assays rely on monoclonal antibodies to bind to this specific protein fragment.

1.90

Answer: B   Heparin therapy

The thrombin clotting time (TCT), also known as the thrombin time (TT), is a coagulation assay, which is usually performed to determine the therapeutic level of the anticoagulant heparin. It is also sensitive in detecting the presence of a fibrinogen abnormality. Within the realm of coagulation assays, the TCT is one of the most procedurally simple. After liberating the plasma from the whole blood by centrifugation, bovine thrombin is added to the sample of plasma. The clot is formed and is detected optically or mechanically by a coagulation instrument. The time between the addition of the thrombin and the clot formation is recorded as the thrombin clotting time. The reference interval of the TCT is generally < 21 s, depending on the method and the endemic patient population. Results outside of reference interval indicate heparin therapy, hypofibrinogenaemia, hyperfibrinogenaemia or lupus anticoagulant.

SECTION 2: CARDIOVASCULAR PHYSIOLOGY – ANSWERS

cardiovascular

2.1

Answer: B   AV node

The atrioventricular node (abbreviated AV node) is the tissue between the atria and the ventricles of the heart, which conducts the normal electrical impulse from the atria to the ventricles. The AV node receives two inputs from the atria: posteriorly via the crista terminalis and anteriorly via the interatrial septum. An important property that is unique to the AV node is *decremental conduction.* This is the property of the AV node that prevents rapid conduction to the ventricle in cases of rapid atrial rhythms, such as atrial fibrillation or atrial flutter. The AV node functions as a critical delay in the conduction system. Without this delay, the atria and ventricles would contract at the same time and blood would not flow effectively from the atria to the ventricles. The delay in the AV node forms much of the PR segment on the ECG. The blood supply of the AV node is from a branch of the right coronary artery in 85–90% of individuals and from a branch of the left circumflex artery in 10–15% of individuals. In certain types of supraventricular tachycardia, a person could have two AV nodes; this will cause a loop in electrical current and uncontrollably rapid heart beat. When this electricity catches up with itself, it will dissipate and return to normal heart-beat speed.

2.2

Answer: D   Total peripheral resistance

The patient in this question is in hypovolaemic shock. In hypovolaemic shock, caused by bleeding, it is necessary to immediately control the bleeding and restore the victim's blood volume by giving infusions of balanced salt solutions. Blood transfusions are necessary for loss of

265

large amounts of blood (eg, greater than 20% of blood volume), but can be avoided in smaller and slower losses. Volume resuscitation will result in reduced sympathetic discharge and adequate ventricular filling resulting in reduced total peripheral resistance with increased cardiac output and cardiac filling pressures.

2.3

Answer: C   *PVR* Increase   *PAP* Decrease

Haemorrhage results in loss of effective blood volume and initiation of sympathetic adrenal discharge. These will result in reduced pulmonary artery pressure and elevation of pulmonary vascular resistance.

2.4

Answer: C   Plasma vasopressin is increased in response to reduced ECF volume

The vascularly generated shock is caused by loss of blood or other fluids (absolute hypovolaemia) or by vasodilatation (relative hypovolaemia). Absolute hypovolaemia is caused by blood loss, plasma loss (burns or other denuding conditions, ascites, hydrothorax etc) or dehydration (water deprivation, severe diarrhoea or vomiting, excessive sweating, intestinal obstruction with luminal fluid accumulation, urinary loss of proteins/salt/water, excessive use of diuretics, hypoaldosteronism etc). Relative hypovolaemia, sometimes with universal vasodilatation, is caused by endotoxins (septic shock from viral or bacterial infections), anaphylactic shock or by a neurogenic vasodilatation (neurogenic shock by severe pains or stress, anaesthetics or brainstem lesions close to the vasoconstrictor centre).

The reduced delivery of oxygen and nutrients to virtually all cells of the body is consequential: The mitochondria synthesise less ATP, the Na^+-K^+ pump operates insufficiently, the metabolic processing of nutrients is depressed, which profoundly depresses muscular contractions and finally digestive enzymes destroy the damaged cells. Glucose transport across the cell membranes in the liver and in the skeletal muscles is depressed, including a severe inhibition of the actions of insulin and other hormones. During progressive shock the metabolism is reduced and so also heat energy, so the body temperature tends to decrease, if the patient is not kept warm. Compensatory mechanisms in shock are called negative feedback mechanisms, because they operate to counteract the fall in blood pressure. Baroreceptor responses and many hormonal control systems, that tend to raise the falling blood pressure, are examples of negative feedback. The gain of a feedback system is defined as the ratio of the response to the stimulus itself. Decompensatory mechanisms exaggerate the primary fall in blood pressure. This is called positive feedback. A positive feedback mechanism can lead to a vicious cycle and death, if its gain is above one. Two examples of positive feedback in shock are ischaemic brainstem depression and cardiac depression.

Mild shock is a condition where compensatory reactions can cure the patient without external help. A latent shock is produced when a healthy blood donor delivers more than the usual 500 ml of blood for transfusion, but the volume is often replaced within an hour. A number of negative feedback mechanisms oppose the induced changes of shock. The falls in MAP and pulse pressure reduce the stimulation of the high-pressure baroreceptors in the carotid sinus and the aortic arch. The negative stimulation of the cardiovascular control centres in the brainstem enhances the sympathetic tone (and reduces the vagal tone), leading to increased heart rate and contractility as well as to arteriolar and venous constriction mainly in the skin, skeletal muscles and the splanchnic area. The blood flow favours the brain and the heart as long as possible.

Reduced capillary pressure with autotransfusion from the interstitial fluid, thirst and drinking followed by absorption of fluid from the gastrointestinal tract and release of powerful vasoconstrictors such as adrenaline, angiotensin II, vasopressin etc are all compensatory mechanisms that counteract shock.

Catecholamines and enkephalins are released from chromaffin granules in the adrenal medulla. Catecholamines increase the heart rate and the cardiac output by stimulation of the adrenergic β_1-receptors in the myocardium. Catecholamines constrict vessels all over the body by stimulating α_1-receptors located on the surface of vascular smooth muscles.

ADH (vasopressin) is secreted from the posterior pituitary gland in response to shock, because the sinoaortic baroreceptors are understimulated. Vasopressin is a modest vasoconstrictor and a strong antidiuretic hormone. The increased ADH secretion causes increased fluid reabsorption by the kidneys and restores blood pressure and volume.

Renin is secreted from the juxtaglomerular apparatus, when blood pressure and renal perfusion fall drastically. Renin acts on the plasma protein, angiotensinogen, to form inactive angiotensin I, which is transformed to the powerful vasoconstrictor, angiotensin II by angiotensin converting enzyme, ACE. Angiotensin II is a powerful dipsogen and increases thirst sensation. The rise in normal plasma potassium due to the ischaemia of shock also releases aldosterone, which promotes potassium loss from the kidney by acting on mineralocorticoid receptors on principal cells in the distal tubule of the nephron.

ACTH and β-endorphins are released into the blood from the anterior pituitary gland in response to haemorrhage or other forms of stress. ACTH and endorphins both exaggerate and restrict the development of shock. These opioids depress the brainstem control centres that normally mediate autonomic responses to stress. Hence, naloxone (an opioid antagonist) improves the circulation and increases the rate of survival from life-threatening shock. On the other hand, ACTH has a small aldosterone- and a strong cortisol-stimulating effect.

2.5

Answer: D The skin vessels are constricted

In haemorrhagic shock, blood loss exceeds the body's ability to compensate and provide adequate tissue perfusion and oxygenation. This frequently is due to trauma, but it may be caused by spontaneous haemorrhage (eg, gastrointestinal [GI] bleeding, childbirth), surgery and other causes. Most frequently, clinical haemorrhagic shock is caused by an acute bleeding episode with a discrete precipitating event. Less commonly, haemorrhagic shock may be seen in chronic conditions with subacute blood loss. Well described responses to acute loss of circulating volume exist. Teleologically, these responses act systematically to divert circulating volume away from non-vital organ systems so that blood volume may be conserved for vital organ function. Acute haemorrhage causes a decreased cardiac output and decreased pulse pressure. These changes are sensed by baroreceptors in the aortic arch and atrium. With a decrease in the circulating volume, neural reflexes cause an increased sympathetic outflow to the heart and other organs. The response is an increase in heart rate, vasoconstriction and redistribution of blood flow away from certain non-vital organs such as the skin, gastrointestinal tract and kidneys.

Concurrently, a multisystem hormonal response to acute haemorrhage occurs. Corticotropin-releasing hormone is stimulated directly. This eventually leads to glucocorticoid and β-endorphin release. Vasopressin from the posterior pituitary is released, causing water retention at the distal tubules. Renin is released by the juxtamedullary complex in response to decreased mean arterial pressure, leading to increased aldosterone levels and eventually to sodium and water resorption. Hyperglycaemia commonly is associated with acute haemorrhage. This is due to a glucagon- and growth-hormone-induced increase in gluconeogenesis and glycogenolysis. Circulating catecholamines relatively inhibit insulin release and activity, leading to increased plasma glucose.

In addition to these global changes, many organ-specific responses occur. The brain has remarkable autoregulation that keeps cerebral blood flow constant over a wide range of systemic mean arterial blood pressures. The kidneys can tolerate a 90% decrease in total blood flow for short periods of time. With significant decreases in circulatory volume, intestinal blood flow is dramatically reduced by splanchnic vasoconstriction. Early and appropriate resuscitation may avert damage to individual organs as adaptive mechanisms act to preserve the organism. Age, medications and co-morbid factors all may affect a patient's response to haemorrhagic shock. Failure of compensatory mechanisms in haemorrhagic shock can lead to death. Without intervention, a classic trimodal distribution of deaths is seen in severe haemorrhagic shock. An initial peak of mortality occurs within minutes of haemorrhage due to immediate exsanguination. Another peak occurs after 1 to several hours due to progressive decompensation. A third peak occurs days to weeks later due to sepsis and organ failure (see also answer to 2.4).

cardiovascular

2.6

Answer: B   Baroceptor reflex

In cardiovascular physiology, the baroreflex or baroreceptor reflex is one of the body's homeostatic mechanisms for maintaining blood pressure. It provides a negative feedback loop in which an elevated blood pressure reflexively causes blood pressure to decrease; similarly, decreased blood pressure depresses the baroreflex, causing blood pressure to rise. The system relies on specialised neurones (baroreceptors) in the aortic arch, carotid sinuses and elsewhere to monitor changes in blood pressure and relay them to the brainstem. Subsequent changes in blood pressure are mediated by the autonomic nervous system. Baroreceptors include those in the auricles of the heart and vena cavae, but the most sensitive baroreceptors are in the carotid sinuses and aortic arch. The carotid sinus baroreceptors are innervated by the glossopharyngeal nerve (CN IX); the aortic arch baroreceptors are innervated by the vagus nerve (CN X). Baroreceptor activity travels along these nerves, which contact the nucleus of the tractus solitarius (NTS) in the brainstem.

The baroreceptors are stretch-sensitive mechanoreceptors. When blood pressure rises, the carotid and aortic sinuses are distended, resulting in stretch and therefore activation of the baroreceptors. Active baroreceptors fire action potentials ('spikes') more frequently than inactive baroreceptors. The greater the stretch, the more rapidly baroreceptors fire action potentials. These action potentials are relayed to the NTS, which uses spike frequency as a surrogate measure of blood pressure. Increased activation of the NTS inhibits the vasomotor centre and stimulates the vagal nuclei. The end result of baroreceptor activation is inhibition of the sympathetic nervous system and activation of the parasympathetic nervous system.

The sympathetic and parasympathetic branches of the autonomic nervous system have opposing effects on blood pressure. Sympathetic activation leads to increased contractility of the heart, increased heart rate, venoconstriction and arterial vasoconstriction, which tend to increase blood pressure by elevating both total peripheral resistance and cardiac output. Conversely, parasympathetic activation leads to a decrease in heart rate and a minor decrease in contractility, resulting in a decreased cardiac output and therefore a tendency to decrease blood pressure.

By coupling sympathetic inhibition with parasympathetic activation, the baroreflex maximises its ability to reduce blood pressure. Sympathetic inhibition leads to a drop in total peripheral resistance and cardiac output, while parasympathetic activation leads to a depressed heart rate and reduced cardiac contractility. The combined effects will dramatically decrease blood pressure. Similarly, coupling sympathetic activation with parasympathetic inhibition allows the baroreflex to elevate blood pressure effectively. Sympathetic activation increases total peripheral resistance and elevates cardiac output, the latter being enhanced by inhibition of the parasympathetic nervous system.

Baroreceptors are tonically active at mean arterial pressures (MAP) above approximately 70 mmHg, called the baroreceptor set point. When MAP falls below the set point, baroreceptors are essentially silent. The baroreceptor set point is not fixed; its value may change with changes in blood pressure that persist for 1–2 days. For example, in chronic hypertension, the set point will increase; on the other hand, chronic hypotension will result in a depression of the baroreceptor set point. At a MAP below approximately 50 mmHg, baroreceptors are completely silent. The baroreflex may also be responsible for a part of the low-frequency component of heart rate variability, the so called Mayer waves.

2.7

Answer: A   Angiotensin II

Angiotensin is an oligopeptide in the blood that causes vasoconstriction, increased blood pressure and release of aldosterone from the adrenal cortex. It is a powerful dipsogen. It is derived from the precursor molecule angiotensinogen, a serum globulin produced in the liver. It plays an important role in the renin–angiotensin system. Angiotensin I is converted to angiotensin II through removal of two terminal residues by the enzyme angiotensin-converting enzyme (ACE or kininase), which is found predominantly in the capillaries of the lung. ACE is a target for inactivation by ACE inhibitor drugs, which decrease the rate of angiotensin II production. Other cleavage products, seven or nine amino acids long, are also known; they have differential affinity for angiotensin receptors, although their exact role is still unclear. The action of angiotensin II itself is targeted by angiotensin II receptor antagonists, which directly block angiotensin II AT_1 receptors. Angiotensin II is degraded to angiotensin III by angiotensinases that are located in red blood cells and the vascular beds of most tissues. It has a half-life in circulation of around 30 s, while in tissue it may be as long as 15–30 min. Angiotensin II has a number of effects throughout the body. These include:

Cardiovascular effects

- It is a potent direct vasoconstrictor, constricting arteries and veins and increasing blood pressure.

- Angiotensin II has prothrombotic potential through adhesion and aggregation of platelets and production of PAI-1 and PAI-2.

- It has been proposed that angiotensin II could be a cause of vascular and cardiac muscle hypertrophy.

Neural effects

- Angiotensin II increases thirst sensation (dipsogen) through the subfornical organ of the brain, decreases the response of the baroreceptor reflex and increases the desire for salt.

- It increases secretion of ADH in the posterior pituitary and secretion of ACTH in the anterior pituitary.

- It also potentiates the release of noradrenaline by direct action on postganglionic sympathetic fibres.

Adrenal effects

- Angiotensin II acts on the adrenal cortex, causing it to release aldosterone, a hormone that causes the kidneys to retain sodium and lose potassium.

- Elevated plasma angiotensin II levels are responsible for the elevated aldosterone levels present during the luteal phase of the menstrual cycle.

Renal effects

- Angiotensin II has a direct effect on the proximal tubules to increase Na^+ resorption.

- Although it slightly inhibits glomerular filtration by indirectly (through sympathetic effects) and directly stimulating mesangial cell constriction, its overall effect is to increase the glomerular filtration rate by increasing the renal perfusion pressure via efferent renal arteriole constriction.

2.8

Answer: E   Total peripheral resistance

Hypovolaemic shock is the most common type of shock and based on insufficient circulating volume. Its primary cause is loss of fluid from the circulation from either an internal or external source. An internal source may be haemorrhage. External causes may include extensive bleeding, high-output fistulae or severe burns. The management of shock requires immediate intervention, even before a diagnosis is made. Re-establishing perfusion to the organs is the primary goal through restoring and maintaining the blood circulating volume, ensuring oxygenation and blood pressure are adequate, achieving and maintaining effective cardiac function and preventing complications. In hypovolaemic shock, caused by bleeding, it is necessary to control the bleeding immediately and restore the victim's blood volume by giving infusions of balanced salt solutions. Blood transfusions are necessary for loss of large amounts of blood (eg, greater than 20% of blood volume), but can be avoided in smaller and slower losses. Hypovolaemic shock due to burns, diarrhoea, vomiting, etc is treated with infusions of electrolyte solutions that balance the nature of the fluid lost. Sodium is essential to keep the fluid infused in the extracellular and intravascular space while preventing water intoxication and brain swelling. Metabolic acidosis (mainly due to lactic acid) develops as a result of poor delivery of oxygen to the tissues and mirrors the severity of the shock. It is best treated by rapidly restoring intravascular volume and perfusion as above. Inotropic and vasoconstrictive drugs should be avoided, as they may interfere in assessment of blood volume return to normal.

cardiovascular

Adequate resuscitation will result in:

- decreased sympathetic discharge with decreased heart rate and total peripheral resistance
- increased filling pressures, ie right and left atrial pressures
- improved blood pressure and increased baroreceptor discharge
- improved cardiac output/index and stroke volume
- improved thermoregulation
- improved urinary flow
- improved $p_a(O_2)$
- reduced base deficit and lactate
- shift of mixed venous O_2 concentration towards normal
- improved gastric mucosal pH (ie, less acidic)
- core−peripheral temperature gradient narrows
- the patient 'looks better'.

2.9

Answer: A   Atrial fibrillation

Atrial fibrillation (AF) is the most common cardiac arrhythmia. The risk of developing atrial fibrillation increases with age − AF affects 4% of individuals in their 80s. An individual may spontaneously alternate between AF and a normal rhythm (paroxysmal atrial fibrillation) or may continue with AF as the dominant cardiac rhythm without reversion to the normal rhythm (chronic atrial fibrillation). Atrial fibrillation is often asymptomatic, but may result in symptoms of palpitations, fainting, chest pain or even heart failure. These symptoms are especially common when atrial fibrillation results in a heart rate that is either too fast or too slow. In addition, the erratic motion of the atria leads to blood stagnation (stasis), which increases the risk of blood clots that may travel from the heart to

cardiovascular

the brain and other areas. So AF is an important risk factor for stroke, the most feared complication of atrial fibrillation. Atrial fibrillation is diagnosed on an electrocardiogram, an investigation performed routinely whenever irregular heart beat is suspected. Characteristic findings are:

- absence of P-waves

- unorganised electrical activity in their place

- irregularity of RR interval due to irregular conduction of impulses to the ventricles

- if paroxysmal AF is suspected, episodes may be documented with the use of Holter monitoring (continuous electrocardiogram [ECG] recording for 24 hours or longer).

2.10

Answer: C   Pericardial effusion

The QRS complex corresponds to the current that causes contraction of the left and right ventricles, which is much more forceful than that of the atria and involves more muscle mass, so resulting in a greater electrocardiogram (ECG) deflection. Due to this, the atrial repolarisation is rarely seen. The duration of the QRS complex is normally less than or equal to 0.10 s. The Q-wave, when present, represents the small horizontal (left to right) current as the action potential travels through the interventricular septum. Very wide and deep Q-waves do not have a septal origin, but indicate myocardial infarction that involves the full depth of the myocardium and has left a scar. The R- and S-waves indicate the spread of the action potential along the ventricular myocardium itself. Abnormalities in the QRS complex may indicate bundle branch block (when wide), ventricular origin of tachycardia, ventricular hypertrophy or other ventricular abnormalities. The complexes are often small or low-voltage in pericarditis or pericardial effusion.

cardiovascular

2.11

Answer: A   Hypokalaemia

The T-wave represents the repolarisation of the ventricles. The QRS complex usually obscures the atrial repolarisation wave so that it is not usually seen. In most leads, the T-wave is positive:

- Inverted (also described as negative) T-waves can be a sign of disease, although an inverted T-wave is normal in V_1 (and V_2-V_3 in African-Americans/Afro-Caribbeans).

- T-wave abnormalities may indicate electrolyte disturbance, such as hyperkalaemia or hypokalaemia.

- The earliest electrocardiographic finding resulting from acute myocardial infarction is the hyperacute T-wave.

High, tent-shaped T-waves, a small P-wave and a wide QRS complex (that becomes sinusoidal) all suggest hyperkalaemia. This finding alone is an important reason for treatment, as it may forewarn of ventricular fibrillation.

ECG changes associated with hypokalaemia include:

- flattened (notched) T-waves
- U-waves
- ST-segment depression
- prolonged QT interval.

2.12

Answer: A   Hypokalaemia

The U-wave is not always seen. It is quite small and follows the T-wave by definition. It is thought to represent repolarisation of the papillary muscles or Purkinje fibres. Prominent U-waves are most often seen in hypokalaemia, but may be present in hypercalcaemia, thyrotoxicosis or exposure to digitalis, adrenaline and class 1A and 3 anti-arrhythmics, as well as in congenital long-QT syndrome and in the setting of intracranial haemorrhage. An inverted U-wave may represent myocardial ischaemia or left ventricular volume overload.

cardiovascular

2.13

Answer: B   0.12–0.20 s

The PR interval is measured from the beginning of the P-wave to the beginning of the QRS complex. It is usually 0.12–0.20 s. A prolonged PR indicates a first degree heart block, while a shortening may indicate an accessory bundle that depolarises the ventricle early, such as seen in Wolff–Parkinson–White syndrome.

2.14

Answer: D   0.40 s

The QT interval is measured from the beginning of the QRS complex to the end of the T-wave. A normal QT interval is usually about 0.40 s. The QT interval as well as the corrected QT interval are important in the diagnosis of long-QT syndrome and short-QT syndrome. The QT interval varies based on the heart rate and various correction factors have been developed to correct the QT interval for the heart rate.

2.15

Answer: C   0.08 s

The ST segment connects the QRS complex and the T-wave. This segment ordinarily lasts about 0.08 s and is usually level with the PR segment. Upward or downward displacement (ST-segment elevation or ST-segment depression) may indicate coronary ischaemia or myocardial infarction.

2.16

Answer: C   Decreased firing rate of cardiac sympathetic fibres

Cardiac sympathetic nerves show decreased action potential frequency as a result of carotid sinus pressure or massage. The increased pressure at the sinus baroreceptors causes an increase in the firing rate of the afferent carotid sinus nerve that inhibits the medullary vasomotor centre. Consequently, both a decrease

cardiovascular

in sympathetic tone and an increase in efferent vagal discharge contribute to the fall in heart rate and arterial blood pressure following massage or a stroke to the carotid sinus. When performing this manoeuvre on your patients or peers, be prepared for cardiac sinus arrest and avoid vigorous massage, which might dislodge an embolus and cause permanent neurological damage.

2.17

Answer: D   Increased sympathetic activity via renal nerves

Renin, also known as angiotensinogenase, is a circulating enzyme released mainly by juxtaglomerular cells in the juxtaglomerular apparatus (JGA) of the kidneys in response to low blood volume or low body NaCl content, mediated through the rapid release of prostaglandins. Although it has hormone-like actions, it cleaves a protein precursor in the circulation rather than working on a cellular target so it is not truly a hormone. Sympathetic activation of membrane β_1 and α_1-adrenergic receptors on JGA cells also causes renin release, probably by altering tubular sodium content or macula densa function. The normal concentration in human plasma is 1.0–2.5 ng/ml/h. Fifteen per cent of patients with essential hypertension have elevated plasma renin levels, while 85% of patients with essential hypertension have normal or decreased plasma renin levels. Reasons for this difference are not well understood. The primary structure of renin precursor consists of 406 amino acids with a pre- and a prosegment carrying 20 and 46 amino acids respectively. Mature renin contains 340 amino acids and has a mass of 37 kDa. Renin activates the renin–angiotensin system by cleaving angiotensinogen, produced in the liver, to yield angiotensin I, which is further converted into angiotensin II by ACE, the angiotensin-converting enzyme. This is a membrane-bound enzyme present on the surface of the vascular endothelium of blood vessels throughout the body. The lung is the primary organ responsible for angiotensin II conversion, due to the large endothelial surface area of the many capillaries used in gas exchange. Angiotensin II then constricts blood vessels, increases the secretion of ADH and aldosterone and stimulates the hypothalamus to activate the thirst reflex, leading to increased blood pressure.

2.18

Answer: A   Inhibition of parasympathetic nerves increases heart rate

Heart rate will increase whenever sympathetic firing rate increases or parasympathetic firing rate decreases, since the cardiac atria receive tonic input from both sympathetic and parasympathetic nerves. In humans, the ventricles are not innervated by parasympathetic nerves and the strength of contraction increases with increasing preload (Frank–Starling mechanism), increasing the sympathetic firing rate. With few exceptions, blood vessels are not innervated by parasympathetic nerves and there is little effect of changes in parasympathetic tone on total peripheral resistance.

2.19

Answer: D   L-type Ca^{2+} channels

The cardiac myocyte action potential is characterised by a rapid depolarisation due to opening of fast Na^+ channels and a more slowly developing plateau phase lasting about 200 ms. The plateau is due to opening of slowly inactivating high-threshold dihydropyridine-sensitive L-type Ca^{2+} channels. This action potential spreads rapidly across the myocardium, because cardiac myocytes are electrically coupled via gap junctions. A subclass of K^+ channels (namely inwardly rectifying K^+ channels) determine the cardiac resting membrane potential. Opening of Na^+ channels causes the rapid upstroke of the action potential. Fast inactivating low-threshold dihydropyridine-insensitive t-type Ca^{2+} channels are activated at thresholds intermediate between I_{Na} and I_{Ca-L} and contribute to the inward current of late stage phase 4 depolarisation in sinus node and His/Purkinje cells. Cl^- channel activity is increased by adrenergic stimulation and contributes to repolarisation of the action potential.

2.20

Answer: A   18 mmHG/min/l

Total peripheral resistance =
Mean arterial pressure/Cardiac output

If central venous pressure is negligibly small compared with mean arterial pressure, we can calculate the peripheral resistance from the data given. The key in obtaining a correct answer is being able to determine mean arterial pressure from systolic pressure P_S and diastolic blood pressure P_D. Because of the particular shape of the pressure curve, this is not simply the arithmetic mean, but rather:

> Mean arterial pressure = $P_D + 1/3 (P_S - P_D)$,
> ie, $70 + 20 = 90$ mmHg.

Therefore:

> Total peripheral resistance = 90 mmHg/5 l per min
> = 18 mmHg × min/l.

2.21

Answer: D   100 ml

For calculation of cardiac stroke volume in this case we apply the Fick principle. Developed by Adolf Eugene Fick (1829–1901), the Fick principle is a technique for measuring cardiac output. It is derived by applying the law of conservation of mass ('what comes in must go out'):

$$VO_2 = Q \times (C_A(O_2) - C_v(O_2))$$

where VO_2 equals O_2 consumption ('what comes in'), Q is cardiac output and C_AO_2 and C_vO_2 are arterial and mixed venous O_2 content, respectively. First, we calculate cardiac output:

> 300 ml O_2/min = Q × (20–15) ml O_2/100 ml blood
>
> 300 ml O_2/min = Q × 5 ml O_2/100 ml blood
> Q = 6000 ml blood/min.

Next, we calculate stroke volume using the formula:

> stroke volume = cardiac output ÷ heart rate

Plugging in our value of 6000 ml/min for cardiac output and 60/min for heart rate yields:

> stroke volume = 6000 ml/min ÷ 60/min stroke volume
> = 100 ml.

2.22

Answer: D   Eleration in systemic arterial pressure from 100 to 130 mmHg

The brain autoregulates and consequently an increase in blood pressure is offset by an increase in local vascular resistance to maintain constant cerebral blood flow. Cerebral blood flow will increase when $p_a(O_2)$ is decreased to < 50 mmHg or when $p_a(CO_2)$ increases above normal. A decrease in arterial oxygen or an increase in arterial CO_2 would therefore cause vasodilatation and decreased resistance to cerebral blood flow. A decrease in viscosity would also increase blood flow. Cerebral blood flow is closely linked to brain parenchymal metabolism and intense activity during a seizure results in large, widespread increases in blood flow.

2.23

Answer: D   Loss of sympathetic tone

With few exceptions, blood vessels are not innervated by parasympathetic nerves and there is little effect of parasympathetic tone on total peripheral resistance. In contrast, sympathetic nerve activity contributes to the basal vascular smooth muscle tone and cutting these nerve fibres results in immediate vasodilatation of the affected extremity. While hypersensitivity to circulating catecholamines will develop over time, this does not contribute to the vasodilatation. Adrenaline and noradrenaline release from the adrenal medulla is regulated by its direct sympathetic innervation (preganglionic cholinergic fibres from the splanchnic nerve) and not affected by sympathetic fibres to the extremities or circulating catecholamines.

2.24

Answer: E   4000 ml/min

For calculation of cardiac output in this patient, the Fick principle will have to be applied. Fick's principle states that the uptake of a substance by an organ equals the arteriovenous difference of the substance multiplied by the blood flowing through the organ.

cardiovascular

Measuring pulmonary arterial (ie, mixed venous) oxygen content, aortic oxygen content and oxygen uptake, the pulmonary blood flow can be calculated. Assuming there are no intracardiac shunts, pulmonary blood flow, systemic blood flow and cardiac output are the same.

$$\text{Cardiac output} = \text{oxygen uptake}/(\text{aortic} - \text{mixed venous oxygen content})$$

$$= 200 \text{ ml/min}/(15 \text{ ml O}_2/100 \text{ ml} - 10 \text{ ml O}_2/100 \text{ ml})$$

$$= 200 \text{ ml/min}/(5 \text{ ml O}_2/100 \text{ ml})$$

$$= 200 \text{ ml/min}/0.05$$

$$= 4000 \text{ ml/min}.$$

The cardiac output of this patient is significantly below normal (~6000 ml/min). If your calculation was 1333 ml/min or 2000 ml/min, you probably forgot to subtract oxygen concentrations. When measuring cardiac output by Fick's method, it is important to use pulmonary arterial oxygen content rather than peripheral vein oxygen content, since different organs vary widely in their oxygen extraction.

2.25

Answer: B   Cardiac stroke volume

Trained athletes have a larger heart volume (muscular hypertrophy) compared to untrained people. This results in a significantly higher stroke volume at rest and an increased cardiac reserve (maximal cardiac output during exercise). Under resting conditions, however, the cardiac output of trained and untrained people is nearly the same and this is due to a correspondingly lower resting heart rate. It is not uncommon to find resting heart frequencies of 40–50 beats/min in trained athletes. Oxygen consumption and respiratory rate at rest are little affected by athletic training.

2.26

Answer: C Kidneys

During resting conditions, approximately 15% of the cardiac output goes to the brain, 15% to the muscles, 30% to the gastrointestinal (GI) tract and 20% to the kidneys. However, when normalised by organ weight, the kidneys receive the largest specific blood flow (400 ml/min × 100 g) at rest and are particularly vulnerable during haemorrhagic shock. The brain also receives relatively high specific blood flow (50 ml/min × 100g). Blood flow through the skin varies between 1 and 100 ml/min × 100 g and serves temperature regulation. Heart muscle not surprisingly also has a relatively high resting specific blood flow (60 ml/min × 100 g), which may increase fivefold during exercise. Skeletal muscles have low specific blood flow (2 to 3 ml/min × 100 g) at rest, which may increase up to 20-fold during strenuous exercise.

2.27

Answer: E Increased PR interval

Damage to the AV node resulting from ischaemia or inflammation may increase the PR interval from a normal value of about 0.12–0.20 s to as much as 0.25–0.40 s. If conduction through the AV node becomes severely impaired, complete block of impulses may occur, in which case the atria and ventricles will beat independently (see *also answer* to 2.1).

2.28

Answer: B 1.5–4.0 m/s

Purkinje fibres work with the sinoatrial node (SA node) and the atrioventricular node (AV node) to control the heart rate. During the ventricular contraction portion of the cardiac cycle, the Purkinje fibres carry the contraction impulse from the left and right bundle branches to the myocardium of the ventricles. This causes the muscle tissue of the ventricles to contract and force blood out of the heart – either to the pulmonary circulation (from the right ventricle) or to the systemic circulation (from the left ventricle). The impulse through the Purkinje fibres is associated with the QRS complex. The rate of conduction of action potentials in Purkinje fibres is about six times greater than the velocity in normal cardiac muscle.

2.29

Answer: E   Ventricular repolarisation

The T-wave in the normal electrocardiogram is an upward deflection representing ventricular repolarisation and occurs during the latter half of ventricular systole (*see also* answer to 2.11).

2.30

Answer: A   Beginning of diastole

Cardiac diastole is the period of time when the heart relaxes after contraction in preparation for refilling with circulating blood. Ventricular diastole is when the ventricles are relaxing, while atrial diastole is when the atria are relaxing. Together they are known as complete cardiac diastole. At the beginning of diastole, the ventricular muscle relaxes, allowing the ventricular pressure to decrease greatly. When the pressure in the left ventricle drops to below the pressure in the left atrium, the mitral valve opens and the left ventricle fills with blood that was accumulating in the left atrium. Likewise, when the pressure in the right ventricle drops below that in the right atrium, the tricuspid valve opens and the right ventricle fills with blood that was accumulating in the right atrium.

2.31

Answer: C

Ventricular systole is the contraction of the muscles of the left and right ventricles. In an electrocardiogram, electrical systole of the ventricles begins at the beginning of the QRS complex. The closing of the mitral and tricuspid valves (known together as the atrioventricular valves) at the beginning of ventricular systole cause the first part of the 'lub–dub' sound made by the heart as it beats. Formally, this sound is known the first heart tone or S_1.

The second part of the 'lub–dub' (the second heart tone or S_2), is caused by the closure of the aortic and pulmonic valves at the end of ventricular systole. As the left ventricle empties, its pressure falls below the pressure in the aorta and the aortic valve closes. Similarly, as the pressure in the right ventricle falls below the pressure in the pulmonary artery, the pulmonic valve closes.

2.32

Answer: D   Pulmonary artery

Normal haemodynamic parameters – adult

Parameter	Equation	Normal range
Arterial blood pressure (BP)	Systolic (SBP) Diastolic (DBP)	90–140 mmHg 60–90 mmHg
Mean arterial pressure (MAP)	SBP + (2 × DBP)/3	70–105 mmHg
Systolic pressure variation (SPV)	(SPmax − SPmin)*	< 5 mmHg unlikely to be preload responsive > 5 mmHg likely to be preload responsive
Pulse pressure variation (PPV)	(PPmax − PPmin)/ [(PPmax + PPmin)/2] × 100*	< 10% unlikely to be preload responsive > 13–15% likely to be preload responsive
Stroke volume variation (SVV)	(SVmax − SVmin)/ [(SVmax + SVmin)/2] × 100*	< 10% unlikely to be preload responsive > 13–15% likely to be preload responsive
Right atrial pressure (RAP)		2–6 mmHg
Right ventricular pressure (RVP)	Systolic (RVSP) Diastolic (RVDP)	15–25 mmHg 0–8 mmHg
Pulmonary artery pressure (PAP)	Systolic (PASP) Diastolic (PADP)	15–25 mmHg 8–15 mmHg
Pulmonary artery wedge pressure (PAWP)		6–12 mmHg

Parameter	Equation	Normal range
Left atrial pressure (LAP)	[???]	6–12 mmHg
Cardiac output (CO)	HR × SV/1000	4.0–8.0 l/min
Cardiac index (CI)	CO/BSA	2.5–4.0 l/min per m^2
Stroke volume (SV)	CO/HR × 1000	60–100 ml/beat
Stroke volume index (SVI)	CI/HR × 1000	33-47 ml/m^2 per beat
Systemic vascular resistance (SVR)	80 × (MAP–RAP)/CO	800–1200 dynes × s/cm^5
Systemic vascular resistance index (SVRI)	80 × MAP–RAP)/CI	1970–2390 dynes × s/cm^5 per m^2
Pulmonary vascular resistance (PVR)	80 × (MPAP–PAWP)/CO	<250 dynes × s/cm^5
Pulmonary vascular resistance index (PVRI)	80 × (MPAP–PAWP)/CI	255–285 dynes × s/cm^5 per m^2

*Averaged over 10 s of blood pressure (BP) data updated every four beats.

Normally in right-heart chambers O_2 saturation is 75% while in left-heart chambers O_2 saturation is 95%. Based on the values given in the table above it is clear that in this vignette the values obtained are for pulmonary artery.

cardiovascular

2.33

Answer: A　Atrial septal defect

Atrial septal defect (ASD) is a form of congenital heart disease that enables communication between the left and right atria via the interatrial septum. The interatrial septum is the tissue that divides the right and left atria. Without this septum or if there is a defect in this septum, it is possible for blood to travel from the left side of the heart to the right side of the heart or from the right side of the heart to the left side of the heart. This results in the mixing of arterial and venous blood. The mixing of arterial and venous blood may or may not be haemodynamically significant, if even clinically significant. This mixture of blood may or may not result in what is known as a 'shunt'. The amount of shunting present, if any, dictates haemodynamic significance. It should be noted, however, that a 'right-to-left-shunt' typically poses the more dangerous scenario.

In unaffected individuals, the chambers of the left side of the heart make up a higher pressure system than the chambers of the right side of the heart. This is because the left ventricle has to produce enough pressure to pump blood throughout the entire body, while the right ventricle only has to produce enough pressure to pump blood to the lungs.

In the case of a large ASD (>9 mm), which may result in a clinically remarkable left-to-right shunt, blood will shunt from the left atrium to the right atrium, causing excessive interatrial communication (In the case of haemodynamically significant ASD (Qp : Qs > 1.5 : 1), the patient is often found to be notably symptomatic and ASD repair may be indicated). This extra blood from the left atrium may cause a volume overload of both the right atrium and the right ventricle which, if left untreated, can result in enlargement of the right side of the heart and ultimately heart failure. At cardiac catheterisation O_2 saturation in the right atrium, right ventricle and pulmonary artery will be very high – up to 90%.

Any process that increases the pressure in the left ventricle can cause worsening of the left-to-right shunt. This includes hypertension, which increases the pressure that the left ventricle has to generate to open the aortic valve during ventricular systole and coronary artery disease, which increases the stiffness of the left ventricle, thereby increasing the filling pressure of the left ventricle during ventricular

cardiovascular

diastole. The right ventricle will have to push out more blood than the left ventricle due to the left-to-right shunt. This constant overload of the right side of the heart will cause an overload of the entire pulmonary vasculature.

Eventually the pulmonary vasculature will develop pulmonary hypertension to try to divert the extra blood volume away from the lungs. The pulmonary hypertension will cause the right ventricle to face increased afterload in addition to the increased preload that the shunted blood from the left atrium to the right atrium caused. The right ventricle will be forced to generate higher pressures to try to overcome the pulmonary hypertension. This may lead to right ventricular failure (dilatation and decreased systolic function of the right ventricle) or elevations of the right-sided pressures to levels greater than the left-sided pressures. When the pressure in the right atrium rises to the level in the left atrium, there will no longer be a pressure gradient between these heart chambers and the left-to-right shunt will diminish or cease.

If left uncorrected, the pressure in the right side of the heart will be greater than that in the left side of the heart. This will cause the pressure in the right atrium to be higher than the pressure in the left atrium. This will reverse the pressure gradient across the ASD and the shunt will reverse; a right-to-left shunt will exist. This phenomenon is known as Eisenmenger's syndrome. Once right-to-left shunting occurs, a portion of the oxygen-poor blood will get shunted to the left side of the heart and ejected to the peripheral vascular system. This will cause signs of cyanosis.

2.34

Answer: B   Pulmonary artery

Developed by Adolf Eugene Fick (1829–1901), the Fick principle is a technique for measuring cardiac output. The following variables are measured:

- VO_2 consumption per minute using a spirometer (with the subject re-breathing air) and a CO_2 absorber.

- C_vO_2 the oxygen content of blood taken from the pulmonary artery (representing venous blood).

- C_AO_2 the oxygen content of blood from a cannula in a peripheral artery (representing arterial blood).

The Fick principle relies on the observation that the total uptake of (or release of) a substance by the peripheral tissues is equal to the product of the blood flow to the peripheral tissues and the arterial–venous concentration difference (gradient) of the substance. In the determination of cardiac output, the substance most commonly measured is the oxygen content of blood and the flow calculated is the flow across the pulmonary system. This gives a simple way to calculate the cardiac output:

Cardiac output = Oxygen consumption ÷ Arteriovenous oxygen difference.

Assuming there are no shunts across the pulmonary system, the pulmonary blood flow equals the systemic blood flow. Measurement of the arterial and venous oxygen content of blood involves the sampling of blood from the pulmonary artery (low oxygen content) and from the pulmonary vein (high oxygen content). In practice, sampling of peripheral arterial blood is a surrogate for pulmonary venous blood. In reality, this method is rarely used these days due to the difficulty of collecting and analysing the gas concentrations. However, by using an assumed value for oxygen consumption, cardiac output can be closely approximated without the cumbersome and time-consuming oxygen consumption measurement. This is sometimes called an assumed Fick determination. A commonly used value for O_2 consumption at rest is 125 ml O_2 per minute per square metre of body surface area.

2.35

Answer: D   Tetralogy of Fallot

The tetralogy of Fallot (TOF) is a congenital heart defect that classically has four anatomical components. It is the most common cyanotic heart defect and the most common cause of blue baby syndrome. It was described in 1672 by Niels Stensen and in 1888 by the French physician Etienne Fallot, for whom it is named.

As classically described, tetralogy of Fallot involves four heart malformations that present together:

- A ventricular septal defect (VSD): a hole between the two bottom chambers (ventricles) of the heart. The defect is centred around the 'outlet septum', the most superior aspect of the septum, and in the majority of cases is single and large. In some cases septal hypertrophy can narrow the margins of the defect.

- Pulmonary stenosis: right ventricular outflow tract obstruction, a narrowing at (valvular stenosis) or just below (infundibular stenosis) the pulmonary valve. The stenosis is mostly the result of hypertrophy of the septoparietal trabeculae; however, the deviated outlet septum is believed to play a role. The degree of stenosis varies between individuals with TOF and is the primary determinant of symptoms and severity. This malformation is infrequently described as subpulmonary stenosis or subpulmonary obstruction.

- Overriding aorta: defined as when the aortic valve is not restricted to the left ventricle, so having biventricular connections. The aortic root can be moved anteriorly or override the septal defect, but it is still to the right of the root of the pulmonary artery. The degree of override is quite variable, with between 5 and 95% of the valve being connected to the right ventricle.

- Right ventricular hypertrophy: The right ventricle is more muscular than normal, causing a characteristic coeur-en-sabot (boot-shaped) appearance as seen by chest X-ray. Due to the misarrangement of the external ventricular septum, the right ventricular wall increases in size to deal with the increased obstruction to the right outflow tract. This feature is now generally agreed to be a secondary anomaly, as the level of hypertrophy generally increases with age.

Tetralogy of Fallot occurs in approximately 3–6 per 10 000 births and represents 5–7% of congenital heart defects. Its cause is thought to be due to environmental or genetic factors or a combination. It is associated with chromosome 22 deletions and diGeorge syndrome. It occurs slightly more often in males than in females. Embryology studies show that it is a result of anterior malalignment of the conal septum, resulting in the clinical combination of a VSD, pulmonary stenosis and an overriding aorta. Right ventricular hypertrophy results from this combination, which causes resistance to blood flow from the right ventricle.

Tetralogy of Fallot results in low oxygenation of blood due to mixing of oxygenated and deoxygenated blood in the left ventricle through the VSD and preferential flow of both oxygenated and deoxygenated blood from the ventricles through the aorta because of obstruction to flow through the pulmonary valve. This is known as a right-to-left shunt. Children with tetralogy of Fallot may develop acute severe cyanosis or hypoxic 'tet spells'. The precise mechanism of these episodes is in doubt, but presumably results from an increase in resistance to blood flow to the lungs with increased preferential flow of desaturated blood to the body.

The primary symptom is low blood oxygen saturation with or without cyanosis from birth or developing in the first year of life. Without cyanosis, the condition is referred to as 'pink tet'. Other symptoms include a heart murmur, which may range from almost imperceptible to very loud, difficulty in feeding, failure to gain weight, retarded growth and physical development, dyspnoea on exertion, clubbing of the fingers and toes and polycythaemia. Tet spells are characterised by a sudden, marked increase in cyanosis, with syncope, and may result in hypoxic brain injury and death. Tetralogy of Fallot is treated on two levels: with immediate emergency care for hypoxic or 'tet' spells and with palliative surgery in the form of Blalock–Taussig shunt (BT shunt) followed by corrective surgery or, occasionally, with corrective surgery as the primary modality of treatment.

2.36

Answer: B   Is related to body surface area

Cardiac index is a haemodynamic measure based on the cardiac output, which is the amount of blood the left ventricle ejects into the systemic circulation in one minute, measured in litres per minute

cardiovascular

(l/min). Cardiac output can be indexed to a patient's body size by dividing by the body surface area (called the BSA) to yield the cardiac index. The normal cardiac index is 2.5–3.5 l/min per m². It correlates better with body surface area than with body weight.

2.37

Answer: C   Pulsus paradoxus

A pulsus paradoxus, also paradoxic pulse and paradoxical pulse, is an exaggeration of the normal variation in the pulse during respiration, in which the pulse becomes weaker as one inhales and stronger as one exhales. It is a sign that is indicative of several conditions, including cardiac tamponade and lung diseases (eg asthma, COPD). The paradox in pulsus paradoxus is that, on clinical examination, one can detect extra beats on cardiac auscultation, during inspiration, when compared with the radial pulse. It results from an accentuated decrease of the blood pressure, which leads to the (radial) pulse not being palpable and may be accompanied by an increase in the jugular venous pressure height (Kussmaul sign). As is usual with inspiration, the heart rate is increased, due to the increased venous return. Pulsus paradoxus is quantified using a blood pressure cuff and stethoscope, by measuring the variation of the pressure in systole with respiration. Normal systolic blood pressure variation (with respiration) is considered to be 10 mmHg. Pulsus paradoxus is an inspiratory reduction in systolic pressure > 10 mmHg. It has been shown to be predictive of the severity of cardiac tamponade.

2.38

Answer: E   Stimulation of respiratory centre

The carotid body (or carotid glomus) is a small cluster of chemoreceptors and supporting cells located near the bifurcation of the carotid artery. It measures changes in the composition of arterial blood flowing past it, including the partial pressures of oxygen and carbon dioxide and is also sensitive to changes in pH and temperature. The chemoreceptors responsible for sensing changes in blood gasses are called glomus cells. While the central chemoreceptors in the brainstem are highly sensitive to CO_2, the carotid body is a peripheral chemoreceptor that provides afferent input to the respiratory centre that is highly O_2-dependent. Below an oxygen partial pressure of 60 mmHg, the carotid body cells release dopamine and trigger excitatory postsynaptic potentials in synapsed neurones leading to the respiratory centre. This event is mediated by a unique potassium channel that is responsive to the partial pressure of O_2. The peripheral chemoreceptor's input is secondary to CO_2-sensitive cells in the central chemoreceptors in healthy patients, but is the primary driver of ventilation in individuals who suffer from chronic hypercapnia (as in emphysema). It gives feedback to the medulla oblongata via the afferent branches of the glossopharyngeal nerve (IX). The medulla, in turn, regulates breathing and blood pressure.

2.39

Answer: C   Heart rate decreases

The systemic cardiovascular response to exercise depends on whether the muscle contractions are primarily isometric or primarily isotonic with the performance of external work. With the start of an isometric muscle contraction, heart rate rises. This increase still occurs if the muscle contraction is prevented by local infusion of a neuromuscular blocking drug. The increase is largely due to decreased vagal tone, although increased discharge of the cardiac sympathetic nerves plays some role. Within a few seconds of the onset of an isometric muscle contraction, systolic and diastolic pressures rise sharply. Stroke volume changes relatively little and blood flow to the steadily contracting muscles is reduced as a result of compression of their blood vessels.

2.40

Answer: B   SV = 32 ml, EOV = 150 ml, ESV = 118 ml, EF = 21%

Stroke volume (SV) is the volume of blood ejected from a ventricle with each beat of the heart. Its value is obtained by subtracting end-systolic volume (ESV) from end-diastolic volume (EDV) for a given ventricle.

cardiovascular

End-diastolic volume (EDV) is the volume of blood in a ventricle at the end of filling (diastole). Because greater EDVs cause greater distension of the ventricle, EDV is often used synonymously with preload, which refers to the length of the sarcomeres in cardiac muscle before contraction (systole). An increase in EDV increases the preload on the heart and, through the Frank–Starling mechanism of the heart, increases the amount of blood ejected from the ventricle during systole (stroke volume). EDV is usually about 120–130 ml but sometimes it can reach 200–250 ml in the normal heart. Because nearly two-thirds of the blood in the systemic circulation is stored in the venous system, end-diastolic volume is closely related to venous compliance. Increasing venous compliance elevates the capacitance of the veins, reducing venous return and therefore end-diastolic volume. Decreasing venous compliance has the opposite effect. For example, activation of the baroreceptor reflex (occurring, for instance, in acute haemorrhage) causes venoconstriction, which decreases venous compliance, improves venous return and therefore increases end-diastolic volume.

End-systolic volume (ESV) is the volume of blood in the ventricles just after systole (at the end of the cardiac ejection period and immediately preceding the beginning of ventricular relaxation). It is a measurement of the adequacy of cardiac emptying, related to systolic function. ESV is usually about 50–60 ml but sometimes as little as 10–30 ml in the normal heart.

Ejection fraction (EF or E_f) is the fraction of blood pumped out of a ventricle with each heart beat. The term ejection fraction applies to both the right and left ventricles; one can speak equally of the left ventricular ejection fraction and the right ventricular ejection fraction. Without a qualifier, the term ejection fraction refers specifically to that of the left ventricle: it is the fraction of the end-diastolic volume that is ejected with each beat; ie, it is SV divided by EDV.

In a healthy 70-kg man, the SV is approximately 70 ml and the left ventricular EDV is 120 ml, giving an ejection fraction of 70/120 or 58%. Right ventricular volumes being roughly equal to those of the left ventricle, the ejection fraction of the right ventricle is normally equal to that of the left ventricle within narrow limits.

Healthy individuals typically have ejection fractions greater than

0.55. However, normal values depend upon the modality being used to calculate the ejection fraction. Damage to the myocardium, such as that sustained during myocardial infarction, impairs the heart's ability to eject blood and therefore reduces ejection fraction. This reduction in the ejection fraction can manifest itself clinically as heart failure. The ejection fraction is one of the most important predictors of prognosis; those with significantly reduced ejection fractions typically have a poorer prognosis. In the clinical vignette the choice B is the correct option as myocardial infarction, by causing systolic dysfunction, is likely to reduce stroke volume and ejection fraction and increase ESV.

2.41

Answer: A   Fatty acids

Mammalian hearts have an abundant blood supply, numerous mitochondria and a high content of myoglobin, a muscle pigment that may function as an O_2 storage mechanism. Normally, less than 1% of the total energy liberated is provided by anaerobic metabolism. During hypoxia, this figure may increase to nearly 10%; but, under totally anaerobic conditions, the energy liberated is inadequate to sustain ventricular contractions. Under basal conditions, 35% of the caloric needs of the human heart are provided by carbohydrate, 5% by ketones and amino acids and 60% by fat. However, the proportions of substrates utilised vary greatly with the nutritional state. After ingestion of large amounts of glucose, more lactate and pyruvate are used; during prolonged starvation, more fat is used. Circulating fatty acids normally account for almost 50% of the lipid utilised. In untreated diabetics, the carbohydrate utilisation of cardiac muscle is reduced and that of fat increased.

2.42

Answer: E   Within physiological limits, the heart pumps all the blood that comes to it

The Frank–Starling law of the heart states that the more the heart is filled during diastole, the greater will be the amount of blood pumped into the aorta; that is, within physiological limits, the heart can pump all the blood that comes to it without excessive damming of blood in the veins. The ability of stretched muscle to contract with greater force is characteristic of all striated muscles. Stretching the muscle is believed to increase interdigitation of the actin and myosin filaments and so to facilitate a more forceful contraction.

2.43

Answer: C   0.2

The relationship between flow, pressure difference and resistance is as follows:

flow = pressure difference ÷ resistance.

Flow in any portion of the vascular system is equal to the effective perfusion pressure in that portion divided by the resistance. The effective perfusion pressure is the mean intraluminal pressure at the arterial end minus the mean pressure at the venous end. So, by substituting the values in the above equation:

resistance = (60 − 20)/200 = 0.2 mmHg/ml per min.

2.44

Answer: A   1 PRU

The relation between the flow in a long narrow tube, the viscosity of the fluid and the radius of the tube is expressed mathematically in the Poiseuille–Hagen formula:

$$F = (P_A - P_B) \times (\pi/8) \times (1/\eta) \times (r^4/l)$$

where

F = flow

$P_A - P_B$ = pressure difference between the two ends of the tube

η = viscosity

r = radius of tube

L = length of tube.

Since flow is equal to pressure difference divided by resistance (R),

$R = 8\eta L \div \pi r^4$

So as the diameter of a vessel changes, the resistance of the vessel changes in inverse proportion to the fourth power of the diameter. Therefore, increasing the diameter of a vessel to twice the initial diameter would decrease the vessel resistance to one-sixteenth of the initial resistance.

2.45

Answer: B   Arterioles

The arterioles are often called the resistance vessels of the body because they account for about half the resistance of the entire systemic circulation. The arteriolar wall has a thick smooth muscle coat in relation to the size of the vessel and it is innervated richly by the autonomic nervous system.

2.46

Answer: A   Has the highest rate of automatic discharge

The sinoatrial node (SA) is about the size of a 5p coin and is located at the junction of the inferior vena cava and the right atrial wall. It contains few contractile elements and is composed primarily of small, round cells ('P' cells). These cells exhibit spontaneous depolarisation on a fairly regular basis, caused by an increase in Na^+ (via slow channels) and Ca^{2+} conductance, coupled to a progressive decrease in K^+ conductance (decreased permeability). The sum of these concomitant conductance changes results in depolarisation of this tissue. This depolarisation during phase 4 is the 'pacemaker potential' and is also referred to as diastolic depolarisation. When threshold is reached, a slow-type action potential is elicited, which spreads from the nodal tissue into the atrial tissue, where it initiates a 'fast'-type action potential. The latter action potential is conducted throughout the atria via internodal tracts. The rate at which this depolarisation occurs determines the rate at which the heart will be depolarised and so contract (heart rate). As the SA node has the highest rate of automatic discharge; it is thus the pacemaker.

cardiovascular

2.47

Answer: B   A failure of the atrioventricular (AV) node to conduct

A heart block can be a blockage at any level of the electrical conduction system of the heart. Blocks that occur within the sinoatrial node (SA node) are described as SA nodal blocks. Blocks that occur within the atrioventricular node (AV node) are described as AV nodal blocks. Blocks that occur below the AV node are known as infra-Hisian blocks (named after the bundle of His). Clinically speaking, most of the important heart blocks are AV nodal blocks and infra-Hisian blocks. Complete failure of the AV node to conduct results in third-degree heart block, also known as complete heart block or third-degree AV block. It is a defect of the electrical system of the heart, in which the impulse generated in the SA node does not propagate to the ventricles. Because the impulse is blocked, an accessory pacemaker below the level of the block will typically activate the ventricles. This is known as an escape rhythm. Since this accessory pacemaker activates independently of the impulse generated at the SA node, two independent rhythms can be noted on the electrocardiogram (ECG). One will activate the atria and create the P-waves, typically with a regular P to P interval. The second will activate the ventricles and produce the QRS complex, typically with a regular R to R interval. The PR interval will be variable, as the hallmark of complete heart block is no apparent relationship between P-waves and QRS complexes.

2.48

Answer: D   The stroke volume would be increased

If a strip of muscle is passively stretched, it will exhibit an increasing amount of tension disproportionate to the amount of stretch. This passive tension is related to non-contractile elements that comprise the series and parallel elastic components in the muscle fibre. At any given length, if the muscle is stimulated to contract isometrically (ie the muscle is not allowed to shorten), it will develop an additional amount of tension, which is a function of the initial fibre length. At lengths shorter or longer than this, developed tension (active) decreases. At lengths where there is little or no overlap of actin and myosin, active tension is zero, even though there may still be

cardiovascular

passive tension. These principles were first promulgated for skeletal muscle and later applied to cardiac muscle by O. Frank in 1895 for the frog heart, followed (1914) by Starling for the dog heart–lung preparation. The concept, known as Starling's Law of the Heart, relates that, within physiological limits, the force generated by the contracting heart, as reflected by cardiac output or stroke volume, is increased if the muscle fibres have been stretched previously.

If cardiac parameters of length and tension are used, there is an optimal end-diastolic volume (EDV) at which the work output (pressure developed or volume pumped) of the heart is maximal. At lower or higher volumes or filling pressures (preload), the amount of developed tension or work produced, such as measured by stroke volume, is reduced. So, an increase in right atrial pressure, caused by an increase in venous pressure, causes increased right ventricular end-diastolic volume, increased right ventricular end-diastolic pressure and increased stroke volume.

2.49

Answer: C   Increased contractility of the heart

Inotropism means contractility. Positive inotropism means increased contractility. Most commonly, the inotropic state is used in reference to various drugs that affect the strength of contraction of heart muscle (myocardial contractility). However, it can also refer to pathological conditions. For example, ventricular hypertrophy can increase inotropic state, while myocardial infarction can decrease it. Positive inotropic agents increase myocardial contractility and are used to support cardiac function in conditions such as decompensated congestive heart failure, cardiogenic shock, septic shock, myocardial infarction, cardiomyopathy, etc. Examples of positive inotropic agents include digoxin, adrenaline, dopamine, dobutamine, calcium and milrinone.

cardiovascular

2.50

Answer: A   Determined by the stroke volume

Pulse pressure is the change in blood pressure seen during a contraction of the heart. Formally it is the systolic pressure minus the diastolic pressure. It can be calculated by stroke volume/compliance. Usually, the resting pulse pressure in healthy adults, sitting position, is about 40 mmHg. The pulse pressure increases with exercise due to increased stroke volume, healthy values being up to pulse pressures of about 100 mmHg, simultaneously as total peripheral resistance drops during exercise. In healthy individuals the pulse pressure will typically return to normal within about 10 min.

For most individuals, during exercise, the systolic pressure progressively increases while the diastolic remains about the same. In some very aerobically athletic individuals, the diastolic will progressively fall as the systolic increases. This behaviour facilitates a much greater increase in stroke volume and cardiac output at a lower mean arterial pressure and enables much greater aerobic capacity and physical performance. The diastolic drop reflects a much greater fall in total peripheral resistance of the muscle arterioles in response to the exercise (a greater proportion of red versus white muscle tissue).

If the usual resting pulse pressure is measured as less than 40 mmHg, the most common reason is an error of measurement. If the pulse pressure is genuinely low, eg, 25 mmHg or less, the cause may be low stroke volume, as in congestive heart failure and/or shock, a serious issue. This interpretation is re-inforced if the resting heart rate is relatively rapid, eg, 100–120 (in normal sinus rhythm), reflecting increased sympathetic nervous system activity.

If the usual resting pulse pressure is consistently greater than 40 mmHg, eg, 60 or 80 mmHg, the most likely basis is stiffness of the major arteries, aortic regurgitation, an extra path for the blood to travel from the arteries to the veins (arteriovenous fistula or malformation), hyperthyroidism or some combination. (A chronically increased stroke volume is also a technical possibility, but very rare in practice.) Some drugs for hypertension have the side-effect of increasing resting pulse pressure irreversibly. A high resting pulse pressure is harmful and tends to accelerate the normal ageing of body organs, particularly the heart, the brain and kidneys.

2.51

Answer: D   6.25 l/min

To calculate cardiac output from the available data we apply the Fick principle. The Fick principle involves measuring:

- whole-body oxygen consumption (VO_2) per minute using a spirometer (with the subject re-breathing air) and a CO_2 absorber

- the oxygen content of blood taken from the pulmonary artery (representing venous blood)

- the oxygen content of blood from a cannula in a peripheral artery (representing arterial blood).

From these values, we know that:

$$VO_2 = (CO \times C_AO_2) - (CO \times C_VO_2)$$

where CO = cardiac output, C_A = oxygen concentration of arterial blood and C_V = oxygen concentration of venous blood.

This allows us to say:

$$CO = VO_2/C_AO_2 - C_VO_2$$

$$CO = 500/0.24 - 0.16$$

$$CO = 500/0.8$$

$$CO = 6.25 \text{ l/min.}$$

2.52

Answer: D   90 ml

To calculate stroke volume from the available data we apply the Fick principle first to calculate cardiac output. The Fick principle involves measuring:

- whole-body oxygen consumption (VO_2) per minute using a spirometer (with the subject re-breathing air) and a CO_2 absorber

- the oxygen content of blood taken from the pulmonary artery (representing venous blood)

- the oxygen content of blood from a cannula in a peripheral artery (representing arterial blood).

From these values, we know that:

$$VO_2 = (CO \times C_AO_2) - (CO \times C_VO_2)$$

where CO = cardiac output, C_AO_2 = oxygen concentration of arterial blood and C_VO_2 = oxygen concentration of venous blood.

This allows us to say:

$$CO = VO_2 / C_AO_2 - C_VO_2$$

$$CO = 500/0.24 - 0.16$$

$$CO = 500/0.8$$

$$CO = 6.25 \text{ l/min.}$$

Next:

cardiac output = stroke volume × heart rate

stroke volume = 6.25/70 × 1000

stroke volume = 90 ml approximately.

2.53

Answer: B   2.0 resistance units (mmHg/l per min)

Pulmonary vascular resistance (PVR) is calculated by using the formula:

PVR = (Mean pulmonary artery pressure – Pulmonary capillary wedge pressure) ÷ Cardiac output.

To calculate PVR from the available data we apply the Fick principle first to calculate cardiac output. The Fick principle involves measuring:

- whole-body oxygen consumption (VO_2) per minute using a spirometer (with the subject re-breathing air) and a CO_2 absorber

- the oxygen content of blood taken from the pulmonary artery (representing venous blood)

- the oxygen content of blood from a cannula in a peripheral artery (representing arterial blood).

From these values, we know that:

$$VO_2 = (CO \times C_AO_2) - (CO \times C_VO_2)$$

where CO = cardiac output, C_A = oxygen concentration of arterial blood and C_VO_2 = oxygen concentration of venous blood.

This allows us to say:

$$CO = VO_2/ C_AO_2 - C_VO_2$$

$$CO = 500/0.24-0.16$$

$$CO = 500/0.8$$

$$CO = 6.25 \text{ l/min.}$$

Next:

Mean pulmonary artery pressure = Diastolic pressure + 1/3(Systolic pressure − Diastolic pressure).

Substituting the values we get:

Mean pulmonary artery pressure = 15 + 1/3(25 − 15)

Mean pulmonary artery pressure = 15 + 3.33 = 18.33.

Finally:

PVR = 18.3−5/6.25 = 13.5/5.25 = 2.0 resistance units (mmHg/l per min) approximately.

2.54

Answer: A   A localised region of ventricular myocardium

Myocardial infarction involving the conduction system of the heart will result in arrhythmias. Injured heart tissue following myocardial infarction conducts electrical impulses more slowly than normal heart tissue. The difference in conduction velocity between injured and uninjured tissue can trigger re-entry or a feedback loop that is believed to be the cause of many lethal arrhythmias. The most serious of these arrhythmias is ventricular fibrillation, an extremely fast and chaotic heart rhythm that is the leading cause of sudden cardiac death. Another life-threatening arrhythmia is ventricular tachycardia, which may or may not cause sudden cardiac death. However, ventricular tachycardia usually results in rapid heart rates that prevent the heart from pumping blood effectively. Cardiac output and blood pressure may fall to dangerous levels, which is particularly bad for the patient experiencing acute myocardial infarction.

2.55

Answer: A   Slowing the heart

Stimulation of the vagus nerve (parasympathetic) causes a negative inotropic effect that includes:

- a shift of the ventricular function curve to the right
- reduced peak systolic pressure
- reduced rate of contraction and relaxation (dP/dt and $-dP/dt$).

These effects appear to be mediated through cGMP, which speeds the breakdown of cAMP. Acetylcholine, the parasympathetic neurotransmitter, also inhibits the release of noradrenaline, the sympathetic neurotransmitter, from sympathetic fibres. It also slows down conduction through the cardiac conduction pathway and results in bradycardia.

2.56

Answer: C   60 ml

Stroke volume is calculated by using the following formula:

cardiac output = stroke volume × heart rate.

Cardiac output is calculated by using the following formula based on the Fick principle:

$$VO_2 = CO \times (C_AO_2 - C_VO_2)$$

where VO_2 = oxygen consumption, CO = cardiac output, C_AO_2 = arterial oxygen content and C_VO_2 = mixed venous oxygen content, respectively.

Substituting the values in this formula we get:

300 ml/min = CO × (20 − 15) ml/100 ml

CO = 300 × 100/5 ml/min

CO = 6000 ml/min.

Next, stroke volume is calculated as follows:

6000 ml/min = stroke volume × 100 beats/min

stroke volume = 6000/100 ml/min

stroke volume = 60 ml/min.

2.57

Answer: E   Tissue cooling

If the blood supply (flow) to a given tissue bed is maintained constant and tissue metabolism is altered, oxygen levels in venous blood will change in an appropriate and predictable way. If, for instance, the tissue is cooled while blood flow is held constant, oxygen levels in venous blood from that particular vascular bed will increase. Part of the reason is that the tissue is being oversupplied with blood for the oxygen needs at that time, therefore oxygen extraction decreases. On the other hand, warming the tissue increases oxygen requirements and, again if flow is held constant, oxygen extraction increases and venous oxygen levels fall. Catecholamines, thyroxine and other agents that increase tissue metabolism have similar effects. Note that, for the manipulations described, the blood supply to the tissue is not permitted to change. Under normal physiological conditions cooling causes blood flow to decrease, while warming increases the flow.

2.58

Answer: B   15%

The brain is the least tolerant of all the body organs to ischaemia. Interruption of cerebral blood flow for as little as 5 s may cause fainting (syncope), while even transient decreases in blood flow result in dizziness. The brain is encased in the rigid cranium and fluids (that comprise about 80% of all tissues) are incompressible. This means that the total volume within the cranial cavity must remain constant. As a result, an increase in arterial vascular volume associated with arteriolar dilatation at one site must be accompanied by a decrease in volume at some other site. The decrease in volume may occur in veins, cerebral ventricles (cerebrospinal fluid) or at other points within the cranium. The brain comprises about 2.5% of the total body weight and receives 15% of the cardiac output. Oxygen extraction is relatively high, however, with venous oxygen levels approximating 13 vol%, an arteriovenous oxygen difference of 7 vol%. These values are similar to those found in resting skeletal muscle.

2.59

Answer: E   Peak in early diastole

The angioarchitecture and physiology of the myocardium result in several unique aspects of the coronary circulation. One of these is the anatomical considerations of the blood supply itself. Perfusion pressure is generated by the heart itself. Because arterial pressure is, in general, closely regulated, short-term fluctuations in coronary inflow pressure are minimal. Alterations in the level of cardiac work (changes in arterial blood pressure or afterload) are accompanied by changes in coronary blood flow that parallel the changes in oxygen requirements. This is another example of active hyperaemia. During systole and diastole, the two main coronary vessels are exposed to changing extravascular pressures. During isovolumic contraction of the left ventricle (systole), extravascular compression causes flow in vessels supplied by the left coronary artery to fall to zero or even become retrograde. With the onset of diastole, removal of the compression results in a large inflow into these vessels early in diastole. Flow parallels aortic pressure during the remainder of the cycle. In the right ventricle, maximal flow occurs during systole because extravascular pressures in the wall of this structure do not exceed aortic pressure during systole. The flow profile in the right ventricle closely resembles the pressure profile in the aorta. Most of the flow to the left ventricle occurs during diastole. Changes in heart rate (that increases cardiac work) restrict coronary inflow because rate increases occur primarily at the expense of the diastolic interval. The increased metabolism, however, causes coronary resistance vessels to dilate, overriding the effect of extravascular compression. The net result is that coronary blood flow increases as heart rate increases. In hearts with limited blood flow, such as may occur with coronary plaque, increased rate may cause chest pain (angina) because flow cannot increase to meet the increased oxygen demand.

In summary, left coronary flow is greater than right coronary flow due to the fact that the mass and the work output of the left ventricle are greater than those of the right. Total coronary flow is determined by the oxygen needs of the myocardium. Peak left coronary flow occurs early in diastole, while peak right coronary flow occurs during systole. Again, since left coronary flow is greater than right coronary flow, total coronary flow is greater during diastole than systole.

2.60

Answer: A   2%

The skin comprises 4–5% of the total body weight and receives about 2% of the cardiac output. The arteria–venous oxygen difference is small (3 vol%), indicating that most of the blood flow is non-nutrient flow.

SECTION 3: RESPIRATORY PHYSIOLOGY – ANSWERS

3.1

Answer: D   Change in lung volume divided by change in distending pressure $(p_{alv} - p_{pl})$

p_{alv} is ambient atmospheric pressure or zero reference pressure and p_{pl}, is a negative intrapleural pressure that becomes even more negative during inspiration. The lungs will expand to a higher volume during inhalation as a result of an increase in the transpulmonary pressure or distending pressure $(p_{alv} - p_{pl})$. Static compliance is measured under conditions of no airflow (stepwise changes in volume with no airflow during measurement of distending pressure). With each increase in distending pressure there is a corresponding increase in lung volume. Compliance is $\Delta V/\Delta P$. Distending pressure divided by change in lung volume gives the lung volume divided by recoil pressure (p_{alv}/p_{pl}) equals compliance only during the first linear part of the lung distension/pressure relationship. Generally speaking, V/P does not equal $\Delta V/\Delta P$. Change in elastic recoil pressure is only part of the compliance calculation.

3.2

Answer: A   Cannot be measured directly with a spirometer

The volume of air remaining in the lungs after a maximal effort to exhale all the air possible is the residual volume. Therefore, this volume is not part of the vital capacity and cannot be measured directly by a spirometer, which measures only changes in volume. Since you cannot voluntarily change your lung volume below the residual volume, the spirometer cannot measure it. Other methods (eg, body plethysmography, inert gas dilution) must be used to measure residual volume. Expiratory reserve volume is vital capacity

respiratory

minus inspiratory capacity and the resting volume of the lungs is the sum of residual volume and expiratory reserve volume. Lungs will recoil inward until the recoil pressure $(p_{alv} - p_{pl})$ equals zero, a volume significantly below the residual volume.

3.3

Answer: A   100 ml

In respiratory physiology, dead space is air that is inhaled by the body in breathing, but does not partake in gas exchange. In adults, it is usually in the range of 150 ml. Not all the air we breathe in is able to be used for the exchange of oxygen and carbon dioxide. About a third of every resting breath is exhaled exactly as it came into the body. Because of dead space, taking deep breaths more slowly (eg ten 500-ml breaths per minute) is more effective that taking shallow breaths quickly (eg, 20 250-ml breaths per minute). Although the amount of gas per minute is the same (5 l/min), a large proportion of the shallow breaths is dead space and does not allow oxygen to get into the blood. Dead space can be enlarged (and better envisaged) by breathing into a long tube. Even though one end of the tube is open to the air, when one inhales, it is mostly the carbon dioxide from expiration. Using a snorkel increases a diver's dead space in the airways (though usually not significantly). Dead space can be divided into two components: 'anatomical' and 'physiological'.

Anatomical dead space is the gas in the conducting areas of the respiratory system, such as the mouth and trachea, where the air doesn't come to the alveoli of the lungs. It is normally about 150 ml (or 2.2 ml per kilogram of body weight). This is about a third of the resting tidal volume (450–500 ml). Anatomical dead space is the volume of the conducting airways. It may be measured by Fowler's method, a nitrogen wash-out technique. It increases with an increase in tidal volume and is dependent on posture.

Physiological dead space is equal to the anatomical dead space plus the alveolar dead space. Alveolar dead space is the area in the alveoli that does receive air to be exchanged, but there is not enough blood flowing through the capillaries for exchange to be effective. It is normally very small (less than 5 ml) in healthy individuals. It can increase dramatically in some lung diseases. Physiological dead space can be measured by Bohr's method.

The product of tidal volume (volume moved in or out with each breath) times the frequency or breathing rate (number of breaths/min) is the total ventilation per minute (also called minute ventilation). In this clinical vignette, the total ventilation is 600 ml times 12 breaths/min = 7200 ml/min. As stated in the problem, the alveolar ventilation (air ventilating the respiratory zone for gas exchange each minute) is 6000 ml/min. The difference is that part of the total ventilation going only to non-exchanging conducting airways = 1200 ml/min or 100 ml per breath at 12 breaths/min. This 100 ml is the dead space volume.

3.4

Answer: B   Lung to collapse inward and the chest wall to spring outward

The response to a stab wound that punctures the lung demonstrates the elasticity of the lung and chest wall. The tendency of the lung to collapse is normally balanced by the tendency of the chest wall to spring out. So, intrapleural pressures are subatmospheric. Introduction of air in this space allows the lung to collapse and not to expand outward. At the same time the chest wall will spring outward, not inward. Lung collapse obviously results in very low lung volume.

3.5

Answer: E   Pulmonary oedema

Normally, O_2 is transferred from air spaces to blood via a perfusion-limited process. So, O_2 moves across the alveolar–capillary membrane by a process of simple diffusion and the amount of gas taken up depends entirely on the amount of blood flow. Processes that impair diffusion of O_2 transform the normal relationship to a diffusion-limited process. So, if O_2 must move a greater distance because of a thickened barrier, as would occur with increased extravascular lung water (pulmonary oedema) or cell components (interstitial fibrosis or asbestosis), the diffusion process is limited. Chronic obstructive lung diseases have little effect on pulmonary diffusion capacity. Breathing a hyperbaric gas mixture would increase the driving force and may overcome diffusion limitation in patients with mild fibrosis

respiratory

or interstitial oedema. Increasing the ventilatory rate will not have this effect and will only serve to maintain a high gradient of O_2 from air to blood. Strenuous, but not mild, exercise decreases passage time and may also favour diffusion limitation.

3.6

Answer: D   Transection of the afferent fibres of the vagus and glossopharyngeal nerves results in prolonged inspiration and shortened expiration

Afferent fibres from pulmonary mechanoreceptors are carried with the vagal and glossopharyngeal nerves to the brainstem and serve to limit inspiration. The respiratory centre of the central nervous system consists of a diffuse group of neurones whose inherent activity is not abolished even after all known afferent stimuli have been eliminated. Although sectioning the brain and observing respiratory changes is a useful approach to locating important areas of respiratory regulation, this approach interferes with many complex pathways that may interact. Nonetheless, transection of the brain above the pons has little effect – an apneustic centre may be located in the pons. Transection above the centre results in prolonged inspiration, but not prolonged expiration. Apparently, a pneumotaxic centre in the upper pons together with vagal afferents limit inspiration. The medullary centre is capable of initiating and maintaining respiration even if separated from the pons.

3.7

Answer: D   Arterial CO_2 pressure ($p_A(CO_2)$) will double

The relationship between alveolar ventilation (V_A) and alveolar CO_2 pressure ($p_A(CO_2)$) is represented as:

$$V_A = (VCO_2/p_A(CO_2)) \times K$$

where K is a constant such that $p_A(CO_2) = F_A(CO_2) \cdot K$. $F_A(CO_2)$ is the fraction of alveolar CO_2. Since VCO_2 is constant if CO_2 production remains unchanged, $p_A(CO_2)$ will double if V_A is halved. In normal people, alveolar CO_2 pressure ($p_A(CO_2)$ is virtually identical to arterial

CO_2 pressure ($p_a(CO_2)$). Therefore, $p_a(CO_2)$ will also double if V_A is halved. On the other hand, alveolar CO_2 pressures ($p_A(CO_2)$ would decrease if ventilation were increased. Unless inspired air is enriched with O_2, arterial O_2 pressure ($p_a(O_2)$) and alveolar O_2 pressure ($p_A(O_2)$) will decrease.

3.8

Answer: A   Anatomical right-to-left shunting

Breathing 100% O_2 should increase the $p_a(O_2)$ to almost 670 mmHg in healthy people (same as alveolar $p_A(O_2)$). Diffusion abnormalities and ventilation/perfusion inequality are also common causes of hypoxaemia. Breathing 100% O_2 will greatly relieve the hypoxaemia in these cases, but not if the patient has an anatomic right-to-left shunt (for example, a ventricular septal defect). One hundred per cent O_2 also greatly increases the $p_a(O_2)$ in profound hypoventilation. The $p_a(O_2)$ will greatly increase in the normal individual as well. In abnormalities of diffusion (eg alveolar wall thickening) the $p_a(O_2)$ will be below 670 mmHg, but not as low as 125 mmHg. In ventilation/perfusion abnormalities, $p_a(O_2)$ will be quite high in all communicating air spaces after 100% O_2 and both alveolar and arterial $p(O_2)$ will be quite high. Only in true right-to-left shunting would breathing 100% O_2 not substantially elevate the $p_a(O_2)$, which could be as low as 125 mmHg. The small rise over normal $p_a(O_2)$ comes mainly from a small amount of additional dissolved O_2 in blood passing through ventilated areas.

3.9

Answer: D   30 mmHg

Bohr's equation states that:

$$V_D/V_T = (p_A(CO_2) - p_E(CO_2))/p_A(CO_2)$$

where $p_E(CO_2)$ is mixed expired CO_2, $p_A(CO_2)$ is alveolar CO_2 pressure. So in a normal person, $p_a(CO_2)$ is virtually identical to $p_A(CO_2)$. So:

$$V_D/V_T = (p_a(CO_2)) - p_E(CO_2)/ p_a(CO_2).$$

respiratory

Since by Fowler's method, $V_D/V_T = 0.25$, in the patient described in the question:

$$(p_a(CO_2) - p_E(CO_2)/\ p_a(CO_2) = (40 - p_E(CO_2)/40 = 0.25.$$

Therefore:

$$p_E(CO_2) = 30 \text{ mmHg}.$$

If considerable inequality of blood flow and ventilation were present, $p_E(CO_2)$ could be much less than 30 mmHg and the patient's physiological dead space would exceed the anatomical dead space.

3.10

Answer: C   Tidal volume, vital capacity and expiratory reserve volume

Vital capacity is the sum of inspiratory reserve volume, tidal volume and expiratory reserve volume. Therefore, to calculate inspiratory reserve volume, the tidal volume and expiratory volume have to be subtracted from the vital capacity. All of these values can be measured by spirometry. The other choices are not sufficient to calculate inspiratory reserve volume. Residual volume can not be measured by spirometry.

3.11

Answer: C   Is a subject in a clinical research experiment who has been breathing a gas mixture of 10% oxygen and 90% nitrogen for a few minutes

Breathing a low-oxygen gas mixture is similar to being at high altitude, but if this is done for only a few minutes, there will be no time for renal compensation. The hypoxia stimulates hyperventilation, which lowers the $p(CO_2)$. The slightly lowered bicarbonate is due to buffering by non-bicarbonate buffers. Decreased $p(CO_2)$ results in decreased H_2CO_3. Decreased H_2CO_3 results in the following reaction being pulled to the right:

$$HCO_3^- + H^+ \rightarrow H_2CO_3^- \rightarrow H_2O + CO_2$$

thus lowering the plasma bicarbonate to slightly below normal.

Had there been time for renal compensation, the bicarbonate would have been much lower. Severe chronic lung disease or an overdose of heroin would have caused respiratory acidosis due to abnormally high arterial $p(CO_2)$ (not low $p(CO_2)$, which this subject has). A lowlander at high altitude for 2 weeks would have had both low $p(O_2)$, a low $p(CO_2)$ like this subject, but would have had an abnormally low plasma bicarbonate and a more nearly normal pH, due to re-compensation in the form of bicarbonate secretion. Acute aspirin overdose in adults usually presents first with a respiratory alkalosis, which includes a low $p(CO_2)$, not a low $p(O_2)$.

3.12

Answer: B   Decrease to < 100 mmHg even though the F_iO_2 is still around 0.2

Even though the cabin of the aeroplane described in the question is pressurised, the barometric pressure decreased to 523 mmHg. So, the F_iO_2 remains the same (0.2), but inspired $p(O_2)$ decreases, since it is the product of F_iO_2 and barometric pressure. Water vapour pressure remains at 47 mmHg as long as body temperature is normal and so $p(O_2)$ of humidified alveolar air must be less than that at sea level. Although a decrease in $p_A(CO_2)$ due to some hyperventilation may slightly enhance $p_A(O_2)$, this is not sufficient to prevent the decrease in $p_A(O_2)$ due to the drop in barometric pressure. Since cabin pressure is less than at sea level, alveolar O_2 will also be lower.

3.13

Answer: D   Is normal and due to shunted blood

Shunted blood is blood that bypasses ventilated parts of the lung and directly enters the arterial circulation. In normal people, this is largely due to mixing of arterial blood with bronchial venous and some myocardial venous blood, which drains into the left heart. Diffusion limitation, although finite, is usually immeasurably small, as is reaction velocity with haemoglobin. Unloading of CO_2 may affect alveolar oxygen partial pressure, but would have no effect on the difference between alveolar and arterial $p(O_2)$. A large ventricular septal defect would result in a significantly lower arterial O_2 compared with alveolar O_2.

respiratory

3.14

Answer: D   The gene that is abnormal in cystic fibrosis encodes a cAMP regulated Cl⁻ channel

Cystic fibrosis (CF) is caused by a mutation in a gene called the cystic fibrosis transmembrane conductance regulator (*CFTR*). This gene encodes a cAMP-regulated Cl⁻ channel. Since Cl⁻ flux via this channel plays different roles in different epithelia, it is not surprising that the symptoms of cystic fibrosis are quite diverse. The volume-absorbing airway epithelium in cystic fibrosis patients shows increased Na⁺ reabsorption, probably because lack of CFTR increases the transepithelial potential difference. This results in a thick, dehydrated mucus predisposing to airway infections. This is in contrast to sweat glands, where cystic fibrosis patients secrete nearly normal volumes of sweat into the acinus, but are unable to absorb NaCl from sweat as it moves through the sweat duct. Therefore, the Na⁺ and Cl⁻ content of sweat are both elevated in cystic fibrosis patients. Lack of Cl⁻ and water secretion in gastrointestinal epithelia can lead to severe constipation and obstruction of the small and large bowels. Impairment of the Cl⁻/HCO_3^- exchange in pancreatic ductal epithelium results in water and enzyme retention and may eventually destroy the pancreas. Cystic fibrosis is more common in Whites than in African-Americans and is one of the most common genetic disorders, occurring in 1 of 2000 White births. The abnormal gene is not located on the X chromosome, but on chromosome 7 (autosomal recessive). Sodium channels are not defective in cystic fibrosis.

3.15

Answer: B   Decrease tidal volume

Respiratory alkalosis is due to hyperventilation, which lowers CO_2. Decreasing tidal volume will reduce alveolar ventilation and correct the respiratory alkalosis. Assuming a dead space of 150 ml, alveolar ventilation in this patient is:

450 ml × 12/min = 5400 ml/min.

If the tidal volume were decreased from 600 to 300 ml and the frequency increased from 12 to 24 per minute, then the alveolar ventilation would decrease to:

150 ml × 12/min = 1800 ml/min

even though the minute ventilation remained unchanged (12 × 600 ml/min = 24 × 300 ml/min).

The fraction of O_2 in the respiratory air does not affect respiratory volumes or frequencies in a mechanically ventilated patient. Increasing minute ventilation or decreasing dead space would increase alveolar ventilation and worsen respiratory alkalosis. PEEP is positive pressure applied during the expiratory phase to prevent the collapse of alveoli and to increase functional residual capacity of the lungs. It is used primarily to improve arterial oxygenation in severely hypoxic patients.

3.16

Answer: D   Increases bicarbonate concentration in the urine

Acetazolamide is an inhibitor of carbonic anhydrase, an enzyme found in large quantities in the brush border of the proximal tubule. This enzyme has two important functions. In the tubular lumen it promotes the dissociation of H_2CO_3 into H_2O and CO_2 and thereby helps to recover filtered bicarbonate. Inside the epithelial cells it promotes the formation of H_2CO_3. Inhibition of this enzyme therefore increases bicarbonate concentration in the urine and results in a mild metabolic acidosis that counteracts the effect of respiratory alkalosis caused by hyperventilation in an oxygen-poor environment. Acetazolamide has been shown to relieve mild cases of altitude sickness in some people. However, it is not an immediate fix for altitude sickness; it speeds up acclimatisation, which in turn helps to relieve symptoms. This may take up to a day or two and requires waiting without any further rapid ascent. It is often advisable to descend if even mild altitude sickness is experienced. If serious sickness is encountered, descent is considered mandatory unless other circumstances present greater danger. Metabolic alkalosis would worsen the symptoms of mountain sickness. Acetazolamide has no direct effect on respiratory drive. Hydrogen concentration in the urine plays only a minor role in acid–base regulation by the kidneys. Most of the excess hydrogen is excreted in the form of non-titratable acid NH_4^+.

respiratory

3.17

Answer: D   20 ml oxygen / 100 ml blood

In a normal person each 100 ml of blood contains about 15 g of haemoglobin and each gram of haemoglobin can bind with about 1.34 ml of oxygen when it is 100% saturated ($15 \times 1.34 = 20$ ml O_2/100 ml blood). The haemoglobin in venous blood leaving the peripheral tissues is about 75% saturated with oxygen, so the amount of oxygen transported by haemoglobin in venous blood is about 15 ml O_2/100 ml blood. Therefore, about 5 ml of oxygen is normally transported to the tissues in each 100 ml of blood. At a $p(O_2) > 100$ mmHg only 3 ml of oxygen will dissolve in every litre of plasma. If the $p(O_2)$ of oxygen in arterial blood ($p_A(O_2)$) is increased significantly (by breathing 100% oxygen) then a small amount of extra oxygen will dissolve in the plasma (at a rate of 0.003 ml O_2/100 ml of blood per mmHg $p(O_2)$) but there will normally be no significant increase in the amount carried by haemoglobin, which is already > 95% saturated with oxygen.

3.18

Answer: A   In the form of bicarbonate ions

Dissolved carbon dioxide reacts with water inside red blood cells to form carbonic acid. This reaction is catalysed by a protein enzyme in the red cells called carbonic anhydrase. Most of the carbonic acid immediately dissociates into bicarbonate ions and hydrogen ions, the hydrogen ions in turn combining with haemoglobin. Approximately 23% of the carbon dioxide produced in the tissues combines directly with haemoglobin to form carbaminohaemoglobin and an additional 7% is transported in the dissolved state in the water of the plasma and cells.

3.19

Answer: D   Decreases in the blood dioxide tension

The blood–brain barrier is almost totally impermeable to hydrogen ions, so that increases in the blood hydrogen ion concentration have relatively little effect on the hydrogen ion concentration in the vicinity of the respiratory centre. Carbon dioxide, on the other hand, permeates the blood–brain barrier with ease and immediately reacts with water to form hydrogen ions. So, more hydrogen ions are released in the respiratory centre when the blood carbon dioxide concentration increases than when the blood hydrogen ion concentration increases. Unlike the effects of carbon dioxide and hydrogen ion concentration, oxygen lack does not directly stimulate the respiratory centre. Instead, it excites special nerve receptors called chemoreceptors located in minute carotid and aortic bodies that lie, respectively, in the carotid bifurcations and along the aorta.

Mechanical stimulation of the lungs can trigger certain reflexes, as discovered in animal studies. In humans, these seem to be more important in neonates and ventilated patients, but of little relevance in health. The tone of respiratory muscle is believed to be modulated by muscle spindles via a reflex arc involving the spinal cord. Drugs can greatly influence the control of respiration. Opioids and anaesthetic drugs tend to depress ventilation, especially with regards to carbon dioxide response. Stimulants such as amphetamines can cause hyperventilation. Pregnancy tends to increase ventilation (lowering plasma carbon dioxide tension below normal values). This is due to increased progesterone levels and results in enhanced gas exchange in the placenta. Ventilation is temporarily modified by voluntary acts and complex reflexes such as sneezing, coughing and vomiting.

respiratory

3.20

Answer: C Diaphragm and external intercostals

The diaphragm is critically important in respiration: to draw air into the lungs, the diaphragm contracts, so enlarging the thoracic cavity and reducing intrathoracic pressure (the external intercostals also participate in this enlargement). When the diaphragm relaxes, air is exhaled by elastic recoil of the lung and the tissues lining the thoracic cavity. Contraction of the external intercostals causes the ribs to rotate upward. This increases the volume of the thoracic cavity, causing the lungs to expand. The abdominal muscles and internal intercostals are muscles of expiration.

3.21

Answer: B   Pulmonary compliance

Pulmonary surfactant is a surface-active lipoprotein formed by type II alveolar cells. It decreases the surface tension of the alveolar fluid. Decreased surface tension causes increased pulmonary compliance, which decreases the work required to expand the lungs. The proteins and lipids that comprise surfactant have both a hydrophilic region and a hydrophobic region. By adsorbing to the air–water interface of alveoli with the hydrophilic head groups in the water and the hydrophobic tails facing towards the air, the main lipid component of surfactant, dipalmitoylphosphatidylcholine, reduces surface tension.

3.22

Answer: B   3000 ml/min

Alveolar ventilation is the amount of air reaching the alveoli per minute. It is calculated as follows:

alveolar ventilation = respiratory rate × (tidal volume
  − anatomical dead space volume).

So, substituting the values in the above equation:

alveolar ventilation = 10 × (550 − 250) = 3000 ml/min.

3.23

Answer: D   a twofold increase in tidal volume and a shorter snorkel

Alveolar ventilation is related to respiratory rate, tidal volume and anatomic dead space by the following formula:

alveolar ventilation = respiratory rate × (tidal volume −
  anatomical dead space volume).

As much of the increase in respiratory rate simply moves air back and forth in the anatomical dead space and this does not contribute to alveolar ventilation, according to the above equation it is obvious that a shorter snorkel would decrease the effective anatomical dead space and this, accompanied by a twofold increase in tidal volume, will cause the greatest increase in alveolar ventilation.

3.24

Answer: E   Results from nitrogen bubbles in the body fluids

As a diver breathing 80% nitrogen (N_2) ascends from a dive, the elevated alveolar pressure of N_2 falls. N_2 diffuses from the tissues into the lungs along the partial pressure gradient. If the return to atmospheric pressure (decompression) is gradual, no harmful effects are observed; but if the ascent is rapid, N_2 escapes from solution. Bubbles form in the tissues and blood, causing the symptoms of decompression sickness (the bends, caisson disease). Bubbles in the tissues cause severe pains, particularly around joints, and neurological symptoms that include paraesthesias and itching. Bubbles in the bloodstream, which occur in more severe cases, obstruct the arteries of the brain and spinal cord. Symptoms commonly appear 10–30 min after the diver resurfaces, and they progress. Abnormalities due to damage to the spinal cord are most common, but there can also be major paralyses and respiratory failure. Bubbles in the pulmonary capillaries are apparently responsible for the dyspnoea that divers called 'the chokes', and bubbles in the coronary arteries may cause myocardial damage. Treatment of this condition is prompt recompression in a pressure chamber, followed by slow decompression. Recompression is frequently life-saving. Recovery is often complete, but there may be residual neurological sequelae as a result of irreversible damage to the nervous system.

3.25

Answer: D   Hypoxic hypoxia

Hypoxia is a pathological condition in which the body as a whole (generalised hypoxia) or region of the body (tissue hypoxia) is deprived of adequate oxygen supply. Low oxygen content in the blood is referred to as hypoxaemia. Hypoxia in which there is complete deprivation of oxygen supply is referred to as anoxia. Generalised hypoxia occurs in healthy people when they ascend to high altitude, where it causes altitude sickness and the potentially

respiratory

fatal complications of altitude sickness, high altitude pulmonary oedema and high altitude cerebral oedema. Hypoxia also occurs in healthy individuals when breathing mixtures of gases with a low oxygen content, for example while diving underwater, especially with closed-circuit rebreather systems that control the amount of oxygen in the air breathed in. Altitude training uses mild hypoxia to increase the concentration of red blood cells in the body for increased athletic performance. Hypoxia has several types:

- **Hypoxic hypoxia**, when there is an inadequate supply of oxygen. The term 'hypoxic hypoxia' refers to the fact that hypoxia occurs as a consequence of low partial pressure of oxygen in arterial blood, in contrast to the other causes of hypoxia listed below, in which the partial pressure of oxygen in arterial blood is normal. Hypoxic hypoxia may be due to:

  - low partial pressure of atmospheric oxygen (eg, at high altitude)

  - either sleep apnoea or hypopnoea causing a decrease in oxygen saturation of the blood

  - inadequate pulmonary ventilation (eg, in chronic obstructive pulmonary disease or respiratory arrest)

  - shunts in the pulmonary circulation or a right-to-left shunt in the heart. Shunts can be caused by collapsed alveoli that are still perfused or a block in ventilation to an area of the lung. Whatever the mechanism, blood meant for the pulmonary system is not ventilated and so no gas exchange occurs (the ventilation/perfusion ratio is zero). Normal anatomical shunt occurs in everyone, because of the thebesian vessels, which empty into the left ventricle, and the bronchial circulation, which supplies the bronchi with oxygen.

- **Anaemic hypoxia**, in which arterial oxygen pressure is normal, but total oxygen content of the blood is reduced.

respiratory

- **Hypaemic hypoxia**, when there is an inability of the blood to deliver oxygen to target tissues:

    - carbon monoxide poisoning, which inhibits the ability of haemoglobin to release the oxygen bound to it

    - methaemoglobinaemia in which an abnormal version of haemoglobin accumulates in the blood.

- **Histotoxic hypoxia**, in which the quantity of oxygen reaching the cells is normal, but the cells are unable to effectively use the oxygen due to disabled oxidative phosphorylation enzymes.

- **Ischaemic or stagnant hypoxia**, in which there is a local restriction in the flow of otherwise well-oxygenated blood. The oxygen supplied to the region of the body is then insufficient for its needs. Examples are cerebral ischaemia, ischaemic heart disease and intrauterine hypoxia, which is an unchallenged cause of perinatal death.

Symptoms of generalised hypoxia depend on its severity and speed of onset. In the case of altitude sickness, where hypoxia develops gradually, the symptoms include headaches, fatigue, shortness of breath and nausea. In severe hypoxia or hypoxia of very rapid onset, changes in levels of consciousness, seizures, coma and death occur. Severe hypoxia induces a blue discoloration of the skin, called cyanosis. Haemoglobin is blue when it is not bound to oxygen (deoxyhaemoglobin), as opposed to the rich red colour that it has when bound to oxygen (oxyhaemoglobin)). In cases where the oxygen is displaced by another molecule, such as carbon monoxide, the skin may be 'cherry red' instead of cyanotic. In most tissues of the body, the response to hypoxia is vasodilatation. By widening the blood vessels, the tissue allows greater perfusion. By contrast, in the lungs, the response to hypoxia is vasoconstriction. This is known as 'hypoxic pulmonary vasoconstriction', or 'HPV'. So, from the above discussion it is quite clear that in this vignette the patient has hypoxic hypoxia.

respiratory

3.26

Answer: C   7.28   55   81

Hypoventilation (also known as 'respiratory depression') occurs when ventilation is inadequate (*hypo* means 'below') to perform needed gas exchange. It generally causes an increased concentration of carbon dioxide (hypercapnia) and respiratory acidosis. It can be caused by medical conditions, by holding one's breath or by drugs. As a side-effect of medicines or recreational drugs, hypoventilation may become potentially life-threatening. Many different central nervous system depressant drugs such as alcohol, benzodiazepines, barbiturates and opiates produce respiratory depression when taken in large or excessive doses; however this is most commonly seen as a cause of death with opiates or opioids. Strong opiates or opioids such as heroin and fentanyl are notorious for producing this effect; in an overdose, an individual may cease breathing (go into respiratory arrest). Generally in recreational drug overdose acute respiratory acidosis is seen as is the case in this clinical vignette whereby the $p(CO_2)$ is elevated above the upper limit of the reference range (over 45 mmHg) with an accompanying acidaemia (pH < 7.35). Hypoventilation may be dangerous for those with sleep apnoea.

3.27

Arterial $p(CO_2)$ pH

Answer: D   Increase   Decrease

Respiratory acidosis is acidosis (abnormal acidity of the blood) due to decreased ventilation of the pulmonary alveoli (alveolar hypoventilation), leading to elevated arterial carbon dioxide concentration ($p(CO_2)$). Production of carbon dioxide occurs rapidly and failure of ventilation promptly increases the level of $p(CO_2)$. Alveolar hypoventilation leads to an increased $p(CO_2)$ (ie hypercapnia). The increase in $p(CO_2)$ in turn decreases the HCO_3^-/$p(CO_2)$ and decreases pH. Hypercapnia and respiratory acidosis occur when impairment in ventilation occurs and the removal of CO_2 by the lungs is less than the production of CO_2 in the tissues. Respiratory acidosis can be acute or chronic. In acute respiratory acidosis, the $p(CO_2)$ is elevated above the upper limit of the reference range (over 45 mmHg) with an accompanying acidaemia (pH < 7.35). In chronic respiratory acidosis, the $p(CO_2)$ is elevated above the upper limit of the reference range, with a normal or near-normal pH secondary to renal compensation and an elevated serum bicarbonate ($HCO_3^- > 30$ mmHg). Acute respiratory acidosis occurs when an abrupt failure of ventilation occurs, as is the case in this vignette. This failure in ventilation may be caused by depression of the central respiratory centre by cerebral disease or drugs, inability to ventilate adequately due to neuromuscular disease (eg, myasthenia gravis, amyotrophic lateral sclerosis, Guillain–Barré syndrome, muscular dystrophy) or airway obstruction related to asthma or chronic obstructive pulmonary disease (COPD) exacerbation (*see also* answer to 3.26).

3.28

Answer: B   Compliance of the lung

Acute respiratory distress syndrome (ARDS), also known as adult respiratory distress syndrome (in contrast with infant respiratory distress syndrome) is a serious reaction to various forms of injuries to the lung. A number of clinical conditions are associated with development of ARDS:

- Sepsis and the systemic inflammatory response syndrome (SIRS) are the most common predisposing factors associated with development of ARDS. These conditions may result from the indirect toxic effects of neutrophil-derived inflammatory mediators in the lungs.

- Severe traumatic injury (especially multiple fractures), severe head injury and pulmonary contusion are strongly associated with development of ARDS. Long bone fractures may give rise to ARDS through fat embolism. After severe head injury, ARDS is thought to result from a sudden discharge of the sympathetic nervous system, leading to acute pulmonary hypertension and injury to the pulmonary capillary bed. Pulmonary contusions cause ARDS through direct trauma to the lung.

- Multiple transfusions are another important risk factor for ARDS, independent of the reason for transfusion

respiratory

or the co-existence of trauma. The incidence of ARDS increases with the number of units transfused. Pre-existing liver disease or coagulation abnormalities further contribute to this risk.

- Patients who have nearly drowned can develop ARDS. Development of ARDS is slightly more common with salt-water aspiration than with fresh-water aspiration. Infiltrates and hypoxia develop within 12–24 h of the initial accident. Patients who are symptomatic after 6 h of observation generally do well. Aspiration is particularly damaging to lung tissue, leading to an osmotic gradient that favours movement of water into airspaces of the lung. Aspiration may be visible on chest X-ray, although the chest X-ray may be normal early in the course of the disease.

- Smoke inhalation causes lung tissue damage from direct heat, toxic chemicals and particulate matter carried into the lower lung. Patients with smoke inhalation initially may be asymptomatic. Patients with airway burns and/or exposure to carbon monoxide or toxic fumes should be monitored closely for development of ARDS, even if symptoms initially are absent.

- Overdoses of narcotics (eg heroin), salicylates, tricyclic antidepressants and other sedatives have been associated with development of ARDS. (Overdoses of tricyclic antidepressants are the most common.) This risk is independent of the risk from concurrent aspiration. Other implicated toxins and drugs include tocolytic agents, hydrochlorothiazide, protamine and interleukin-2 (IL-2).

ARDS was first described in 1967 by Ashbaugh, who described a syndrome of severe respiratory failure associated with pulmonary infiltrates, similar to infant hyaline membrane disease. The 1994 American–European Consensus Committee defined ARDS as the acute onset of bilateral infiltrates on chest X-ray, a partial pressure of arterial oxygen ($p_a(O_2)$) to fraction of inspired oxygen $F_i(O_2)$ ratio of less than 200 mmHg and a pulmonary artery occlusion pressure of less than 18 or the absence of clinical evidence of left arterial hypertension. Put simply, ARDS is the presence of pulmonary oedema in the absence of volume overload or depressed left ventricular function. This is distinguished from acute lung injury, which is similar to ARDS with the exception of a $p_a(O_2)/F_i(O_2)$ ratio of less than 300 mmHg.

The development of ARDS starts with damage to the alveolar epithelium and vascular endothelium, resulting in increased permeability to plasma and inflammatory cells into the interstitium and alveolar space. Damage to the surfactant-producing type II cells and the presence of protein-rich fluid in the alveolar space disrupts the production and function of pulmonary surfactant, leading to microatelectasis and impaired gas exchange. Lung compliance decreases and the work of breathing increases. Ultimately, regional variations in pulmonary perfusion, ventilation/perfusion (V/Q) mismatch with shunting of blood through unventilated alveoli and increased alveolar–arterial oxygen gradient occur. Eventually, resorption of alveolar oedema, regeneration of epithelial cells, proliferation and differentiation of type II alveolar cells and alveolar remodelling occur. Some patients have an uncomplicated course and rapid resolution, whereas others may progress to fibrosing alveolitis, which involves the deposition of collagen in alveolar, vascular and interstitial spaces, leading to poor lung compliance. Fibrosing alveolitis has been reported histologically as early as 5–7 days.

3.29

Answer: C   Increased renal excretion of HCO_3^-

High altitude are regions on the Earth's surface (or in its atmosphere) that are high above mean sea level. The composition and temperature of the atmosphere at high altitude are substantially different than at sea level. These differences can affect living organisms, including humans. High altitude is sometimes defined to begin at 1500 m above sea level. At high altitude, atmospheric pressure is lower compared with sea level. This is due to two competing physical effects: gravity, which causes the air to be as close as possible to the ground; and the heat content of the air, which causes the molecules to bounce off each other and expand. The lower atmospheric pressure affects animals and humans, due to the decrease in the partial pressure of

respiratory

oxygen. The percentage saturation of haemoglobin with oxygen determines the content of oxygen in our blood. After the body reaches around 2100 m (7000 feet) above sea level, the saturation of oxyhaemoglobin begins to plummet. Altitude acclimatisation, the physiological adaptations to altitude, can have immediate and long-term effects. The higher up you get the less oxygen there is.

Immediate effects:

- hyperventilation
- fluid loss (due to a decreased thirst drive)
- increase in heart rate
- slightly lowered stroke volume.

Long-term effects:

- lower lactate production (because reduced glucose breakdown decreases the amount of lactate formed)
- compensatory alkali loss in urine
- decrease in plasma volume
- increased erythropoietin release
- increased haematocrit
- increase in red cell mass
- higher concentration of capillaries in striated muscle tissue
- increase in myoglobin
- increase in mitochondria
- increase in aerobic enzyme concentration such as 2,3-DPG
- pulmonary vasoconstriction.

3.30

Answer: D   Respiratory acidosis

This patient had an acidosis with a high $p(CO_2)$ and normal standard bicarbonate—respiratory acidosis. This is a common finding in acute exacerbations of chronic obstructive pulmonary disease. It is usually managed with nebulisers, steroids and antibiotics, and non-invasive ventilation (*see also* answer to 3.27).

3.31

Answer: C   Mixed acidosis

This patient had acidosis with both a high $p(CO_2)$ and a low standard bicarbonate—mixed acidosis. The anion gap is 26 mmol/l (increased). The $p(O_2)$ is lower than expected because the patient was breathing around 70% oxygen. Does this fit with the clinical picture? Yes, he had a lactic acidosis from prolonged fitting and a respiratory acidosis from intravenous diazepam. This disturbance will return to normal with attention to A – airway manoeuvres and oxygen, B – assisted ventilation if needed, C – treatment with fluids.

3.32

Answer: B   Metabolic alkalosis

This patient had alkalosis due to a high standard bicarbonate—metabolic alkalosis. The $p_a(CO_2)$ was appropriately low in compensation. This was hypokalaemic hypochloraemic metabolic acidosis because of potassium and chloride loss from vomiting. Treatment was of the underlying cause (pyloric stenosis) and intravenous sodium chloride with potassium.

3.33

Answer: D   Compensated respiratory alkalosis

This patient had a normal pH but had both a low $p(CO_2)$ and a low standard bicarbonate. How do we know if this was a compensated respiratory alkalosis or a compensated metabolic acidosis? Easy.

respiratory

The history indicates five days of hyperventilation, so this is a compensated respiratory alkalosis. What if this was a diabetic patient who was unwell with fever, vomiting and high glucose? Then it would have been a compensated diabetic ketoacidosis.

3.34

Answer: E   Renal tubular acidosis

This patient had acidosis due to low bicarbonate. The $p(CO_2)$ was appropriately low in compensation. The anion gap was normal (13.5 mmol/l). This makes intra-abdominal ischaemia (which causes lactic acidosis) unlikely. Was this a gastrointestinal problem or a kidney problem? If this were a gastrointestinal problem, you would expect low potassium. This man had diabetic nephropathy, which predisposes to renal tubular acidosis. Type 4 (hyporeninaemic hypoaldosteronism) is typically associated with high potassium and is found in diabetic and hypertensive renal disease.

3.35

Answer: E   Hypoxia by causing an increased respiratory minute volume

This question primarily deals with carotid body and its innervation. While the central chemoreceptors in the brainstem are highly sensitive to CO_2, the carotid body is a peripheral chemoreceptor that provides afferent input to the respiratory centre that is highly O_2-dependent. Below an oxygen partial pressure of 60 mmHg, the carotid body cells release dopamine and trigger excitatory postsynaptic potentials in synapsed neurones leading to the respiratory centre. This event is mediated by a unique potassium channel that is responsive to the partial pressure of O_2. The peripheral chemoreceptor's input is secondary to that of CO_2-sensitive cells in the central chemoreceptors in healthy patients, but is the primary driver of ventilation in individuals who suffer from chronic hypercapnia (as in emphysema). It gives feedback to the medulla oblongata via the afferent branches of the glossopharyngeal nerve (IX). The medulla, in turn, regulates breathing and blood pressure. Blockade of cranial nerves IX bilaterally will block this effect.

3.36

Answer: E   Exercise

The oxygen–haemoglobin dissociation curve plots the proportion of haemoglobin in its saturated form on the vertical axis against the prevailing oxygen tension on the horizontal axis. It is usually a sigmoid plot. Haemoglobin molecules can bind up to four oxygen molecules in a reversible way. Many factors influence the affinity of this binding and alter the shape of the curve, including:

- pH

- the concentration of 2,3-diphosphoglycerate (2,3-DPG)

- temperature

- the type of haemoglobin molecules (adult versus fetal types)

- the presence of poisons, especially carbon monoxide.

The shape of the curve results from the interaction of bound oxygen molecules with incoming molecules. The binding of the first molecule is difficult. However, this facilitates the binding of the second and third molecules and it is only when the fourth molecule is to be bound that the difficulty increases, partly as a result of crowding of the haemoglobin molecule, partly as a natural tendency of oxygen to dissociate.

Left shift of the curve is a sign of haemoglobin's increased affinity for oxygen (eg at the lungs). Similarly, right shift shows decreased affinity, as would appear with an increase in body temperature (also seen after exercise), hydrogen ion, 2,3-diphosphoglycerate (DPG) or carbon dioxide concentration. The 'plateau' portion of the oxyhaemoglobin dissociation curve is the range that exists at the pulmonary capillaries (minimal reduction of oxygen transported until the $p(O_2)$ falls below 60 mmHg). The 'steep' portion of the oxyhaemoglobin dissociation curve is the range that exists at the systemic capillaries (a small drop in systemic capillary $p(O_2)$ can result in the release of large amounts of oxygen for the metabolically active cells). Under normal resting conditions in a healthy individual, the normal position of the curve is at a pH of 7.4. A shift in the position of the curve with a change in pH is called the Bohr effect. The curve

respiratory

shifts to the right (representing a decrease in affinity for O_2) in acute acidosis, increase in $p(CO_2)$, increase in temperature and increase in 2,3-DPG. The curve shifts to the left (representing an increase in affinity for O_2) in acute alkalosis, decrease in $p(CO_2)$, decrease in temperature and decrease in 2,3-DPG.

The oxygen dissociation curve for fetal haemoglobin is to the left of that of adult haemoglobin, to facilitate diffusion of oxygen across the placenta. The oxygen dissociation curve for myoglobin exists even further to the left. Carbon monoxide has a much higher affinity for haemoglobin than oxygen does. In carbon monoxide poisoning, oxygen cannot be transported and released to body tissues, which results in hypoxia.

3.37

Answer: D   Chemical pneumonia

Mendelson's syndrome is characterised by a bronchopulmonary reaction (chemical pneumonia) following aspiration of gastric contents during general anaesthesia due to abolition of the laryngeal reflexes. The main clinical features, which may become evident within 2–5 hours after anaesthesia, consist of cyanosis, dyspnoea, pulmonary wheeze, crepitant rales, bronchi, decreased arterial oxygen tension and tachycardia. Pulmonary oedema can cause sudden death or death may occur later from pulmonary complications. It occurs predominantly in association with obstetric anaesthesia. Mendelson found this complication in 0.15% of 44 016 deliveries.

3.38

Answer: B   Decreased first second forced expiratory volume
(FEV₁)/forced vital capacity (FVC) ratio

Patients suspected of having asthma should undergo pulmonary function testing to confirm and quantify the severity and reversibility of airway obstruction. Pulmonary function data quality is effort-dependent and requires patient education before the test. If it is safe to do so, bronchodilators should be stopped before the test: 6

h for short-acting β-agonists, such as albuterol; 8 h for ipratropium; 12–36 h for theophylline; 24 h for long-acting β-agonists, such as salmeterol and formoterol; and 48 h for tiotropium.

Spirometry should be obtained before and after inhalation of a short-acting bronchodilator. Signs of airway obstruction before bronchodilator inhalation include reduced forced expiratory volume in the first second (FEV₁) and a reduced ratio of FEV₁ to forced vital capacity (FEV₁/FVC). The forced vital capacity (FVC) may also be decreased. Lung volume measurements may show an increase in the residual volume and/or the functional residual capacity because of air trapping. An improvement in FEV₁ of > 12% or > 0.2 l in response to bronchodilator treatment confirms reversible airway obstruction, although absence of this finding should not preclude a therapeutic trial of bronchodilators. Spirometry should be repeated at least yearly in known asthmatics to monitor disease progression. Flow–volume loops should also be reviewed to diagnose or exclude vocal cord dysfunction, a common cause of upper airway obstruction that mimics asthma. Provocative testing, in which inhaled methacholine (or alternatives, such as inhaled histamine, adenosine, bradykinin or exercise testing) is used to provoke bronchoconstriction, is indicated for suspected asthmatics with normal findings on spirometry and flow-volume testing, suspected cough-variant asthma and no contraindications. Contraindications include FEV₁ < 1 l or < 50%, recent myocardial infarction or stroke and severe hypertension (systolic blood pressure [BP] > 200 mmHg; diastolic blood pressure [BP] > 100 mmHg). A decline in FEV₁ of > 20% supports the diagnosis of asthma. However, FEV₁ may decline in response to these drugs in other diseases, such as COPD. Diffusing capacity for carbon monoxide (DLco) testing can help distinguish asthma from COPD. Values are normal or elevated in asthma and usually reduced in COPD, particularly in the setting of emphysema.

3.39

Answer: A   Alveolar hypoventilation

The arterial blood gas analysis shows respiratory acidosis due to CO_2 accumulation (hypercapnia) from a decrease in respiratory rate and/or volume (hypoventilation). Causes of alveolar hypoventilation include conditions impairing central nervous system (CNS)

respiratory

respiratory drive, impaired neuromuscular transmission and other causes of muscular weakness (including effects of anaesthetics and sedatives as is the case in this vignette), and obstructive, restrictive and parenchymal pulmonary disorders. Hypoxia typically accompanies hypoventilation. Hypercapnia lowers arterial pH (respiratory acidosis). Severe acidaemia (pH < 7.2) contributes to pulmonary arteriolar vasoconstriction, systemic vascular dilatation, reduced myocardial contractility, hyperkalaemia, hypotension and cardiac irritability, with the potential for life-threatening arrhythmias. Acute hypercapnia also causes cerebral vasodilatation and increased intracranial pressure, a major problem in patients with acute head injury. Over time, tissue buffering and renal compensation can largely correct the acidaemia. However, sudden increases in $p(CO_2)$ can occur faster than compensatory changes ($p(CO_2)$ rises 3–6 mmHg/min in a totally apnoeic patient).

3.40

Answer: D   Increased total lung capacity

Patients suspected of having emphysema/chronic obstructive pulmonary disease should undergo pulmonary function testing to confirm airway obstruction and to quantify its severity and reversibility. Pulmonary function testing is also useful for following disease progression and monitoring response to treatment. The primary diagnostic tests are FEV_1, which is the volume of air forcefully expired during the first second after a full breath; forced vital capacity (FVC), which is the total volume of air expired with maximal force; and flow–volume loops, which are simultaneous spirometrical recording of airflow and volume during forced maximal expiration and inspiration. Reduction of FEV_1, FVC and the ratio of FEV_1/FVC are the hallmark of airway obstruction. Flow–volume loops show a concave pattern in the expiratory tracing. FEV_1 declines up to 60 ml/year in smokers, compared with a less steep decline of 25–30 ml/year in non-smokers, beginning at about age 30. In middle-aged smokers who already have a low FEV_1, the decline occurs at a more rapid rate. When the FEV_1 falls below about 1 L, patients develop dyspnoea with activities of daily living; when the FEV_1 falls below about 0.8 l, they are at risk of hypoxaemia, hypercapnia and cor pulmonale. FEV_1 and forced vital capacity (FVC) are easily measured with office spirometry and define severity of disease because they correlate with symptoms and mortality. Normal reference values are determined by patient age, sex and height.

Other test abnormalities may include an increased total lung capacity, functional residual capacity and residual volume, which can help distinguish chronic obstructive pulmonary disease (COPD) from restrictive pulmonary disease, in which these measures are diminished; decreased vital capacity; and decreased single-breath diffusing capacity for carbon monoxide (DLco). Decreased DLco is non-specific and is reduced in other disorders that affect the pulmonary vascular bed, such as interstitial lung disease, but can help distinguish COPD from asthma, in which DLco is normal or elevated.

3.41

Answer: E   Is affected by the volume of blood in the pulmonary capillaries

The diffusing capacity for carbon monoxide (DLco) is a measure of the ability of gas to transfer from alveoli to RBCs across the alveolar epithelium and the capillary endothelium. The DLco depends not only on the area and thickness of the blood–gas barrier but also on the volume of blood in the pulmonary capillaries. The distribution of alveolar volume and ventilation also affects the measurement. DLco is measured by sampling end-expiratory gas for carbon monoxide (CO) after a patient inspires a small amount of CO, holds his breath and exhales. Measured DLco should be adjusted for alveolar volume (which is estimated from dilution of helium) and the patient's haematocrit. DLco is reported as ml/min per mmHg and as a percentage of a predicted value.

Conditions that primarily affect the pulmonary vasculature, such as primary pulmonary hypertension and pulmonary embolism, decrease DLco. Conditions that affect the lung diffusely, such as emphysema and pulmonary fibrosis, decrease both DLco and alveolar ventilation (V_A). Reduced DLco also occurs in patients with past lung resection because total lung volume is smaller, but DLco corrects to or even exceeds normal when adjusted for V_A because increased additional vascular surface area is recruited in the remaining lung. Anaemic patients often have lower DLco values that correct when adjusted

respiratory

for Hb. *DL*co may be higher than predicted in patients with heart failure, presumably because the increased pulmonary venous and arterial pressures result in recruitment of additional pulmonary microvessels. *DL*co is also increased in patients with polycythaemia, in part because of increased Hct and because of the vascular recruitment that occurs with increased pulmonary pressures due to increased viscosity. *DL*co is increased in patients with alveolar haemorrhage because RBCs in the alveolar space can also bind CO. *DL*co is also increased in patients with asthma. Although this increase is attributed to presumed vascular recruitment, the actual mechanism is unknown.

3.42

Answer: C   Cheyne–Stokes breathing

Cheyne–Stokes respiration is an abnormal pattern of breathing characterised by periods of breathing with gradually increasing and decreasing tidal volume interspersed with periods of apnoea. In cases of increasing intracranial pressure, it is often the first abnormal breathing pattern to appear. The condition was named after John Cheyne and William Stokes, the physicians who first classified it. It is caused by the failure of the respiratory centre in the brain to compensate quickly for changing serum partial pressure of oxygen and carbon dioxide. This abnormal pattern of breathing can be seen in patients with strokes, head injuries or brain tumours and in patients with congestive heart failure. In some instances, it can occur in otherwise normal people during sleep at high altitudes, where it is an important sign of altitude sickness. It a symptom of carbon monoxide poisoning, along with syncope or coma. Hospice personnel often note the presence of Cheyne–Stokes breathing as a patient nears death and report that patients able to speak after such episodes do not report any distress associated with the breathing, although it is sometimes disturbing to the family. This type of respiration is also often seen after morphine administration.

Biot's respirations, sometimes also called cluster respiration, is an abnormal pattern of breathing characterised by groups of quick, shallow inspirations followed by regular or irregular periods of apnoea. It is distinguished from ataxic respiration by having more regularity and similar-sized inspirations, whereas ataxic respirations are characterised by completely irregular breaths and pauses. As the breathing pattern deteriorates, it merges with ataxic respirations. It is caused by damage to the medulla oblongata due to strokes or trauma or by pressure on the medulla due to uncal or tentorial herniation. It generally indicates a poor prognosis.

Kussmaul breathing is the rapid, deep and laboured breathing of people who have acidosis. Kussmaul breathing is named for Adolph Kussmaul, the nineteenth century German doctor who first noted it. It is also called 'air hunger'. The cause of Kussmaul breathing is respiratory compensation for a metabolic acidosis, most commonly occurring in diabetics in diabetic ketoacidosis. Blood gases in a patient with Kussmaul breathing will show a low $p(CO_2)$ because of a forced increased respiratory rate (blowing off the carbon dioxide). The patient feels an urge to breathe deeply and it appears almost involuntary. The effect can be reproduced, to a degree, by rapidly breathing in the air in a recently emptied plastic soft-drink bottle, which will normally contain a substantial amount of carbon dioxide.

Ondine's curse, congenital central hypoventilation syndrome or primary alveolar hypoventilation, is a respiratory disorder that is fatal if untreated. People afflicted with Ondine's curse classically suffer from respiratory arrest during sleep. This very rare and serious form of central sleep apnoea involves an inborn failure of autonomic control of breathing. About 1 in 200 000 liveborn children have the condition. In 2006, there were only about 200 known cases world-wide. In all cases, episodes of apnoea occur in sleep, but in a few patients, at the most severe end of the spectrum, apnoea also occurs while awake. Patients generally require tracheostomies and lifetime mechanical ventilation on a respirator to survive.

3.43

Answer: A   Adrenocorticotropic hormone (ACTH)

In addition to respiratory functions such as gas exchange and regulation of hydrogen ion concentration, the lungs also:

- influence the concentration of biologically active substances and drugs

- filter out small blood clots formed in veins

respiratory

- serve as a physical layer of soft, shock-absorbent protection for the heart, which the lungs flank and nearly enclose

- ectopically synthesise ACTH (adrenocorticotrophic hormone) and ADH (antidiuretic hormone).

3.44

Answer: D   Respiratory acidosis

Chronic obstructive pulmonary disease (COPD) results in chronic respiratory acidosis. Hypoventilation in COPD involves multiple mechanisms, including decreased responsiveness to hypoxia and hypercapnia, increased ventilation/perfusion mismatch leading to increased dead space ventilation and decreased diaphragm function secondary to fatigue and hyperinflation.

3.45

Answer: A   The alveolar–capillary $p(O_2)$ gradient is increased

During exercise the minute ventilation increases linearly along with the work rate (O_2 consumption) until the anaerobic threshold is reached. Above the anaerobic threshold, minute ventilation increases more steeply as the work rate increases, because the lactic acid that is generated imposes an additional respiratory drive. CO_2 output increases linearly with the work rate until the anaerobic threshold is reached. Above the anaerobic threshold, the CO_2 output increases more steeply because respiration increases. The arterial CO_2 tension declines as the body stores are depleted, because excretion exceeds production. O_2 consumption also increases linearly with the work rate and is exactly dependent on the work performed. The O_2 content of the mixed venous blood decreases. The alveolar–arterial pressure gradient normally remains at 5–10 mmHg during moderate levels of exercise, but widens slightly beyond the anaerobic threshold because the alveolar O_2 tension increases. Finally, the respiratory exchange ratio (volume of expired CO_2 per minute divided by the volume of O_2 that is consumed per minute) never exceeds 1.25 even at maximal levels of exercise. The conversion of HCO_3^- to carbonic acid during the buffering of lactic acid increases the amount of CO_2 that is liberated by the lungs and therefore increases the respiratory exchange ratio.

3.46

Answer: B   Increases still further over the course in the next 1–3 days

The increase in ventilation that occurs immediately following ascent to high altitude is caused by stimulation of the peripheral chemoreceptors by the arterial hypoxaemia. Because of the very high blood flow per tissue mass of the carotid chemoreceptors, they essentially respond to arterial $p(O_2)$. The increase in ventilation is partly inhibited by the resulting fall in $p(CO_2)$, which causes a rise in pH of the cerebrospinal fluid (CSF). This reduces the stimulation of the central chemoreceptors, which works against the increased drive from the peripheral chemoreceptors. However, after a day or so, the pH of the CSF is reduced to some extent by the outward movement of bicarbonate and so this inhibitory effect on the central chemoreceptors is diminished. Consequently, ventilation increases still further over the course of the next 1–3 days. The increase in ventilation is not caused by the reduced work of breathing the less dense air, though it is true that the work of breathing is reduced to some extent at high altitude. If a subject is asked to breathe as fast and as deeply as they can for 15 s, it can be shown that the amount of air that is exhaled is greater at high altitude than at sea level, but this does not cause increased ventilation.

3.47

Answer: A   Decreased arterial O_2 concentration

Carbon monoxide poisoning causes some of the haemoglobin in the blood to be combined with CO to give carboxyhaemoglobin. As a result, there is a decreased arterial O_2 concentration. However, it is important to realise that this does not decrease the arterial $p(O_2)$. In this respect, carbon monoxide poisoning is similar to anaemia where again the arterial $p(O_2)$ is typically normal but the arterial oxygen concentration is reduced. There is an increase in the affinity of the

respiratory

haemoglobin for oxygen as indicated by the leftward shift of the oxygen dissociation curve. So, carbon monoxide poisoning causes a fall in tissue $p(O_2)$ for two reasons: first, less oxygen is carried in the arterial blood and second the unloading is impeded by the higher haemoglobin affinity. Ventilation is unaffected in mild carbon monoxide poisoning; the chemoreceptors respond primarily to the arterial $p(O_2)$ and, because this is normal, ventilation remains essentially unchanged. The word 'mild' is included in the question because with very severe carbon monoxide poisoning there may be brain damage, which may alter ventilation.

3.48

Answer: E $p(O_2)$ of mixed venous blood is reduced

A patient with anaemia and normal lungs typically has a normal arterial $p(O_2)$. Because the position of the oxygen dissociation curve is typically normal, the arterial oxygen saturation is also normal. If the oxygen consumption and cardiac output are normal, the arterial–venous O_2 concentration difference will also be normal. As a matter of fact, cardiac output is sometimes reflexly increased in anaemia and if this occurs, the arterial–venous O_2 concentration difference will be decreased. Although the arterial $p(O_2)$ is typically normal, the $p(O_2)$ of mixed venous blood must fall. This is because the venous oxygen concentration falls to a very low level as the normal amount of oxygen is extracted and so the venous $p(O_2)$ is abnormally low.

3.49

Answer: B   Improves matching of ventilation and blood flow in some lung diseases

Suppose a lobe or lobule of lung is poorly ventilated because of partial bronchial obstruction. The resulting alveolar hypoxia will reduce the blood flow through the mechanism of hypoxic pulmonary vasoconstriction. The result is improvement in the matching of ventilation and blood flow. Although the mechanism of hypoxic pulmonary vasoconstriction is not fully understood, we know that central nervous connections are not required because

respiratory

the phenomenon can be demonstrated in isolated lungs. Reducing the $p(O_2)$ of the blood entering the lung results in much less vasoconstriction than reducing the $p(O_2)$ of alveolar gas. Hypoxic pulmonary vasoconstriction is important in the perinatal period. When the newborn baby makes the transition from placental to air breathing, it is important for pulmonary vascular resistance to fall precipitously within a few seconds. As a consequence, pulmonary blood flow dramatically increases from its value of only about 15% of the cardiac output in utero. The increase in pulmonary blood flow is assisted by closure of both the ductus arteriosus and the foramen ovale. Hypoxic pulmonary vasoconstriction is reversible unless it is long-standing.

3.50

Answer: A   At high altitude

Pulmonary vascular resistance increases at high altitude as a result of the global alveolar hypoxia. The exact mechanism is still unknown but is apparently a local effect on the smooth muscle of the pulmonary arterial wall. The increase causes right ventricular hypertrophy with characteristic electrocardiogram (ECG) changes. Pulmonary vascular resistance during space flight would, if anything, decrease as blood flow becomes more uniform. Anaemia would decrease viscosity – a term in the resistance formula. With exercise, pulmonary arterial pressure tends to rise causing recruitment and distension of pulmonary vessels leading to a fall in pulmonary vascular resistance. Inspiring 100% oxygen would also cause the pulmonary vascular resistance to drop.

3.51

Answer: E   Ventilation/perfusion ratio

The pathophysiological changes that follow pulmonary embolism (PE) involve derangements in pulmonary haemodynamics, gas exchange and mechanics. The change in cardiopulmonary function is proportional to the extent of obstruction, which varies with the size and number of emboli obstructing the pulmonary arteries and with the patient's pre-embolic cardiopulmonary status. The resulting

respiratory

physiological changes may include pulmonary hypertension with right ventricular failure and shock, dyspnoea with tachypnoea and hyperventilation, arterial hypoxaemia and pulmonary infarction. Tachypnoea, often with dyspnoea, almost always occurs after a PE. It appears to be due to stimulation of juxtacapillary receptors in the alveolar capillary membrane by swelling of the alveolar interstitial space. This stimulation increases reflex vagal afferent activity, which stimulates medullary respiratory neurones. Consequent alveolar hyperventilation is manifested by a lowered $p_a(CO_2)$. After occlusion of the pulmonary artery, areas of the lung are ventilated but not perfused, resulting in wasted ventilation with increased ventilation/perfusion ratio – the physiological hallmark of PE – contributing further to the hyperventilatory state. Depletion of alveolar surfactant within hours after the embolic event results in diminished lung volume and compliance. Reduced lung volume secondary to atelectasis or infarction after pulmonary emboli (PE) may be manifest on the chest X-ray by diaphragmatic elevation. Diminished lung volume and possibly lowered airway $p(CO_2)$ may induce bronchoconstriction, leading to expiratory wheezing. Arterial hypoxaemia typically occurs with diminished arterial O_2 saturation ($S_a(O_2)$ from 94 to 85%), but $S_a(CO_2)$ may be normal. Hypoxaemia is due to right-to-left shunting in areas of partial or complete atelectasis not affected by embolisation. Ventilation/perfusion imbalance probably also contributes to hypoxaemia. The mechanisms responsible for the ventilation/perfusion imbalance and atelectasis are not fully defined. In massive PE, severe hypoxaemia may result from right atrial hypertension that causes right-to-left shunting of blood through a patent foramen ovale. Low venous O_2 tension may also contribute to development of arterial hypoxaemia.

3.52

Answer: D   On the carotid and aortic chemoreceptors

The carotid and aortic bodies are able to monitor the physically dissolved O_2 and CO_2 and the H^+ concentration of arterial blood. These chemoreceptors are stimulated by a decline in the $p(O_2)$, especially when it falls below 60 mmHg. They are also stimulated by an increase in the arterial blood H^+ concentration (decreased pH) or an increase in physically dissolved CO_2 (or $p(CO_2)$). While it is not clear precisely how increases in H^+ or CO_2 or decreases in the $p(O_2)$ stimulate the chemoreceptors, the peripheral chemoreceptors are the only sensors capable of detecting a fall in the $p(O_2)$. So, the peripheral chemoreceptors account for increases in ventilation resulting from hypoxia. However, these chemoreceptors only detect levels of physically dissolved O_2 and not the O_2 that is chemically attached to haemoglobin. In contrast to the peripheral receptors, the central chemoreceptors are not sensitive to changes in the $p_a(O_2)$ of cerebral blood or cerebrospinal fluid.

3.53

Answer: E   Increased residual volume

The best diagnostic test for evaluating patients with suspected chronic obstructive pulmonary disease (COPD) is lung function measured with spirometry. Key spirometrical measures may be obtained with a portable office spirometer and should include forced vital capacity (FVC) and the normal forced expiratory volume in the first second of expiration (FEV_1). The ratio of FEV_1 to forced vital capacity (FEV_1/FVC) normally exceeds 0.75. Patients with COPD typically present with obstructive airflow. A FEV_1/FVC ratio of less than 70% in a patient with a postbronchodilator FEV_1 of less than 80% of the predicted value is diagnostic for COPD. Severity is further stratified based on symptoms and FEV_1 values. A patient with severe disease has an FEV_1 of less than 50% of the predicted value; values below 30% of the predicted value represent very severe disease. Beyond office spirometry, complete pulmonary function testing may show increased total lung capacity, functional residual capacity and residual volume. A substantial loss of lung surface area available for effective oxygen exchange causes diminished carbon monoxide diffusion in the lung (*DL*co) in patients with emphysema. This finding may help distinguish COPD from asthma, because patients with asthma typically have normal *DL*co values.

respiratory

respiratory

3.54

Answer: B   Lung compliance

The development of acute respiratory distress syndrome (ARDS) starts with damage to the alveolar epithelium and vascular endothelium, resulting in increased permeability to plasma and inflammatory cells which pass into the interstitium and alveolar space, resulting in lung oedema. Damage to the surfactant-producing type II cells and the presence of protein-rich fluid in the alveolar space disrupt the production and function of pulmonary surfactant, leading to microatelectasis and impaired gas exchange. The pathophysiological consequences of lung oedema in ARDS include a decrease in lung volumes, compliance and large intrapulmonary shunts (blood perfusing unventilated segments of the lung). A fall in the residual volume is uniformly present and contributes to ventilation/perfusion inequality. It has been hypothesised that a defective surfactant may be partially responsible for the small lung volumes and that it may worsen oedema accumulation in ARDS (as increases in alveolar surface tension have been shown to increase lung water content by lowering interstitial hydrostatic pressure and increasing). The decrease in lung compliance is secondary to the increased lung recoil pressure of the oedematous lung, which clinically increases the work of breathing and leads to respiratory muscle fatigue.

3.55

Answer: D   Lungs

Hypoxic pulmonary vasoconstriction is a local response to hypoxia resulting primarily from constriction of small muscular pulmonary arteries in response to reduced alveolar oxygen tension. This unique response of pulmonary arterioles results in a local adjustment of perfusion to ventilation. This means that if a bronchiole is obstructed, the lack of oxygen causes contraction of the pulmonary vascular smooth muscle in the corresponding area, shunting blood away from the hypoxic region to better-ventilated regions. Skeletal muscle, heart, kidney and gut arteries all dilate under hypoxic conditions, resulting in increased blood flow to these organs.

3.56

Answer: A   2%

The bronchial circulation is part of the systemic circulation and receives about 2% of the cardiac output from the left heart. Bronchial arteries arise from branches of the aorta, intercostal, subclavian or internal mammary arteries. The bronchial arteries supply the tracheobronchial tree with both nutrients and O_2. Vascular pressures in the bronchial circulation are similar to those in other systemic vascular beds. About a third of the venous drainage from the bronchial circulation is via the azygos, hemiazygos and intercostal veins, which return bronchial venous blood to the right atrium. However, about two-thirds of bronchial capillary blood is thought to drain into anastomoses or communicating vessels that empty into the pulmonary veins. This vascular connection between the bronchial and pulmonary circulation is called the bronchopulmonary circulation. This communicating circulation adds a small volume of poorly oxygenated bronchial venous blood to the freshly oxygenated blood in the pulmonary vein.

3.57

Answer: A   10 ml

The total volume of fluid present in the intrapleural space is estimated to be only 2–10 ml. A small amount of protein is present in intrapleural fluid. At end expiration, mean intrapleural pressure (p_{pl}) is about 5 cm H_2O below atmospheric pressure (-5 cmH_2O) and p_{pl} becomes more subatmospheric with inspiration such that, at end inspiration of a typical tidal volume, p_{pl} may be -10 cmH$_2$O. The magnitude of the subatmospheric or 'negative' intrapleural pressure reflects the tendency of the lung to recoil or pull away from the inner chest cage. Because the intrapleural fluid is a liquid that cannot be expanded or contracted, it results in a 'negative' intrapleural pressure that becomes more 'negative' with lung inflation.

respiratory

3.58

Answer: A   +10 cmH$_2$O

Many pulmonary disorders can alter compliance of the lung, chest cage or both. So, a measurement of compliance can be a useful clinical assessment of a patient's respiratory system. To determine compliance of the respiratory system, changes in transmural pressures ($p_{in} - p_{out}$) immediately across the lung or chest cage (or both) are measured simultaneously with changes in lung or thoracic cavity volume. Changes in lung or thoracic cage volume are determined using a spirometer with transmural pressures measured by pressure transducers. For the lung alone, transmural pressure is calculated as the difference between alveolar (p_A; inside) and intrapleural (p_{pl}; outside) pressure. To calculate chest cage compliance, transmural pressure is p_{pl} (inside) minus atmospheric pressure (p_B; outside). For the combined lung–chest cage, transmural pressure or transpulmonary pressure is computed as:

$$p_A - p_B$$

p_A pressure is determined by having the subject deeply inhale a measured volume of air from a spirometer. The subject then exhales measured air volumes in several steps. After each expired air volume, the subject seals his or her mouth around a manometer and completely relaxes the respiratory muscles with the glottis open. The pressure recorded at the mouth is called relaxation or recoil pressure because the respiratory muscles are relaxed. In addition, the pressure measured at the mouth is the same as alveolar pressure (p_A) because the airway is open to the alveoli and no air flow is present (static conditions). Intrapleural pressure is approximated by convincing the subject swallow a balloon, attached to a pressure transducer, into the oesophagus. Oesophageal pressure closely reflects average intrapleural or intrathoracic pressure.

3.59

Answer: A   Enhanced alveolar stability

Because pulmonary surfactant lowers surface tension as alveolar radius decreases, alveolar pressure (p_A) is typically lower in smaller than in larger-radius alveoli during lung inflation. This causes smaller-radius alveoli to fill with air before the larger-radius alveoli, because opening or expanding pressures are lower. In addition, atelectasis (alveolar collapse) is prevented at end expiration because surface tension is low in alveoli with small radii. Surfactant also promotes alveolar stability along with alveolar interdependence. Surfactants also aid in keeping alveoli 'dry' because, if alveoli had a high surface tension, it would tend to draw fluid into the alveoli. Overall, the presence of surfactant lowers the muscle work necessary to inflate the lung. At the same time, surface tension increases as alveoli inflate, which contributes to lung recoil.

3.60

Answer: B   Increase in airway CO_2

The autonomic nervous system innervates the smooth muscle and secretory glands that surround the airway lumen from the trachea to the alveolar ducts. Parasympathetic cholinergic fibres (acetylcholine as transmitter) of the vagus nerve trunk stimulate constriction of airway smooth muscle and increase secretion of glandular mucus. So, increased parasympathetic stimulation tends to narrow the airway lumen from greater muscle contraction and mucus secretion to increase airway resistance. Sympathetic adrenergic fibres, especially those mediated via β_2-adrenergic receptors, cause smooth muscle relaxation and inhibit mucus gland secretion. So, sympathetic stimulation tends to reduce airway resistance.

Various chemical irritants, like smoke and dust, stimulation of arterial chemoreceptors or release of histamine and certain prostaglandins, can also evoke airway constriction. In addition, a local decrease in airway CO_2 may cause bronchoconstriction, while an increase in airway CO_2 can evoke bronchodilatation.

3.61

Answer: A   Elastance

The forces of elastance (compliance), frictional resistance and inertia have been identified as the forces that oppose lung inflation and deflation. About 60–66% of the total work performed by the respiratory muscles is used to overcome the elastic or compliance

respiratory

characteristics of the lung–chest cage, 30–35% is used to overcome frictional resistance and only 2–5% of the work is used for inertia. However, this partitioning of the opposing forces is altered by changes in tidal volume or breathing frequency.

3.62

Answer: C   500 ml

The vessels of the pulmonary circulation are very compliant (easily distensible) and so typically accommodate about 500 ml of blood in an adult man. This large lung blood volume can serve as a reservoir for the left ventricle, particularly during periods when left ventricular output momentarily exceeds venous return. So, cardiac output can be increased rapidly by drawing upon pulmonary blood volume without depending on an instantaneous increase in venous return. Because of this function, the lung is sometimes referred to as an 'accessory' heart.

3.63

Answer: C   15 mmHg

The hydrostatic pressure of the pulmonary circulation refers to the actual pressure inside pulmonary vessels relative to atmospheric pressure. Hydrostatic (blood pressure) in the pulmonary vascular bed is low compared with that of similar systemic vessels. The mean pulmonary arterial pressure is about 15 mmHg (ranging from about 13 to 19 mmHg) and is much lower than the average systemic arterial pressure of 90 mmHg. The pressure drop between pulmonary artery and capillary is small compared with that of systemic vessels because the lung lacks high resistance arterioles. The lack of arterioles minimises active regulation of lung blood flow distribution. In addition, there may be little damping of the arterial pressure pulse associated with right heart ejection (systole). During late diastole, blood flow in some lung capillaries, particularly at the lung apex, may momentarily cease.

3.64

Answer: A   10 mmHg

Driving pressure is the difference between inflow and outflow pressure. For the pulmonary circulation, this is the difference between pulmonary arterial (p_a) and left atrial pressure (p_{LA}). Normally, mean driving pressure is about 10 mmHg, computed by subtracting p_{LA} (5 mmHg) from p_A (15 mmHg). This is in contrast to a mean driving pressure of nearly 100 mmHg in the systemic circulation, where right atrial pressure is subtracted from aortic pressure. In the pulmonary circulation, a small driving pressure is adequate because of the relatively low resistance to blood flow:

$$\text{pulmonary driving pressure} = p_a - p_{LA}.$$

3.65

Answer: D   Nitric oxide

In the body, nitric oxide (known as the 'endothelium-derived relaxing factor' or 'EDRF', before its chemical structure was elucidated) is synthesised from arginine and oxygen by various nitric oxide synthase (NOS) enzymes and by sequential reduction of inorganic nitrate. The endothelium of blood vessels uses nitric oxide to signal the surrounding smooth muscle to relax, so dilating the artery and increasing blood flow. The production of nitric oxide is noted to be increased in high-altitude populations, which helps to avoid hypoxia in thin air. Nitric oxide is a key biological messenger, playing a role in a variety of biological process. These include blood vessel dilatation, neurotransmission, modulation of the hair cycle and penile erection. Nitric oxide is also generated by macrophages and neutrophils as part of the human immune response. It is toxic to bacteria and other human pathogens. Many bacterial pathogens have evolved mechanisms for nitric oxide resistance. Nitric oxide can contribute to reperfusion injury when excessive amounts produced during reperfusion (following a period of ischaemia) react with superoxide to produce the damageing free radical, peroxynitrite. Inhaled nitric oxide has been shown to help survival and recovery from Paraquat poisoning, which produces lung-tissue-damaging superoxide and hinders NOS metabolism.

respiratory

SECTION 4:
FLUIDS, ELECTROLYTES AND ACID–BASE PHYSIOLOGY – ANSWERS

4.1

Answer: E   Increase extracellular volume and decrease intracellular volume

Infusion of hypertonic sodium chloride solution increases both intracellular and extracellular osmolarity while increasing extracellular fluid volume and decreasing intracellular fluid volume by causing osmosis of water out of the cells into the extracellular compartment.

4.2

Answer: C   Her intracellular fluid volume will be greater

Sweating causes fluid loss and salt loss, mainly from the extracellular compartment. Replenishing the fluid volume (without replacement of the salt) will restore the total body water, but extracellular fluid volume will be reduced because of osmosis of water from the extracellular compartment into the intracellular compartment.

4.3

Answer: C   0 mmHg

The rate of filtration at any point along a capillary depends on a balance of forces sometimes called Starling's forces after the physiologist who first described their operation in detail. One of these forces is the hydrostatic pressure gradient (the hydrostatic pressure in the capillary minus the hydrostatic pressure of the interstitial fluid) at that point. The interstitial fluid pressure varies from one organ to another and there is considerable evidence that it is subatmospheric (about −2 to −3 mmHg) in subcutaneous tissue. It is positive in the liver and kidneys and is as high as 6 mmHg in the brain. The other force is the osmotic pressure gradient across the capillary wall (colloid osmotic pressure of plasma minus colloid osmotic pressure of interstitial fluid). This component is directed inward. So:

$$\text{fluid movement} = k[(p_c - p_i) - (\pi_c - \pi_i)]$$

where

k = capillary filtration coefficient

p_c = capillary hydrostatic pressure

p_i = interstitial hydrostatic pressure

π_c = capillary colloid osmotic pressure

π_i = interstitial colloid osmotic pressure.

In this question the net hydrostatic pressure across capillary wall is calculated as:

$1 \times$ [capillary hydrostatic pressure (17) − interstitial fluid hydrostatic pressure (−3)] − [plasma colloid osmotic pressure (28) − interstitial fluid colloid osmotic pressure (8)] = 0 mmHg

4.4

Answer: A   Increased plasma colloid osmotic pressure

Increased capillary permeability, increased capillary pressure, increased interstitial fluid colloid osmotic pressure and lymphatic blockage would increase fluid movement into the interstitial spaces. Increased plasma colloid osmotic pressure, however, would oppose fluid movement from the capillaries into the interstitial compartment.

fluids

4.5

Answer: D   An increase in the molecular weight of the substance

The rate of diffusion of a substance is proportional to the difference in the concentration of the diffusing substance between the two sides of the membrane, the temperature of the solution, the permeability of the membrane and, in the case of ions, the electrical potential difference between the two sides of the membrane.

4.6

Answer: A   Transport fluid and proteins away from the interstitium to the blood

The lymphatic system performs all of the functions listed as options, but removal of fluid and proteins (especially proteins) is the most important physiological function. In the absence of a lymphatic system, the interstitial fluid protein concentration would increase greatly, causing widespread extracellular oedema.

4.7

Answer: D   Efferent arteriolar constriction

Constriction of efferent arterioles decreases peritubular capillary hydrostatic pressure, allowing greater amounts of fluid to be reabsorbed by the peritubular capillaries. Also, increased efferent arteriolar resistance reduces renal plasma flow while increasing glomerular filtration rate; this raises the filtration fraction and the concentration of protein in peritubular capillaries, thereby causing greater amounts of fluid to be reabsorbed. Decreased plasma protein concentration, decreased plasma colloid osmotic pressure, decreased filtration fraction and increased peritubular capillary hydrostatic pressure all lead to decreased peritubular capillary reabsorption.

fluids

4.8

Answer: C   Glomerular filtration rate

If a substance passes through the glomerular membrane with perfect ease, the glomerular filtrate contains virtually the same concentration of the substance as does the plasma and if the substance is neither secreted nor reabsorbed by the tubules, all of the filtered substance continues on into the urine. Therefore, the plasma clearance of the substance is equal to the glomerular filtration rate. Inulin clearance is commonly used as a measure of glomerular filtration rate because it is freely filtered, but neither secreted nor reabsorbed by the kidney tubules.

4.9

Answer: E   200 ml/min

The glomerular filtration rate is equal to the inulin clearance because inulin, a low-molecular-weight polysaccharide, is freely filtered into Bowman's capsule but is not reabsorbed or secreted. The clearance (C) of any substance can be calculated as follows: $C = (U \times V)/P$, where U and P are the urine and plasma concentrations of the substance, respectively and V is the urine flow rate. So, glomerular filtration rate = $(1.0 \times 2.0)/0.01 = 200$ ml/min.

4.10

Answer: D   88 ml/min

The clearance (C) of any substance can be calculated as follows: $C = (U \times V)/P$, where U and P are the urine and plasma concentrations of the substance, respectively and V is the urine flow rate. So, glomerular filtration rate = $(0.220 \times 2.0)/0.005 = 88$ ml/min. (Values in mmol/l changed to mol/l by dividing by 1000.)

fluids

4.11

Answer: D   Glucose

Under normal conditions the renal clearance of glucose is zero, since glucose is completely reabsorbed in the renal tubules and not excreted.

4.12

Answer: C   Distal end of the ascending loop of Henlé

Fluid in the distal end of the ascending limb of loop of Henlé is hypotonic regardless of the state of hydration because of the active reabsorption of sodium chloride but not water, which is impermeant in this tubular segment. In dehydration, the late distal convoluted tubule and the collecting duct become more and more hypertonic in the presence of ADH (antidiuretic hormone), which increases permeability of these tubular segments. The glomerular filtrate and proximal tubule have the same tonicity as plasma.

4.13

Answer: D   Increased urinary volume and a very dilute urine

Destruction of the supraoptic nuclei of the brain removes the source of ADH and therefore makes the distal tubule and collecting ducts impermeable to water. For this reason water fails to be reabsorbed in these parts of the tubules, causing a large volume of diluted urine.

4.14

Answer: A   Increased secretion of K+ by the distal and collecting tubules

The majority of potassium (K+) in the body is stored intracellularly at about 40–50 mmol/kg. Only about 2% is distributed in the extracellular fluid compartment. The relative distribution of K+ in the intracellular fluid vs extracellular fluid can be affected by insulin/glucose (which tends to move K+ into cells) or acid–base balance (acidosis tends to keep K+ out of cells). Usual dietary intake

fluids

of K$^+$ varies from 80 to 150 mmol/day. Dietary intake of K$^+$ in excess of daily requirements must be excreted in urine and stools ('what goes in must come out'). The renal handling of K$^+$ is similar to sodium in many ways, except there is secretion in addition to filtration, reabsorption and excretion. In the glomerulus, K$^+$ is freely filtered and, in the proximal tubule, it is reabsorbed like sodium and water (isotonic reabsorption due to facilitated transport with Na$^+$, TF/UF = 1). In the loop of Henlé, the thin descending limb is impermeable to K$^+$, while the thin ascending limb is permeable to K$^+$. In the thick ascending limb of loop of Henlé, K$^+$ reabsorption occurs secondary to Na$^+$/K$^+$/2Cl$^-$ pump action. If Cl$^-$ reabsorption is blocked, K$^+$ reabsorption will be blocked as well. Secretion of K$^+$ occurs in the cortical collecting duct, whereas both secretion and reabsorption occur in the medullary collecting duct. K$^+$ reabsorption is linked to Na$^+$ reabsorption up to, but not including, the distal tubules. From the distal tubule and on, K$^+$ is secreted and can be influenced by factors such as aldosterone. Very distally, K$^+$ handling (secretion and reabsorption) becomes independent of Na$^+$, enabling the body to make minor corrections to stay in Na$^+$ and K$^+$ balance.

4.15

Answer: D   40   25.0   7.41

Blood pH is normally maintained at 7.36–7.44. pH is a logarithmic scale. A change in pH of 0.3 units is equivalent to a doubling of hydrogen ion concentration. pH is maintained by biological buffering mechanisms involving:

- proteins
- bicarbonate
- haemoglobin
- blood gas analyser measures
- partial pressure of oxygen ($p(O_2)$)
- partial pressure of carbon dioxide ($p(CO_2)$)
- pH.

Other variables are derived using Henderson–Hasselbalch equation.

Table: Variables derived from a blood gas analyser

Variable	Normal value
Temperature	37 °C
pH	7.36–7.44
Partial pressure CO_2 ($p(CO_2)$)	4.6–5.6 kPa (35–45 mmHg)
Partial pressure O_2 ($p(O_2)$)	10.0–13.3 kPa (80–100 mmHg)
Bicarbonate	22–26 mmol/l
Total carbon dioxide	24–28 mmol/l
Standard bicarbonate (SBC)	22–26 mmol/l
Base excess (BE)	−2 to +2 mmol/l
Standard base excess (SBE)	−3 to +3 mmol/l
Oxygen saturation	>95%
Haemoglobin	11.5–16.5 g/dl

4.16

Answer: C   35   17.5   7.32

Metabolic acidosis is a clinical disturbance characterised by a relative increase in total body acid. It can be induced by two basic mechanisms, as follows: an inability of the kidneys to excrete the dietary hydrogen (H^+) load and an increase in the generation of H^+ that is due to the addition of H^+ (lactic acid or ketoacids) or to the loss of bicarbonate (HCO_3^-) due to inappropriate wasting by the kidney or the gastrointestinal tract. Metabolic acidosis most commonly stimulates the central and peripheral chemoreceptors that control respiration, resulting in an increase in alveolar ventilation, which results in a compensatory respiratory alkalosis leading to a decrease in $p(CO_2)$.

4.17

Answer: E   60   37.5   7.42

Respiratory acidosis is a clinical disturbance that is due to alveolar hypoventilation. Production of carbon dioxide occurs rapidly and failure of ventilation promptly increases the partial arterial pressure of carbon dioxide ($p(CO_2)$). The reference range for $p(CO_2)$ is 35–45 mmHg. Alveolar hypoventilation leads to an increased $p(CO_2)$ (ie hypercapnia). The increase in $p(CO_2)$ in turn decreases the HCO_3^-/ $p(CO_2)$ and decreases pH. Hypercapnia and respiratory acidosis

fluids

occur when impairment in ventilation occurs and the removal of CO_2 by the lungs is less than the production of CO_2 in the tissues. In fully compensated respiratory acidosis, the plasma pH and $[H^+]$ are returned to nearly normal in the face of increased $p(CO_2)$ because of the compensatory rise in $[HCO_3^-]$ that occurs as a result of increased renal production of HCO_3^-.

4.18

Answer: A   29   22.0   7.50

Alkalosis, by definition, is a pathological state that causes or tends to cause an increase in blood pH. Hence, one can have an alkalosis with normal pH if compensation has occurred; alkalaemia is defined as a blood pH above 7.44. The term 'respiratory' in respiratory alkalosis refers to the primary respiratory mechanism responsible for the change. Hypocapnia (low $p(CO_2)$) develops whenever CO_2 elimination by the lungs exceeds tissue production. One or more of three basic mechanisms usually underlie respiratory alkalosis:

- hypoxia
- metabolic acidosis
- direct central nervous system stimulation of respiration.

In respiratory acid–base disturbances, changes in ventilation, and hence $p(CO_2)$, represent the primary disturbance and compensation occurs by alterations in plasma bicarbonate.

In chronic respiratory alkalosis, increased urinary bicarbonate excretion resists the pH change caused by hypocapnia. This renal compensation begins within several hours and takes several days for the maximal response. In acute respiratory alkalosis, an initial small decrease may occur in plasma bicarbonate concentration because of chemical mass action. Hypocapnia leads to increased formation of carbonic acid, to lowered plasma hydrogen ion concentration (alkalaemia) and to concomitant reduced plasma bicarbonate concentration. This is quantitatively less profound than renal compensation and is not related to change in bicarbonate excretion.

Formulae for estimating appropriate compensation in simple respiratory alkalosis (limit of compensation is [HCO$_3^-$] of approximately 15) include the following:

- acute alkalosis – change in pH = (change in $p(CO_2)$) × 0.08

- chronic alkalosis – change in pH = (change in $p(CO_2)$) × 0.003.

In uncompensated respiratory alkalosis plasma [HCO$_3^-$] is near normal.

4.19

Answer: B   33   32.0   7.61

In combined respiratory and metabolic alkalosis, there are two primary disturbances: decreased $p_a(CO_2)$ because of hyperventilation and increased plasma [HCO$_3^-$] either because of ingestion of base or loss of [H$^+$] (for example, vomiting of gastric acid). This leads to marked decrease in plasma [H$^+$].

4.20

Answer: D   Potassium

In normal circumstances more than 90% of the filtered load of K is reabsorbed by the proximal tubules and loops of Henlé and almost all K appearing in the urine has been secreted by the late distal tubules and collecting tubules. So the rate of excretion is usually independent of the rate of filtration, but is closely tied to the rate of secretion and control of K excretion is largely accomplished by control of the secretion rate. Around 65–70% of the filtered potassium is reabsorbed along with water in the proximal tubule and the concentration of potassium in the tubular fluid varies little from that of the plasma. The mechanisms involved are not completely understood. A large fraction of the reabsorption probably occurs by passive diffusion via the paracellular route. In addition a transport mechanism for K may exist in the apical membrane of tubular cells. In the thick ascending limb of the loop of Henlé, potassium

fluids

is transported out of the tubular fluid by the $Na^+-K^+-2Cl^-$ co-transporter. Some of this recycles back into the tubular fluid via K channels in the apical membrane but a fraction of it moves into the interstitial fluid. Approximately 20% of the filtered potassium is reabsorbed here. Note that transport out of the thick ascending limb establishes the potential for countercurrent trapping of potassium in the medulla in a manner similar to that for Na and NH_3. Potassium may be reabsorbed in the collecting tubule, perhaps by the H^+/K^+-ATPase mechanism. Both reabsorption and secretion can occur in this segment. Which process prevails depends upon the factors affecting each. Potassium is added to the tubular fluid by principal cells in the late distal tubule and in the cortical collecting tubule. K enters the secreting cells from the blood via the Na^+/K^+-ATPase pump. It then diffuses from the cell down the electrochemical gradient through K channels that exist in the luminal or apical membrane into the tubular fluid. The electrical gradient across the apical membrane opposes the exit of K from the cell but that gradient is reduced by the Na flux through the epithelial Na^+ channel (ENaC) in that membrane. So the chemical gradient dominates. A K–Cl co-transporter (symport) may also exist in the apical membrane and transport both K and Cl from the cell into the lumen.

4.21

Answer: E   Protein concentration

Interstitial fluid (or tissue fluid or intercellular fluid) is a solution that bathes and surrounds the cells of multicellular animals. It is the main component of the extracellular fluid, which also includes plasma, lymph and transcellular fluid. On average, a person has about 11 litres of interstitial fluid providing the cells of the body with nutrients and a means of waste removal. Plasma and interstitial fluid are very similar. Plasma, the major component in blood, communicates freely with interstitial fluid through pores and intercellular clefts in capillary endothelium. Interstitial fluid consists of a water solvent containing amino acids, sugars, fatty acids, coenzymes, hormones, neurotransmitters, salts, as well as waste products from the cells.

The composition of tissue fluid depends upon the exchanges between the cells in the tissue and the blood. This means that tissue

fluids

fluid has a different composition in different tissues and in different areas of the body. Not all of the contents of the blood pass into the tissue, which means that tissue fluid and blood are not the same. Red blood cells, platelets and plasma proteins cannot pass through the walls of the capillaries. The resulting mixture that does pass through is essentially blood plasma without the plasma proteins. Tissue fluid also contains some types of white blood cell, which help combat infection.

4.22

Answer: A   Equal

The Henderson–Hasselbalch (frequently misspelled *Henderson–Hasselbach*) equation in chemistry describes the derivation of pH as a measure of acidity (using K_a, the acid dissociation constant) in biological and chemical systems. The equation is also useful for estimating the pH of a buffer solution and finding the equilibrium pH in acid–base reactions.

Two equivalent forms of the equation are:

$$pH = pK_a + log_{10} [A^-]/[HA]$$

or

$$pH = pK_a + log_{10} [base]/[acid].$$

Here, pK_a is $-log_{10}(K_a)$ where K_a is the acid dissociation constant, that is:

$$pK_a = -log_{10}(K_a) = -log_{10} ([H_3O^+][A^-]/[HA])$$

for the reaction:

$$HA + H_2O \approx A^- + H_3O^+$$

In these equations, A^- denotes the ionic form of the relevant acid. Bracketed quantities such as [base] and [acid] denote the molar concentration of the quantity enclosed. Maximum buffering capacity is found when $pH = pK_a$ or when the number of free anions to undissociated acid is equal and buffer range is considered to be at a $pH = pK_a \pm 1$.

fluids

4.23

Answer: E Prolonged vomiting

Potassium is one of the body's major ions. Nearly 98% of the body's potassium is intracellular. The ratio of intracellular to extracellular potassium is important in determining the cellular membrane potential. Small changes in the extracellular potassium level can have profound effects on the function of the cardiovascular and neuromuscular systems. The kidney determines potassium homeostasis and excess potassium is excreted in the urine. The reference range for serum potassium level is 3.5–5 mEq/l, with total body potassium stores of approximately 50 mEq/kg (ie approximately 3500 mEq in a 70-kg person). Hypokalaemia is defined as a potassium level less than 3.5 mEq/l. Moderate hypokalaemia is a serum level of 2.5–3 mEq/l. Severe hypokalaemia is defined as a level less than 2.5 mEq/l. Hypokalaemia may result from conditions as varied as renal or gastrointestinal (GI) losses, inadequate diet, transcellular shift (movement of potassium from serum into cells) and medications. The important causes of hypokalaemia are:

Renal losses:

- renal tubular acidosis
- hyperaldosteronism
- magnesium depletion
- leukaemia (mechanism uncertain).

GI losses:

- vomiting or nasogastric suctioning
- diarrhoea
- enemas or laxative use
- ileal loop.

Medication effects:

- diuretics (most common cause)
- β-adrenergic agonists
- steroids

fluids

- theophylline

- aminoglycosides.

Transcellular shift:

- insulin

- alkalosis.

Malnutrition or decreased dietary intake, parenteral nutrition.

4.24

Answer: C   Diffusion through channels between endothelial cells

Capillaries are the smallest of the body's blood vessels, measuring 5–10 μm. They connect arterioles and venules and they are the blood vessels that most closely interact with tissues. The walls of capillaries are composed of only a single layer of cells, the endothelium. This layer is so thin that molecules such as oxygen, water and lipids can pass through it by diffusion and enter the tissues. Waste products such as carbon dioxide and urea can diffuse back into the blood to be carried away for removal from the body. Capillary permeability can be increased by the release of certain cytokines. Ion channels are pore-forming proteins that help to establish and control the small voltage gradient that exists across the plasma membrane of all living cells by allowing the flow of ions down their electrochemical gradient. An ion channel is an integral membrane protein or more typically an assembly of several proteins. Such 'multi-subunit' assemblies usually involve a circular arrangement of identical or homologous proteins closely packed around a water-filled pore through the plane of the membrane or lipid bilayer. The pore-forming subunit(s) are called the alpha subunit, while the auxiliary subunits are denoted beta, gamma and so on. While some channels permit the passage of ions based solely on charge, the archetypal channel pore is just one or two atoms wide at its narrowest point. It conducts a specific species of ion such as sodium or potassium and conveys them through the membrane in single file – nearly as quickly as the ions move through free fluid. In some ion channels, passage through the pore is governed by a 'gate', which may be opened or closed by chemical or electrical signals, temperature or mechanical force, depending on the variety of channel.

fluids

4.25

Answer: C   Severe diarrhoea

Severe diarrhoea, by causing fluid loss and loss of bicarbonate, will cause marked dehydration and metabolic acidosis.

4.26

Answer: B   It has a protein content of 20 mg/100 ml

Normal cerebrospinal fluid (CSF) is clear and colourless. It may be cloudy in infections; straw- or yellow-coloured if there is excess protein, as may occur with cancer or inflammation; blood-tinged if there was recent bleeding; or yellow to brown (xanthochromic) if caused by an older instance of bleeding. A series of laboratory tests analyse the CSF for a variety of substances to rule out possible medical disorders of the central nervous system. The following are normal values for commonly tested substances:

- CSF pressure: 50–180 mmH$_2$O
- glucose: 2/3 of plasma value: 50–80 mg/dl
- protein: 15–50 mg/dl
- leukocytes (white blood cells) total less than 5 per ml
- lymphocytes: 60–70%
- monocytes: 30–50%
- neutrophils: none.

Normally, there are no red blood cells in the CSF unless the needle passes though a blood vessel on route to the CSF. If this is the case, there should be more red blood cells in the first tube collected than in the last.

4.27

Answer: A   It is actively secreted by the choroid plexus

Cerebrospinal fluid (CSF), *liquor cerebrospinalis*, is a clear body fluid that occupies the subarachnoid space in the brain (the space between the arachnoid and pia layers of the meninges). It is a very pure saline solution with microglia and acts as a 'cushion' or buffer for the cortex. Cerebrospinal fluid also occupies the ventricular system of the brain and the spinal cord. It is a prime example of the separation of brain function from the rest of the body, as all CSF is generated locally in the brain. It is actively secreted by the choroid plexus, which is formed by specialised ependymal cells. The choroid plexus enters the lateral ventricles through the choroid fissure, along the line of the fimbria/fornix and the 3rd and 4th ventricles through their roofs. The CSF formed by the choroid plexuses in the ventricles, circulates through the interventricular foramina into the 3rd ventricle and then via the mesencephalic duct (cerebral aqueduct) into the 4th ventricle through two lateral apertures (foramina of Luschka) and one median aperture (foramen of Magendie). It then flows through the cerebromedullary cistern down the spinal cord and over the cerebral hemispheres. It is then allowed to flow into the venous system by the arachnoid granulations. The cerebrospinal fluid is produced by the ventricles (mostly the lateral ventricles) at a rate of 500 ml/day. Since the volume that may be contained by the brain is 150 ml, it is frequently replaced, exceeding amounts getting into the blood. This continuous flow through the ventricular system into the subarachnoid space and finally exiting into the venous system provides something of a 'sink' that reduces the concentration of larger, lipo-insoluble molecules penetrating into the brain and CSF. The CSF contains approximately 0.3% plasma proteins, (or 15–40 mg/dl, depending on sampling site). CSF from the lumbar region contains **15–45 mg/dl protein** (lower in children) and 50–80 mg/dl glucose (two-thirds of blood glucose). Protein concentration in cisternal and ventricular cerebrospinal fluid (CSF) is lower. Normal CSF contains **0–5 mononuclear cells**. The CSF pressure, measured at lumbar puncture, is 100–180 mmH$_2$O (8–15 mmHg) with the patient lying on the side and 200–300 mmH$_2$O with the patient sitting up. It has a lower pH than arterial blood. The CSF has many putative roles, including mechanical protection of the brain, distribution of neuroendocrine factors and facilitation of pulsatile cerebral blood flow (*see also* answer to 4.26).

fluids

4.28

Answer: C It breaks down in areas of brain that are infected

The blood–brain barrier (abbreviated BBB, not to be confused with the blood–cerebrospinal fluid barrier, a function of the choroid plexus) is a membrane that controls the passage of substances from the blood into the central nervous system. It is a physical barrier between the local blood vessels and most parts of the central nervous system and stops many substances from travelling across it. Throughout the body, the walls of the capillaries are made up of endothelial cells separated by small gaps. These gaps allow soluble chemicals within tissues to pass into the bloodstream, where they can be carried throughout the body and subsequently pass out of the blood into different tissues. In the brain, these endothelial cells are packed more tightly together, due to the existence of zonulae occludentes (tight junctions) between them, blocking the passage of most molecules. The blood–brain barrier blocks all molecules except those that cross cell membranes by means of lipid solubility (such as oxygen, carbon dioxide, ethanol and steroid hormones) and those that are allowed in by specific transport systems (such as sugars and some amino acids). Substances with a molecular mass higher than 500 Da generally cannot cross the blood–brain barrier, while smaller molecules often can. Many drugs are unable to pass the barrier, since 98% of them are heavier than 500 Da. In addition, the endothelial cells metabolise certain molecules to prevent their entry into the central nervous system; the most-studied example of this is L-DOPA. In addition to tight junctions acting to prevent transport between epithelial cells, there are two mechanisms to prevent passive diffusion through the cell membranes. Glial cells surrounding capillaries in the brain pose a secondary hindrance to hydrophilic molecules and the low concentration of interstitial proteins in the brain prevent access by hydrophilic molecules. The blood–brain barrier protects the brain from the many chemicals flowing around the body. Many bodily functions are controlled by hormones, which are detected by receptors on the plasma membranes of targeted cells throughout the body. The secretion of many hormones is controlled by the brain, but these hormones generally do not penetrate the brain from the blood, so to control the rate of hormone secretion effectively there are specialised sites where neurones can 'sample' the composition of the circulating

fluids

blood. At these sites, the blood–brain barrier is 'leaky'. These sites include three important 'circumventricular organs': the subfornical organ, the area postrema and the organum vasculosum of the lamina terminalis (OVLT).

4.29

Answer: D   Is relatively rich in glucose

The extracellular fluid (ECF) includes all fluids outside the cells. This fluid can be divided into three fluid departments:

- interstitial (in the tissue spaces) fluid

- blood plasma and lymph

- specialised compartments called *transcellular fluid*, eg cerebrospinal fluid, synovial fluid, humours of the eye, pleural, peritoneal and pericardial fluid and glandular fluids.

The extracellular fluid surrounds all the cells in the body and is in equilibrium with the intracellular fluid. So, its composition must remain fairly constant even though substances are passing into and out of the cells. The interstitial fluid, though called a fluid, is in a reality a gel-like composition made up of:

- water

- proteoglycan molecules (high-molecular-weight mucopolysaccharides) and collagen.

Advantages of a gel-matrix in contrast to just a fluid:

- proteoglycan molecules keep cells apart – easier diffusion of substances

- prevents fluid from pooling to the lower extremities

- hinders the spread of bacteria and other micro-organisms.

The extracellular fluid constitutes 40% of total body water, with intracellular fluid comprising the remaining 60%. It is relatively rich in glucose. In humans, the normal glucose concentration of extracellular fluid that is regulated by homeostasis is approximately

fluids

5 mmol. The pH of extracellular fluid is tightly regulated by buffers around 7.4. It contains more Na^+, Cl^-, HCO_3^- and less K^+, Ca^{2+}, Mg^{2+}, PO_4^{3-}, SO_4^{2-} and amino acids compared with intracellular fluid.

4.30

Answer: A   Crystalline amino acids

Total parenteral nutrition (TPN), is the practice of feeding a person intravenously, circumventing the gut. It is normally used following surgery, when feeding by mouth or using the gut is not possible, when a person's digestive system cannot absorb nutrients due to chronic disease or, alternatively, if a person's nutrient requirement cannot be met by enteral feeding (tube feeding) and supplementation. It has been used for comatose patients, although enteral feeding is usually preferable and less prone to complications. Short-term TPN may be used if a person's digestive system has shut down (for instance because of peritonitis) and they are at a low enough weight to cause concerns about nutrition during an extended hospital stay. Long-term TPN is occasionally used to treat people suffering the extended consequences of an accident or surgery. The preferred method of delivering TPN is with a medical infusion pump. A sterile bag of nutrient solution, between 500 ml and 4 l, is provided. The pump infuses a small amount (0.1–10 ml/h) continuously to keep the vein open. Feeding schedules vary, but one common regimen ramps up the nutrition over a few hours, levels off the rate for a few hours and then ramps it down over a few more hours, to simulate a normal set of meal times. The nutrient solution consists of water, glucose, salts, amino acids, vitamins and sometimes emulsified fats. Long-term TPN patients sometimes suffer from lack of trace nutrients or electrolyte imbalances. Because increased blood sugar commonly occurs with TPN, insulin may also be added to the infusion. Occasionally, other drugs are also added. Chronic TPN is performed through a Hickman line or a Port-a-Cath (venous access systems). In infants, sometimes the umbilical artery is used. Battery-powered ambulatory infusion pumps are used with chronic TPN patients and usually the pump and a small (100-ml) bag of nutrient to keep the vein open are carried in a waist pouch. Outpatient TPN practices are still being refined. Aside from their dependence on a pump, chronic TPN patients live quite normal lives.

4.31

Answer: A   Anasarca

Anasarca (or 'generalised oedema') is a condition characterised by widespread swelling of the skin due to effusion of fluid into the extracellular space. It is usually caused by either cardiac failure, liver failure or renal failure. It can also be created from the administration of exogenous intravenous fluid. Certain plant-derived anticancer chemotherapeutic agents, such as docetaxel, cause anasarca through a poorly understood capillary leak syndrome. This condition is also called leukophlegmatia.

4.32

Answer: D   Metabolic alkalosis

Metabolic alkalosis is a primary increase in serum bicarbonate (HCO_3^-) concentration. This occurs as a consequence of a loss of H^+ from the body or a gain in HCO_3^-. In its pure form, it manifests as alkalaemia (pH > 7.40). As a compensatory mechanism, metabolic alkalosis leads to alveolar hypoventilation with a rise in arterial carbon dioxide tension ($p_a(CO_2)$), which diminishes the change in pH that would otherwise occur. Normally, arterial $p_a(CO_2)$ increases by 0.5–0.7 mmHg for every 1 mEq/l increase in plasma bicarbonate concentration, a compensatory response that is very quick. If the change in $p_a(CO_2)$ is not within this range, then a mixed acid–base disturbance occurs. For example, if the increase in $p_a(CO_2)$ is more than 0.7 times the increase in bicarbonate, then metabolic alkalosis co-exists with primary respiratory acidosis. Likewise, if the increase in $p_a(CO_2)$ is less than the expected change, then a primary respiratory alkalosis is also present. The first clue to metabolic alkalosis is often an elevated bicarbonate concentration that is observed when serum electrolytes are obtained. Remember that an elevated serum bicarbonate concentration may also be observed as a compensatory response to primary respiratory acidosis. However, a bicarbonate concentration greater than 35 mEq/l is almost always caused by metabolic alkalosis. Calculation of the serum anion gap may also help to differentiate between primary metabolic alkalosis and the metabolic compensation for respiratory acidosis. The anion gap is frequently elevated to a modest degree in metabolic alkalosis because of the increase in the negative charge of albumin and the enhanced production of lactate. However, the only definitive way to diagnose metabolic alkalosis is by performing a simultaneous blood gases analysis, which reveals elevation of both pH and $p_a(CO_2)$ and increased calculated bicarbonate.

4.33

Answer: B   45 l, 30 l, 15 l

The total body water (TBW) content of humans is approximately 60% of body weight. Two-thirds is located in the intracellular and one-third in the extracellular compartment. So, in a 75-kg individual, TBW = 60 × 75/100 = 45 l. Intracellular content = 2/3 × 45 = 30 l and extracellular content = 1/3 × 45 = 15 l.

4.34

Answer: C   Nothing per oral regimen

In this patient the cause for hypokalaemia is insufficient consumption of potassium as he is nil-by-mouth with no intravenous supplementation.

4.35

Answer: E   Increased level of angiotensin II

Thirst is the basic need or instinct of humans or animals to drink. It arises from a lack of fluids and/or an increase in the concentration of certain osmolites such as salt. If the water volume of the body falls below a certain threshold or the osmolite concentration becomes too high, the brain signals thirst. The osmolite concentration in the blood is measured with specialised sensors in the hypothalamus, notably in two circumventricular organs that lack an effective blood–brain barrier, the organum vasculosum of the lamina terminalis and the subfornical organ. These areas project to the supraoptic nucleus and paraventricular nucleus, which contain neurones that secrete the antidiuretic hormone, vasopressin, from their nerve endings in the posterior pituitary, but also project to other hypothalamic areas, including especially the median preoptic nucleus, to trigger thirst. Continuous dehydration can cause myriad problems, but is most often associated with neurological problems such as seizures and renal problems. Excessive thirst, known as polydipsia, along with excessive urination, known as polyuria, may be an indication of diabetes. Angiotensin II is a hormone that is a powerful dipsogen (ie it stimulates thirst) that acts via the subfornical organ.

4.36

Answer: D   Severe diarrhoea or vomiting

The electrolyte disturbance hyponatraemia exists in humans when the sodium level in the plasma falls below 135 mmol/l. At lower levels water intoxication may result, an urgently dangerous condition. Hyponatraemia is an abnormality that can occur in isolation or, as most often is the case, as a complication of other medical illnesses. Severe hyponatraemia may cause osmotic shift of water from the plasma into the brain cells. Typical symptoms include nausea, vomiting, headache and malaise. As the hyponatraemia worsens, confusion, diminished reflexes, convulsions, stupor or coma may occur. Since nausea is, itself, a stimulus for the release of ADH (the water-retaining hormone), the potential for a vicious circle of hyponatraemia and its symptoms exists.

4.37

Answer: B   Metabolic acidosis

Sodium bicarbonate injection is indicated in the treatment of metabolic acidosis, which may occur in severe renal disease, uncontrolled diabetes, circulatory insufficiency due to shock or severe dehydration, extracorporeal circulation of blood, cardiac arrest and severe primary lactic acidosis. Sodium bicarbonate is further indicated in the treatment of certain drug intoxications, including barbiturates (where dissociation of the barbiturate protein complex is desired), in poisoning by salicylates or methyl alcohol and in haemolytic reactions requiring alkalinisation of the urine to diminish nephrotoxicity of blood pigments. Sodium bicarbonate also is indicated in severe diarrhoea, which is often accompanied by

fluids

a significant loss of bicarbonate.

Treatment of metabolic acidosis should, if possible, be superimposed on measures designed to control the primary cause of the acidosis – eg insulin in uncomplicated diabetes, blood volume restoration in shock. However, since an appreciable time interval may elapse before all of the ancillary effects are brought about, therapy is indicated to minimise risks inherent to the acidosis itself. Caution with bicarbonate therapy is indicated because of its potential complications, including the following:

- volume overload
- hypokalaemia
- CNS acidosis
- hypercapnia
- tissue hypoxia via leftward shift of the haemoglobin–oxygen dissociation curve
- alkali stimulation of organic acidosis (lactate)
- overshoot alkalosis.

4.38

Answer: B   Increase in extracellular fluid volume

In medicine, saline is a solution of sodium chloride in sterile water, used commonly for intravenous injection. Sodium chloride (NaCl) is ordinary salt. Saline solutions are available in various concentrations for different purposes. Normal saline is the solution of 0.9% w/v of NaCl (this nomenclature is confusing – 'normal sodium chloride' to a chemist means a concentration of 5.85% w/v, also expressed as 1 N NaCl$_{(aq)}$). It contains 154 mEq/l of Na$^+$ and Cl$^-$. It has a slightly higher degree of osmolality (ie more solute per litre) than blood (hence, though it is referred to as being isotonic with blood in clinical contexts, this is a technical inaccuracy): about 300 mOsm/l. Normal saline is therefore used frequently in intravenous drips for patients who cannot take fluids orally and have developed severe dehydration. Normal saline is typically the first fluid used when dehydration is severe enough to threaten the adequacy of blood

fluids

circulation and is the safest fluid to give quickly in large volumes. Other concentrations of saline are frequently used for other purposes, such as supplying extra water to a dehydrated patient or supplying the daily water and salt needs ('maintenance' needs) of a patient who is unable to take them by mouth. Because infusing a solution of low osmolality can cause problems, intravenous solutions with reduced saline concentrations typically have dextrose (glucose) added to maintain a safe osmolality while providing less sodium chloride. As the molecular weight (MW) of dextrose is greater, this has the same osmolality as normal saline but contributes less sodium to the circulation. Because dextrose monohydrate (MW 198, in contrast to MW 180 for glucose) is the commercial form of dextrose used in these preparations, 5% dextrose actually contains only 4.5 g/dl of glucose.

Concentrations commonly used include:

- half-normal saline (0.45% NaCl), often with 'D5' (5% dextrose), contains 77 mEq/l of Na+ and Cl− and 4.5 g/l glucose.

- quarter-normal saline (0.22% NaCl) has 39 mEq/l of Na+ and Cl− and always contains 5% dextrose for osmolality reasons.

- dextrose (glucose) 4% in 0.18% saline is used sometimes for maintenance replacement.

The amount of normal saline infused depends largely on the needs of the patient (eg ongoing diarrhoea or heart failure) but is typically between 1.5 and 3 litres a day for an adult.

4.39

Answer: D Metabolic acidosis with some respiratory compensation

With arterial blood pH of 7.33, the patient clearly has an acidosis. The first question you should ask yourself is, 'Is it respiratory or non-respiratory (metabolic)?' If it were respiratory, the $p_a(CO_2)$ would have been above normal. Since it is lower than normal, this indicates the acidosis is metabolic with some respiratory compensation in response to the acidaemia; uncompensated metabolic acidosis would show normal $p_a(CO_2)$. It is unlikely that the metabolic acidosis is due to diabetic ketoacidosis; if this were the case, you would expect glucose to be present in the urine.

4.40

Answer: A   Decreased ability to produce adequate urinary NH_4^+ excretion

In healthy subjects on a normal diet, about 70 mEq of hydrogen ion is produced each day (largely from oxidation of sulphur-containing amino acids). This would produce a progressive metabolic acidosis if the H^+ were not excreted in the urine as NH_4^+ and $H_2PO_4^-$. Both are decreased in the later stages of renal failure (eg from chronic glomerulonephritis). Since NH_4^+ excretion plays the major role in disposing of daily H^+, a deficiency in ammonium excretion explains the metabolic acidosis (probably simply a reflection of the diminished number of functioning nephrons). Hypoventilation or hyperventilation are not the cause of this patient's acidosis. Excess β-hydroxybutyric and acetoacetic acids (ie ketoacidosis) is unlikely in this patient. Decreased catabolism of methionine and cysteine also could not account for the metabolic acidosis.

fluids

SECTION 5:
RENAL PHYSIOLOGY –
ANSWERS

5.1

Answer: B   It is freely filtered and partially secreted

Clearance is defined as the volume of plasma cleared of a given substance per unit time. The formula to calculate the clearance of a substance is given as:

$$C_x = (U_x \times V)/P_x$$

where C_x is the clearance of substance X, U_x is the urine concentration of substance X, V is the urine flow rate and P_x is the arterial plasma concentration of substance X. So the units of clearance are volume/unit time (usually ml/min).

The clearance principle is utilised to calculate glomerular filtration rate (GFR). Inulin is a polymer of fructose utilised for measuring GFR as it is freely filtered. The normal range of GFR for men and women is:

- men: 97–137 ml/min

- women: 88–128 ml/min.

On the other hand, the clearance of para-aminohippuric acid (PAH) has been calculated to be, on the average, 625 ml/min. This means that a large proportion of the PAH (around 80%) is secreted at the tubules. In fact plasma is cleared of PAH in a single pass through the kidneys. So the clearance of PAH can be utilised to measure the total renal plasma flow. As the substance X in this question has renal clearance greater than inulin but less than PAH, it is freely filtered and partially secreted.

renal

5.2

Answer: D   Para-aminohippuric acid (PAH)

Renal blood flow (RBF) is the volume of blood delivered to the kidney per unit time. In humans, the kidneys together receive roughly 20% of cardiac output, amounting to 1 l/min in a 70-kg adult man. RBF is closely related to RPF, which is the volume of blood plasma delivered to the kidney per unit time. While the terms generally apply to arterial blood delivered to the kidneys, both RBF and RPF can be used to quantify the volume of venous blood exiting the kidney per unit time. In this context, the terms are commonly given subscripts to refer to arterial or venous blood or plasma flow, as in RBF_a, RBF_v, RPF_a and RPF_v. Physiologically, however, the differences in these values are negligible so that arterial flow and venous flow are often assumed to be equal.

Renal blood flow calculations are based on renal plasma flow and haematocrit (Hct). This follows from the fact that haematocrit estimates the fraction of blood consumed by red blood cells. Hence, the fraction of blood that is in the form of plasma is given by 1-Hct:

$$RPF = RBF/(1-Hct).$$

Alternatively:

$$RBF = \frac{RPF}{1-Hct}$$

Renal plasma flow is given by the Fick principle:

$$RPF = (U_x \times V) \div (P_a - P_v).$$

This is essentially a conservation of mass equation that balances the renal inputs (the renal artery) and the renal outputs (the renal vein and ureter). Put simply, a non-metabolisable solute entering the kidney via the renal artery has two points of exit, the renal vein and the ureter. The mass entering through the artery per unit time must equal the mass exiting through the vein and ureter per unit time:

$$RPF_a \times P_a = (RPF_v \times P_v) + (U_x \times V)$$

where P_a is the arterial plasma concentration of the substance, P_v is its venous plasma concentration, U_x is its urine concentration and V is the urine flow rate. The product of flow and concentration gives mass per unit time.

renal

As mentioned previously, the difference between arterial and venous blood flow is negligible, so RPF_a is assumed to be equal to RPF_v, so:

$$RPF_a \times P_a = (RPF_v \times P_v) + (U_x \times V).$$

Rearranging yields the previous equation for RPF:

$$RPF = (U_x \times V) \div (P_a - P_v).$$

Values of P_v are difficult to obtain in patients. In practice, PAH clearance is used instead to calculate the effective renal plasma flow (eRPF). PAH is freely filtered and it is net-secreted by the kidney, so that its venous plasma concentration is approximately zero. Setting P_v to zero in the equation for RPF yields:

$$eRPF = (U_x \times V) \div P_a$$

which is the equation for renal clearance. For PAH, this is commonly represented as:

$$eRPF = (U_{PAH} \div P_{PAH}) \times V.$$

Since the venous plasma concentration of PAH is not exactly zero (in fact, it is usually 10% of the PAH arterial plasma concentration), eRPF usually underestimates RPF by approximately 10%. This margin of error is acceptable considering the ease with which eRPF is measured.

5.3

Answer: C   300

Transport maximum (or T_m) refers to the point at which increases in concentration do not result in an increase in movement of a substance across a membrane. In renal physiology, the concept of transport maximum is often discussed in the context of glucose and para-aminohippuric acid (PAH). For both substances (as with all substances), the quantity excreted can be determined with the following equation:

excretion = (filtration + secretion) − reabsorption.

The body 'wants' to retain glucose and eliminate PAH. However, its ability to do so is proportionate to the channel proteins available for the transmission:

renal

- Glucose is not secreted, so *excretion = filtration – reabsorption*. Both filtration and reabsorption are directly proportional to the concentration of glucose in the plasma. However, reabsorption has a transport maximum of about 300 mg/dl in healthy nephrons, while filtration has effectively no limit (within reasonable physiological ranges). So, if the concentration rises above 300 mg/dl, the body cannot retain all the glucose, leading to glucosuria.

- PAH is not reabsorbed, so *excretion = filtration + secretion*. As with glucose, the transfer is at the proximal tubule, but in the opposite direction: from the peritubular capillaries to the lumen. At low levels, all the PAH is transferred, but at high levels, the transport maximum is reached and the PAH takes longer to clear.

In practice, the transport maximum is not all-or-nothing. As the concentration approaches the transport maximum, some of the channels are overwhelmed before others are. For example, with glucose, some sugar appears in the urine at levels much lower than 300 mg/dl. The point at which the effects start to appear is called 'threshold', and the difference between threshold and transport maximum is called 'splay'.

5.4

Answer: A   Acute nephritic syndrome

Acute nephritic syndrome is a group of disorders that cause inflammation of the internal kidney structures (specifically, the glomeruli). This is uncommon in developed countries due to improved hygiene and decreased post-streptococcal and other post-infection glomerulonephritis. However, it is still a common presentation in Third World countries. Children between 2 and 12 are most commonly affected, but it may occur at any age. Men predominate, especially with the serious cases. Predisposing factors/causes include:

renal

- Infections with group A streptococcal bacteria (acute post-streptococcal glomerulonephritis). In warm climates, the disease most commonly follows infected skin lesions and occurs more often in the summer. In cold climates the disease occurs more frequently because of streptococcal throat infection during winter months. The risk of developing acute nephritic syndrome depends on the type of streptococcal bacteria.

- Primary renal diseases: immunoglobulin A nephropathy, membranoproliferative glomerulonephritis, idiopathic rapidly progressive crescentic glomerulonephritis.

- Secondary renal diseases: subacute bacterial endocarditis, infected ventriculo–peritoneal shunt, glomerulonephritis with visceral abscess, glomerulonephritis with bacterial, viral or parasitic infections.

- Multisystem diseases: systemic lupus erythematosus (SLE), Wegener's granulomatosis, Goodpasture's syndrome, microscopic polyarteritis, mixed cryoglobulinaemia, Henoch–Schönlein purpura, haemolytic uraemic syndrome.

- Allergy: acute allergic tubulointerstitial nephritis. The prognosis of post-streptococcal glomerulonephritis (GN) is good. Outcome in SLE, systemic vasculitis and Goodpasture's syndrome is less favourable. The risk of progression to end-stage renal failure with post-streptococcal GN is very small for children but becomes worse with increasing age. In adults, 5% have persistent proteinuria, hypertension and reduced renal function. Some of these may progress to end-stage renal failure.

renal

5.5

Answer: B   75

To calculate the reabsorption rate of substance Z we use the following equation:

excretion = (filtration + secretion) − reabsorption.

As this substance is freely filtered, its filtration rate is equal to that of inulin. So substituting the values in the above equation we get:

25 = (100 + 0) − reabsorption

reabsorption = 100 − 25

reabsorption = 75 mg/min.

5.6

Answer: E   Surreptitious use of diuretics

The laboratory data suggests hypokalaemic metabolic alkalosis. Of all the options given in this question, surreptitious use of diuretics is most likely to cause this picture. Thiazides and loop diuretics enhance sodium chloride excretion in the distal convoluted tubule and the thick ascending loop, respectively. These agents cause metabolic alkalosis by chloride depletion and by increased delivery of sodium ions to the collecting duct, which enhances potassium ion and hydrogen ion secretion. Volume depletion also stimulates aldosterone secretion, which enhances sodium ion reabsorption in the collecting duct and increases hydrogen ion and potassium secretion in this segment. Urine chloride is low after discontinuation of diuretic therapy, while it is high during active diuretic use.

5.7

Answer: D   Plasma renin

The evaluation of a patient in whom hyperaldosteronism is suggested has several distinct stages. The finding of hypertension, hypokalaemia or both most commonly precipitates the decision to screen. The presence of these two features together has a 50% predictive value.

renal

The first step entails confirmation that hyperaldosteronism is present and, if it is not present, exclusion of other conditions that produce a similar picture. The next step involves differentiating primary from secondary causes of hyperaldosteronism. The aldosterone-to-renin ratio (ARR) is the most sensitive means of differentiating primary from secondary causes of hyperaldosteronism. It can be obtained under random conditions of sodium intake. Values obtained in the upright position (standing for 2 h) have greater sensitivity than supine test results. Patients should be normokalemic because hypokalaemia suppresses aldosterone secretion. A ratio of plasma aldosterone (ng/dl) to plasma renin activity (ng/ml/h) of greater than 20 with a plasma aldosterone level greater than 15 ng/dl is highly suggestive of primary aldosteronism. The principle behind this test is that, as aldosterone secretion rises, plasma renin activity (PRA), a measure of the rate of production of angiotensin I from endogenous angiotensinogen, in ex vivo testing should fall because of sodium retention. This negative feedback response should occur when the aldosterone levels are supraphysiological for that individual patient and PRA may fall well before plasma aldosterone is clearly increased. When using this screening test, the aldosterone must be elevated in addition to an elevated ARR because, with the more sensitive PRA assays, having an ARR in excess of 20 without having an elevated aldosterone is possible. The most important factors that can interfere with the diagnostic reliability of the ARR test are drugs and renal impairment. Beta-blockers can reduce PRA levels, leading to a falsely elevated ratio and dihydropyridine calcium antagonists (eg nifedipine) can reduce aldosterone levels, tending to lead to a falsely normal ratio in some patients with primary aldosteronism. Diuretics tend to induce secondary aldosteronism. Spironolactone, an aldosterone receptor antagonist, can raise plasma renin levels. Spironolactone and diuretics should be withheld for 6 weeks and β-blockers and dihydropyridine calcium antagonists should be withheld for 5–7 days before testing. Patients' hypertension can be controlled with diltiazem and α-blockers when testing for primary aldosteronism. Renal impairment can lead to a high aldosterone-to-renin ratio in patients without primary aldosteronism because fluid retention suppresses PRA and hyperkalaemia stimulates aldosterone secretion. After a positive screening test result, subsequent testing is directed at confirming aldosterone secretory autonomy and differentiating an aldosterone-producing adenoma, for which surgery is currently

renal

the first line of treatment, from idiopathic hyperaldosteronism, which is usually treated medically. The possibility of glucocorticoid-remediable aldosteronism, which accounts for approximately 1% of primary aldosteronism, should be kept in mind.

5.8

Answer: E   Nephrotic syndrome

Nephrotic syndrome is a disorder in which the glomeruli have been damaged, causing them to leak protein from the blood into the urine. It is a fairly benign disease when it occurs in childhood, but may lead on to chronic renal failure, especially in adults or be a sign of an underlying serious disease such as systemic lupus erythematosus or a malignancy. The most common sign is excess fluid in the body. This may take several forms:

- puffiness around the eyes, characteristically in the morning

- oedema over the ankles that is pitting (ie leaves a little pit when the fluid is pressed out, which resolves over a few seconds)

- fluid in the pleural cavity causing pleural effusion

- fluid in the peritoneal cavity causing ascites

- renal failure

- hypertension (rarely)

- some patients may notice foamy urine, due to a lowering of the specific gravity by the high amount of proteinuria.

- coagulation abnormalities: renal vein thrombosis is more common than thrombosis in non-renal circulation.

- lower back pain, usually in the kidney or bladder area.

- actual urinary complaints such as haematuria or oliguria are uncommon and are seen commonly in nephritic syndrome.

renal

Laboratory investigations will show:

- proteinuria (nephrotic syndrome is arbitrarily defined as urinary protein loss of greater than 3.5 g/day)

- hypoalbuminaemia (as is the case in this vignette)

- high levels of cholesterol (hypercholesterolaemia), specifically elevated LDL, usually with concomitantly elevated VLDL

- lipiduria.

5.9

Answer: C   Inulin

Glomerular filtration rate (GFR) is the volume of fluid filtered from the renal glomerular capillaries into the Bowman's capsule per unit time. Clinically, this is often measured to determine renal function. There are several different techniques used to calculate or estimate the glomerular filtration rate. The GFR was originally determined by injecting inulin into the plasma. Since inulin is not reabsorbed by the kidney after glomerular filtration, its rate of excretion is directly proportional to the rate of filtration of water and solutes across the glomerular filter. In clinical practice, however, creatinine clearance is used to measure GFR. Creatinine is an endogenous molecule, synthesised in the body, that is freely filtered by the glomerulus (but also secreted by the renal tubules in very small amounts). Creatinine clearance is therefore a close approximation of the GFR. The GFR is typically recorded in millilitres per minute (ml/min). The normal range of GFR for men and women is:

- men: 97–137 ml/min

- women: 88–128 ml/min.

GFR can decrease due to hypoproteinaemia. GFR can increase due to constriction of the efferent arteriole.

renal

5.10

Answer: B   Haemodialysis

The woman in this clinical vignette has developed renal failure as suggested by her laboratory investigations showing raised potassium, BUN and creatinine. She is a candidate for haemodialysis as peritoneal dialysis in the presence of laparotomy will not be a suitable choice. Haemodialysis is a method for removing waste products such as potassium and urea, as well as free water from the blood when the kidneys are incapable of this (ie in renal failure). It is a form of renal replacement therapy. Haemodialysis is typically conducted in a dedicated facility, a special room in either a hospital or a clinic (with specialised nurses and technicians) that specialises in haemodialysis. Although less typical, dialysis can also be done in a patient's home as home haemodialysis. The principle of haemodialysis is the same as other methods of dialysis: it involves diffusion of solutes across a semi-permeable membrane. Haemodialysis utilises countercurrent flow, where the dialysate is flowing in the opposite direction to blood flow in the extracorporeal circuit. Countercurrent flow maintains the concentration gradient across the membrane at a maximum and increases the efficiency of the dialysis. Fluid removal (ultrafiltration) is achieved by altering the hydrostatic pressure of the dialysate compartment, causing free water and some dissolved solutes to move across the membrane along a created pressure gradient. The dialysis solution that is used is a sterilised solution of mineral ions. Urea and other waste products, and also potassium and phosphate, diffuse into the dialysis solution. However, concentrations of sodium and chloride are similar to those of normal plasma to prevent loss. Bicarbonate is added in a higher concentration than plasma to correct blood acidity. A small amount of glucose commonly is also used. Note that this process is different from the related technique of haemofiltration.

5.11

Answer: B   Decreased oncotic pressure

The glomeruli of the kidneys are the parts that normally filter the blood. They consist of capillaries that are fenestrated (leaky, due to little holes called *fenestrae* or windows) and that allow fluid, salts

renal

and other small solutes to flow through, but normally not proteins. In nephrotic syndrome, the glomeruli become damaged due to diabetes, glomerulonephritis or even prolonged hypertension so that small proteins, such as albumin can pass through the kidneys into urine. Nephrotic syndrome is characterised by proteinuria (detectable protein in the urine) and low albumin levels in blood plasma. As a compensation, the liver begins to make more of all its proteins and levels of large proteins (such as α_2-macroglobulin) increase. Oedema usually occurs due to salt and water retention by the diseased kidneys as well as sometimes due to the reduced colloid oncotic pressure (because of reduced albumin in the plasma). Cholesterol levels are also increased and though the mechanism is not fully understood, it is thought to be due to the increased synthesis of lipoproteins in the liver. There is an increased tendency for thrombosis (up to 25%), perhaps due to urinary loss of inhibitors of clotting such as antithrombin III, as well as hypovolaemia due to movement of water from plasma into tissue (causing oedema). Similar loss of immunoglobulins increases the risks of infections and relevant immunisation is recommended against pneumococci, *Haemophilus influenzae* and meningococci.

5.12

Answer: A   Angio-oedema

Angio-oedema, also known by its eponym Quincke's oedema and the older term angioneurotic oedema, is the rapid swelling of the skin, mucosa and submucosal tissues. Apart from the common form, mediated by allergy, it has been reported as a side-effect of some medications, specifically angiotensin-converting enzyme (ACE) inhibitors. Additionally, there is an inherited form, hereditary angio-oedema, which is due to deficiency of the blood protein C1-esterase inhibitor. The outdated term, 'hereditary angioneurotic oedema', referred to the belief that it was a purely stress-related condition brought on by emotional trauma and/or neuroses. This inaccurate portrayal of hereditary angio-oedema caused many sufferers to be wrongly labelled as mentally unstable and they were frequently denied medical treatment for their symptoms. These symptoms are often excruciatingly painful, especially when the swelling occurs deep inside the gastrointestinal (GI) tract, bladder and reproductive

renal

organs. Modern medicine has since debunked the theory, so removing the word 'neurotic' from its name. Cases where angio-oedema progresses rapidly should be treated as a medical emergency as airway obstruction and suffocation can occur. Rapid treatment with adrenaline, often with an Epi-Pen, can be life-saving.

5.13

Answer: D Secondary active transport with sodium

Glucose is an essential substrate for the metabolism of most cells. Glucose transport through biological membranes requires specific transport proteins. Transport of glucose through the apical membrane of renal tubular as well as intestinal epithelial cells depends on the presence of secondary active Na^+–glucose symporters, SGLT-1 and SGLT-2, which concentrate glucose inside the cells, using the energy provided by co-transport of Na^+ ions down their electrochemical gradient.

5.14

Answer: E It will have no amino acids

The proximal tubule is the portion of the duct system of the nephron leading from Bowman's capsule to the loop of Henlé. The most distinctive characteristic of the proximal tubule is its brush border (or 'striated border'). The luminal surface of the epithelial cells of this segment of the nephron is covered with densely packed microvilli forming a border readily visible under the light microscope. The microvilli greatly increase the luminal surface area of the cells, presumably facilitating their reabsorptive function. The cytoplasm of the cells is densely packed with mitochondria, in keeping with the energetic requirements of the cells, reabsorptive activity. The table below summarises the reabsorptive functions of proximal tubule.

renal

Substance	% of filtrate reabsorbed	Comments
Salt and water	Approximately two-thirds	Much of the mass movement of water and solutes occurs in between the cells through the tight junctions via paracellular transport, which in this case is not selective. The solutes are absorbed isotonically, in that the osmotic potential of the fluid leaving the proximal tubule is the same as that of the initial glomerular filtrate or plasma
Organic solutes (primarily glucose and amino acids)	100%	Glucose, amino acids, inorganic phosphate and some other solutes are reabsorbed via secondary active transport through co-transport channels driven by the sodium gradient out of the nephron
Potassium	Approximately 65%	
Urea	Approximately 50%	
Phosphate	Approximately 80%	Parathyroid hormone (PTH) reduces reabsorption of phosphate in the proximal tubules, but because it also enhances the uptake of phosphate from the intestine and bones into the blood, the responses to parathyroid hormone (PTH) cancel each other out and the serum concentration of phosphate remains approximately the same

5.15

Answer: C   H$^+$ secretion occurs by active transport

To maintain normal plasma bicarbonate, the kidney must secrete H$^+$ into the tubular lumen. The processes of H$^+$ secretion and HCO$_3^-$ reabsorption occurs throughout the nephron, except in the ascending limb of the loop of Henlé. H$^+$ secretion permits conservation of HCO$_3^-$ via reclamation of filtered, (ie HCO$_3^-$ reabsorption) and regeneration of HCO$_3^-$ by urinary net acid excretion. H$^+$ secretion into the tubular lumen occurs by active transport and is coupled to Na$^+$ reabsorption; for each H$^+$ secreted, one Na$^+$ and one HCO$_3^-$ are reabsorbed. The renal epithelium secretes approximately 4300 mEq (mmol) of H$^+$ daily. Approximately 85% of

renal

the total H^+ secretion occurs in the proximal tubules. Approximately 10% of the total H^+ secretion occurs in the distal tubules, and about 5% occurs in the collecting ducts. H^+ secretion decreases the pH of the urine by making it more acidic.

5.16

Answer: C   Efferent arteriolar constriction

Increased renal blood flow increases the GFR, while reduced renal blood flow reduces GFR. Afferent arteriolar constriction results in decreased renal blood flow and decreased glomerular pressures, leading to decreased GFR. Efferent arteriolar constriction results in increased resistance to outflow from glomeruli. This results in increased glomerular pressure with resultant increased GFR. Sympathetic stimulation causes preferential afferent arteriolar constriction, which decreases renal blood flow and decreases glomerular pressure, resulting in decreased GFR. Angiotensin II induces contraction of mesangial cells, causing decreased glomerular capillary area with resultant reduction in GFR.

5.17

Answer: E   Proximal convoluted tubule

Glucose is reabsorbed almost 100% via sodium–glucose transport proteins (apical) and GLUT (basolateral) in the proximal convoluted tubule. Glycosuria or glucosuria is a condition of osmotic diuresis typical in those suffering from diabetes mellitus. It leads to excretion of glucose in the urine. Due to a lack of insulin, plasma glucose levels are above normal. This leads to saturation of receptors in the kidneys and occurs at plasma glucose levels above 11 mmol/l. 'Renal glycosuria', also known as 'renal glucosuria', is a rare condition in which glucose is excreted in the urine despite normal or low blood glucose levels. With normal kidney (renal) function, glucose is excreted in the urine only when there are abnormally elevated levels of glucose in the blood. However, in those with renal glycosuria, glucose is abnormally eliminated in the urine due to improper functioning of the renal tubules. In most affected individuals, the condition causes no apparent symptoms (asymptomatic) or serious

renal

effects. When renal glycosuria occurs as an isolated finding with otherwise normal kidney function, the condition is thought to be inherited as an autosomal recessive trait.

5.18

Answer: E   Pre-eclampsia

Pre-eclampsia is said to be present when hypertension arises in pregnancy (pregnancy-induced hypertension) in association with significant protein in the urine. Its cause remains unclear, although the principal cause appears to be a substance or substances from the placenta causing endothelial dysfunction in the maternal blood vessels. While blood pressure elevation is the most visible sign of the disease, it involves generalised damage to the maternal endothelium and kidneys and liver, with the release of vasopressive factors only secondary to the original damage. Pre-eclampsia may develop at varying times within pregnancy and its progress differs among patients; most cases present pre-term. It has no known cure apart from ending the pregnancy (induction of labour or abortion). It may also present up to 6 weeks post partum. It is the most common, dangerous complication of pregnancy and it may affect both the mother and the fetus. Pre-eclampsia is diagnosed when a pregnant woman develops high blood pressure (two separate readings taken at least 6 h apart of 140/90 or more) and 300 mg of protein in a 24-h urine sample (proteinuria). Swelling or oedema, (especially in the hands and face) was originally considered an important sign for a diagnosis of pre-eclampsia, but in current medical practice only hypertension and proteinuria are necessary for a diagnosis. However, unusual swelling, particularly of the hands, feet or face, notable by leaving an indentation when pressed on, can be significant and should be investigated.

5.19

Answer: A   Creatinine clearance

Live donation is split into four groups. Within the living-related (LR) group there are three types. The HLA-identical group comprise usually brothers and sisters with the same genetic make-up. The

renal

1-haplotype mismatch group account for the greatest percentage of live donor transplants and include brother, sister and mother. The 2-haplotype mismatch group also include sister, brother and grandmother. Lastly there is the living-unrelated (LUR) group. The survival rates are definitely better than those of cadaver transplants. There are, however, differences within each of the live donor groups. It is estimated that the half-life of an HLA-identical kidney is between 24 and 26 years and as most patients in this group are around 35 years of age, most will only ever require one transplant in their lifetime. In the 1-haplotype group, half-life is approximately 11–12 years. Patients in this group tend to be slightly older (around 45 years) and it is estimated that approximately 50% of patients have a treatment for life. The half-life of the 2-haplotype and LUR kidney is similar to that of the cadaveric kidney, around 9–10 years, but it is reported that the live-donor group experience fewer rejection episodes, need less immunosuppression and have reduced complications from immunosuppression as a result.

Additionally, graft function following live donation is usually much quicker (normally immediate) compared with cadaver kidneys and fewer problems are experienced with acute tubular necrosis (ATN). This is believed to be associated with shorter delays in transplanting the organ. This is called the cold ischaemic time, in which the kidney, after removal, is perfused to enhance preservation. In live kidney transplantation the organ is transplanted almost immediately, limiting the ischaemic time of the kidney, whereas the cadaveric kidney may have a 12–48-hour delay before being transplanted, so lengthening the ischaemic time and resulting in delayed function of the kidney.

Most problems encountered with live donation are associated with the donor. Firstly, there are the potentially harmful investigative procedures carried out in the assessment phase, the most hazardous being renal angiography, where there is cannulation of the artery and injection of a radio-opaque dye to determine the blood supply to the kidney. Secondly, there are the short-term risks of nephrectomy surgery. According to the literature, there is a mortality rate of between 1 in 1600 and 1 in 3000, but this no more than is associated with any anaesthetic. Other associated risks come with most major abdominal surgery and include haemorrhage, chest and wound infection, pneumothorax, prolonged ileus, thrombosis and, most importantly, pulmonary embolism, which is the most common cause of death following nephrectomy. In the initial postoperative period creatinine clearance may be decreased but this recovers fully over a few weeks to months.

Long-term complications include prolonged wound pain. Initially this is alleviated with the help of opiate analgesia. Hypertension is often noted in the literature as a long-term complication of kidney donation and carries a risk of about 30%, but it is also noted that this is no more than in other people of the same age group. Patients are also told of the possibility of developing proteinuria, which is an early sign of kidney disease; however, many studies have failed to show any significant increase associated with renal impairment. It is therefore necessary for long-term follow-up of these patients to minimise the potential morbidity from associated problems of kidney donation. In clinical terms, live kidney donation is considered to carry a minimal risk and with the benefits for the recipient would seem a potentially valuable source for organ retrieval.

5.20

Answer: B   Form the juxtaglomerular apparatus in combination the macula densa and juxtaglomerular cells

The mesangium is an inner layer of the glomerulus, within the basement membrane surrounding the glomerular capillaries. This term is often used interchangeably with mesangial cells, but in this context refers specifically to the intraglomerular mesangial cells. These cells are phagocytic and secrete the amorphous basement membrane-like material known as the mesangial matrix. They are typically separated from the lumen of the capillaries by endothelial cells. The other type of cells in the mesangium are the extraglomerular mesangial cells. Extraglomerular mesangial cells (or lacis cells) are light-staining cells in the kidney found outside the glomerulus, near the vascular pole and macula densa. Lacis cells form the juxtaglomerular apparatus in combination with two other types of cells: the macula densa of the distal convoluted tubule and juxtaglomerular cells of the afferent arteriole. This apparatus controls blood pressure through the renin–angiotensin–aldosterone system.

renal

5.21

Answer: A   Forms part of juxtaglomerular complex

The distal convoluted tubule (DCT) is a portion of nephron between the loop of Henlé and the collecting duct system. It is partly responsible for the regulation of potassium, sodium, calcium and pH:

- It regulates pH by absorbing bicarbonate and secreting protons (H^+) into the filtrate.

- Sodium and potassium levels are controlled by secreting K^+ and absorbing Na^+. Sodium absorption by the distal tubule is mediated by the hormone aldosterone. Aldosterone increases sodium reabsorption. Sodium and chlorine (salt) reabsorption are also mediated by a group of kinases called WNK kinases. There are four different WNK kinases, WNK1, WNK2, WNK3 and WNK4.

- It also participates in calcium regulation by absorbing Ca^{2+} in response to parathyroid hormone.

- Arginine vasopressin receptor 2 is also expressed in the DCT.

Histologically, cells of the DCT can be differentiated from cells of the proximal convoluted tubule (PCT):

Characteristic	PCT	DCT
Apical brush border	Usually have	Do not have
Eosinophilicity	More	Less
Cytoplasm	More	Less
Visible nuclei	Less likely	More likely

The macula densa of the distal convoluted tubule and juxtaglomerular cells of the afferent arteriole in combination with extraglomerular mesangial cells (or lacis cells) form the juxtaglomerular apparatus.

renal

5.22

Answer: E   Low plasma HCO_3^-

In chronic renal failure as the kidney function decreases:

- there is loss of ability to concentrate urine with resultant low urine specific gravity

- blood pressure is increased due to fluid overload and production of vasoactive hormones, leading to hypertension and congestive heart failure

- urea accumulates, leading to azotaemia and ultimately uraemia (symptoms ranging from lethargy to pericarditis and encephalopathy)

- potassium accumulates in the blood (known as hyperkalaemia with symptoms ranging from malaise to fatal cardiac arrhythmias)

- erythropoietin synthesis is decreased (leading to anaemia causing fatigue)

- fluid volume overload – symptoms may range from mild oedema to life-threatening pulmonary oedema

- hyperphosphataemia due to reduced phosphate excretion, associated with hypocalcaemia (due to vitamin D_3 deficiency) and hyperparathyroidism leads to renal osteodystrophy and vascular calcification

- metabolic acidosis, due to decreased generation of bicarbonate by the kidney, leads to uncomfortable breathing and further worsening of bone health.

CRF patients suffer from accelerated atherosclerosis and have a higher incidence of cardiovascular disease, with a poorer prognosis.

5.23

Answer: C   Renal transplant can be expected to restore abnormal calcium and phosphorous metabolism towards normal

Kidney transplantation or renal transplantation is the organ transplant of a kidney in a patient with end-stage renal disease. Kidney

renal

transplantation is typically classified as deceased-donor (formerly known as cadaveric) or living-donor transplantation depending on the source of the recipient organ. Living-donor renal transplants are further characterised as genetically related (living-related) or non-related (living-unrelated) transplants, depending on whether a biological relationship exists between the donor and recipient. The donor and recipient have to be ABO blood group compatible and should ideally share as many HLA and 'minor antigens' as possible. This decreases the risk of transplant rejection and need for dialysis and a further transplant. The risk of rejection after transplant may be reduced if the donor and recipient share as many HLA antigens as possible, if the recipient is not already sensitised to potential donor HLA antigens and if immunosuppressant levels are kept in an appropriate range.

The new kidney usually begins functioning immediately after surgery, but this may – depending on the quality of the organ – take a few days. Hospital stay is typically for 4–7 days. The glomerular filtration rate should be within the normal range for age and sex of the patient to label the transplant successful. If complications arise, additional medicines may be administered to help the kidney produce urine. Medicines are used to suppress the immune system from rejecting the donor kidney. These medicines must be taken for the rest of the patient's life even if the donor organ is from a living-related donor. The most common medication regimen today is: tacrolimus, mycophenolate and prednisone. Some patients may instead take ciclosporin, rapamycin or azathioprine. Acute rejection occurs in 10–25% of people after transplant during the first 60 days. Rejection does not mean loss of the organ, but may require additional treatment. Rejection involves both cellular and antibody mechanisms. Recent studies have indicated that kidney transplantation is a life-extending procedure and most metabolic and biochemical abnormalities are reversed.

5.24

Answer: A   Acidosis

Acute renal failure (ARF) is a rapid loss of renal function due to damage to the kidneys, resulting in retention of nitrogenous (urea and creatinine) and non-nitrogenous waste products that are normally excreted by the kidney. Depending on the severity and duration of the renal dysfunction, this accumulation is accompanied by metabolic disturbances, such as metabolic acidosis and hyperkalaemia, changes in body fluid balance and effects on many other organ systems. It can be characterised by oliguria or anuria (decrease or cessation of urine production), although *non-oliguric ARF* may occur. It is a serious disease and treated as a medical emergency. Metabolic acidosis and hyperkalaemia, the two most serious biochemical manifestations of acute renal failure, may require medical treatment with sodium bicarbonate administration and antihyperkalaemic measures, and if not appropriately treated can be life-threatening.

5.25

Answer: D   Stress incontinence

Urinary incontinence is the involuntary excretion of urine from one's body. It is often temporary and it almost always results from an underlying medical condition. It has several types. These include:

- Stress incontinence – essentially due to pelvic floor muscle weakness. It is loss of small amounts of urine with coughing, laughing, sneezing, exercising or other movements that increase intra-abdominal pressure and so increase pressure on the bladder. Physical changes resulting from pregnancy, childbirth and menopause often cause stress incontinence and in men it is a common problem following a prostatectomy. It is the most common form of incontinence in women and is treatable. The urethra is supported by fascia of the pelvic floor. If the fascial support is weakened, as it can be in pregnancy and childbirth, the urethra can move downward at times of increased abdominal pressure, resulting in stress incontinence. Stress incontinence can worsen during the week before the menstrual period. At that time, lowered oestrogen levels may lead to lower muscular pressure around the urethra, increasing chances of leakage. The incidence of stress incontinence increases following menopause, similarly because of lowered oestrogen levels. Urine analysis, cystometry and postvoid residual volume are normal.

renal

- Urge incontinence – involuntary loss of urine occurring for no apparent reason while suddenly feeling the need or urge to urinate. The most common cause of urge incontinence are involuntary and inappropriate detrusor muscle contractions.

  - *Idiopathic detrusor over activity* – local or surrounding infection, inflammation or irritation of the bladder.

  - *Neurogenic detrusor over activity* – defective central nervous system (CNS) inhibitory response.

  Medical professionals describe such a bladder as 'unstable', 'spastic', or 'overactive'. Urge incontinence may also be called 'reflex incontinence' if it results from overactive nerves controlling the bladder.

  Patients with urge incontinence can suffer incontinence during sleep, after drinking a small amount of water or when they touch water or hear it running (as when washing dishes or hearing someone else taking a shower).

  Involuntary actions of bladder muscles can occur because of damage to the nerves of the bladder, to the nervous system (spinal cord and brain) or to the muscles themselves. Multiple sclerosis, Parkinson's disease, Alzheimer's disease, stroke and injury – including injury that occurs during surgery – can all harm bladder nerves or muscles.

- Functional incontinence – occurs when a person does not recognise the need to go to the toilet, recognise where the toilet is or get to the toilet in time. The urine loss may be large. Causes of functional incontinence include confusion, dementia, poor eyesight, poor mobility, poor dexterity or unwillingness to toilet because of depression, anxiety or anger. People with functional incontinence may have problems thinking, moving or communicating that prevent them from reaching a toilet. A person with Alzheimer's disease, for example, may not think well enough to plan a timely trip to the toilet. A

renal

person in a wheelchair may be blocked from getting to a toilet in time. Conditions such as these are often associated with age and account for some of the incontinence of elderly women and men in nursing homes.

- Overflow incontinence - sometimes people find that they cannot stop their bladders from constantly dribbling or continuing to dribble for some time after they have passed water. It is as if their bladders were like a constantly overflowing pan – hence the general name overflow incontinence. Overflow incontinence occurs when the patient's bladder is always full, so that it frequently leaks urine. Weak bladder muscles, resulting in incomplete emptying of the bladder, or a blocked urethra can cause this type of incontinence. Autonomic neuropathy from diabetes or other diseases can decrease neural signals from the bladder (allowing for overfilling) and may also decrease the expulsion of urine by the detrusor muscle (allowing for urinary retention). Additionally, tumours and kidney stones can block the urethra. In men, benign prostatic hypertrophy may also restrict the flow of urine. Overflow incontinence is rare in women, although sometimes it is caused by fibroid or ovarian tumours. Spinal cord injuries or nervous system disorders are additional causes of overflow incontinence. Also, overflow incontinence in women can be from increased outlet resistance from advanced vaginal prolapse causing a 'kink' in the urethra or after an anti-incontinence procedure that has overcorrected the problem. Early symptoms include a hesitant or slow stream of urine when water is passed. Anticholinergic medications may worsen overflow incontinence.

- Mixed incontinence – stress and urge incontinence often occur together in women. Combinations of incontinence – and this combination in particular – are sometimes referred to as 'mixed incontinence'.

renal

5.26

Answer: E   Proximal convoluted tubule

Glucose, amino acids, inorganic phosphate and some other solutes are reabsorbed via secondary active transport in the proximal renal tubule through co-transport channels driven by the sodium gradient out of the nephron.

5.27

Answer: D   Renin

In the kidney, the juxtaglomerular cells (JG cells) are cells that synthesise, store and secrete the enzyme renin. They are specialised smooth muscle cells in the wall of the afferent arteriole that delivers blood to the glomerulus. In synthesising renin, they play a critical role in the renin–angiotensin system and so in renal autoregulation, the self-governance of the kidney. In appropriately stained slides, juxtaglomerular cells are distinguished by their granulated cytoplasm.

5.28

Answer: B   Distal convoluted tubule

In the kidney, the macula densa is an area of closely packed specialised cells lining the region of the distal convoluted tubule (DCT) lying next to the glomerular vascular pole. The cells of the macula densa are sensitive to the ionic content and water volume of the fluid in the DCT, producing molecular signals that promote renin secretion by other cells of the juxtaglomerular apparatus. The release of renin is an essential component of the renin–angiotensin–aldosterone system, which regulates blood pressure and volume. The cells of the macula densa cells are taller and have more prominent nuclei than cells surrounding the distal convoluted tubule. The close proximity and prominence of the nuclei cause this segment of the DCT's wall to appear darker in microscopic preparations, hence the name *macula densa*. A decrease in blood pressure results in a decreased concentration of sodium ions in the distal convoluted tubule. (This is due to reduced filtration by the glomerulus: less filtrate is expelled into Bowman's space and the proximal convoluted tubule; the resulting fluid reaching the distal convoluted tubule will have a lower

renal

sodium concentration after the water is removed.) In response, the macula densa cells release prostaglandins, which trigger granular juxtaglomerular cells lining the afferent arterioles to release renin into the bloodstream. The juxtaglomerular cells can also release renin independently of the macula densa, as they are also triggered by baroreceptors lining the arterioles and release renin if a fall in blood pressure in the arterioles is detected.

5.29

Answer: B   Extensive binding of drug to plasma proteins

Renal excretion of drugs will be reduced if they are extensively bound to plasma proteins, as plasma proteins are not filtered under normal conditions. All the rest of the options will either enhance renal excretion of drugs or increase their removal from the body.

5.30

Answer: C   Reduced active transport of sodium

The loop of Henlé is the portion of the nephron that leads from the proximal convoluted tubule to the distal convoluted tubule. It is named after its discoverer, F. G. J. Henlé. The loop has a hairpin bend in the renal medulla. Its primary function uses a countercurrent multiplier mechanism in the medulla to reabsorb water and ions from the urine. It can be divided into four parts:

Descending limb of loop of Henlé	The descending limb has low permeability to ions and urea, while being highly permeable to water
Thin ascending limb of loop of Henlé	The thin ascending limb is not permeable to water, but it is permeable to ions
Medullary thick ascending limb of loop of Henlé	Sodium (Na^+), potassium (K^+) and chloride (Cl^-) ions are reabsorbed by active transport. K^+ is passively transported along its concentration gradient through a K^+ channel in the basolateral aspect of the cells, back into the lumen of the ascending limb. This K^+ 'leak' generates a positive electrochemical potential difference in the lumen. The electrical gradient drives more reabsorption of Na^+, as well as other cations such as magnesium (Mg^{2+}) and, importantly, calcium (Ca^{2+})
Cortical thick ascending limb	The cortical thick ascending limb drains urine into the distal convoluted tubule

renal

The loop of Henlé is supplied by blood in a series of straight capillaries descending from the cortical efferent arterioles. These capillaries (called the vasa recta; *recta* is from the Latin for 'straight') also have a countercurrent exchange mechanism that prevents wash-out of solutes from the medulla, thereby maintaining the medullary concentration. As water is osmotically driven from the descending limb into the interstitium, it readily enters the vasa recta. The low blood flow through the vasa recta allows time for osmotic equilibration and can be altered by changing the resistance of the vessels' efferent arterioles. Also, the vasa recta still have the large proteins and ions that were not filtered through the glomerulus, which provide an oncotic pressure for water to enter the vasa recta from the interstitium.

5.31

Answer: E   A rise in the volume of urine passed in a given time

A normal person filters 25 000 mmol of sodium (Na^+) but excretes 150 mmol of Na^+ per day. Na reabsorption is coupled with absorption of water. If Na^+ excretion is changed by only 5%, this amounts to an excretion of 1250 mmol Na^+ in 9 l of fluid per day. So, even a seemingly small 5% change can lead to a huge difference in the normal ECF volume as well as urine volume.

5.32

Answer: A   Collecting ducts

The collecting duct system is the last component of the kidney to influence the body's electrolyte and fluid balance. In humans, the system accounts for 4–5% of the kidney's reabsorption of sodium and 5% of the kidney's reabsorption of water. At times of extreme dehydration, over 24% of the filtered water may be reabsorbed in the collecting duct system.

The wide variation in water reabsorption levels for the collecting duct system reflects its dependence on hormonal activation. The collecting ducts, particularly the outer medullary and cortical collecting ducts, are largely impermeable to water without the

renal

presence of antidiuretic hormone (ADH or vasopressin):

- in the *absence* of ADH, water in the renal filtrate is left alone to enter the urine, promoting diuresis

- when ADH is *present*, as is the case in this patient with haemorrhage, aquaporins allow for the reabsorption of this water, thereby inhibiting diuresis.

5.33

Answer: E   Urination will occur if inhibition of the external sphincter through spinal reflex pathways is stronger than the voluntary constrictor signals to the external sphincter from the brain

Urination occurs whenever the bladder pressure exceeds the sphincter tone. The external sphincter is a skeletal muscle innervated by motor neurones from the pudendal nerve, not by sympathetic fibres. As the bladder fills, sensory signals from bladder stretch receptors elicit a micturition reflex via parasympathetic fibres originating in the sacral spinal cord. These transient contractions elicit an urge to urinate, but normally urination does not occur unless the external sphincter relaxes. If the lumbar spinal cord is damaged while the sacral segments are intact, micturition reflexes will occur, resulting in spontaneous and uncontrolled bladder emptying (automatic bladder). If the sacral spinal cord is damaged, micturition reflexes are lost and the bladder fills to capacity, resulting in overflow incontinence (atonic bladder). Higher centres in the brainstem keep the micturition reflex inhibited except when micturition is desired.

5.34

Answer: A   Decreased sensitivity of blood vessels to angiotensin

Blood vessels of patients with Bartter's syndrome adapt to the increased angiotensin levels by down regulating their angiotensin II receptors. This explains why these patients usually have normal blood pressure. Patients with Bartter's syndrome have primary elevated renin due to idiopathic hyperfunction of the juxtaglomerular

renal

apparatus. Consequently, these patients have elevated levels of angiotensin II and aldosterone.

5.35

Answer: C   240 mmol/day

About 40% of total plasma Ca^{2+} is bound to proteins and not filtered at the glomerular basement membrane. Therefore, the estimated daily filtered load is 1.5 mmol/l × 160 l/day = 240 mmol/day. The exact amount of free versus total Ca^{2+} depends on the blood pH: free Ca^{2+} increases during acidosis and decreases during alkalosis.

5.36

Answer: B   Of a combination of pore size and negative charges lining the pores

Glomerular pores have a diameter of approximately 8 nm. Albumin, the smallest serum protein (with a molecular weight of 69 000) has a diameter of approximately 6 nm and therefore pore size alone cannot explain the virtual absence of albumin in the urine. However, albumin is prevented from passing through the pores by electrostatic repulsion, since the pores are lined by negative charges and albumin, like most serum proteins, is itself negatively charged. Filtered amino acids and some very-low-weight proteins are reabsorbed in the renal tubules, but this does not explain the virtual absence of protein in the urine of this patient. Urine is usually sterile and filtered proteins are not metabolised.

5.37

Answer: C   Increase the per cent of filtered Na^+ excreted

Both Na^+ and K^+ excretion are tightly regulated. So, as GFR decreases in disease, the percentage of filtered Na^+ or K^+ that is excreted increases to maintain a normal amount of Na^+ or K^+ excretion (assuming Na^+ and K^+ intake remain the same). Substances like creatinine (almost exclusively excreted by glomerular filtration) and urea (some reabsorption) have no adaptive mechanisms to regulate plasma levels. So, a significant decrease in GFR results in significant increases in plasma creatinine and urea (assuming production of both substances remains constant). This is because the amount of substance X that is excreted ($U_x \times V$) equals the amount produced. Furthermore, $U_x \times V$ equals GFR $\times P_x$. If GFR decreases, P_x increases. Because of the increase in per cent filtered Na^+ and K^+ that is excreted, an increase in plasma Na^+ or a decrease in plasma K^+ would not be expected with a GFR that is 50% of normal. (U_x: urine concentration of x, P_x: plasma concentration of x, V: urine volume.)

5.38

Answer: B   Fall, since tubular secretion of potassium is inversely coupled to acid secretion

Secretion of acid and potassium by the renal tubule are inversely related. So, increased excretion of H^+ during renal compensation for respiratory acidosis will result in decreased secretion (or increased retention) of potassium ions, with the result that the body's potassium store rises. An increase in K^+ excretion would be associated with renal compensation for respiratory alkalosis. The filtered load of K^+ depends only on K^+ plasma concentration and glomerular filtration rate, not on plasma pH.

5.39

Answer: E   Substantial increases in renal blood flow

An increase in the rate of renal blood flow (RBF) greatly increases the glomerular filtration rate (GFR). The filtrate formed is derived by ultrafiltration of plasma in the glomerular capillaries. The more plasma available (from increased RBF), the more filtrate is formed. Vasoconstriction of glomerular afferent arterioles would not increase GFR but decrease it, because of a decrease in both RBF and capillary ultrafiltration pressure. Vasoconstriction of vasa recta has no direct impact on GFR, as vasa recta are involved with the countercurrent exchange mechanism. Because of the autoregulatory ability of the kidneys, an increase in mean arterial pressure from 90 mmHg to 140 mmHg would not have much of an effect on either RBF or GFR. Autoregulation acts to maintain a constant blood flow and capillary

renal

pressure by its influence on afferent arteriolar resistance. Strong, acute stimulation of sympathetic activity to the kidneys results in decreased RBF, decreased GFR and may produce renal shutdown with zero urinary output (*see also* answer to 5.16).

5.40

Answer: A　Decreased baroreceptor firing rate

Acute dehydration results in decreased plasma volume and increased plasma osmolarity, since more water than salt is lost in sweat. The decrease in plasma volume leads to an inhibition of the baroreceptors and a lower firing rate. The increase in plasma osmolarity leads to increased ADH secretion and high plasma ADH levels, which increases water permeability of collecting duct cells. Therefore more water is reabsorbed by the kidneys and renal water excretion is low.

5.41

Answer: B　Primary aldosteronism

Most patients with primary aldosteronism (Conn's syndrome) have an adrenal adenoma. The increased plasma aldosterone concentration leads to increased renal Na^+ reabsorption, which results in plasma volume expansion. The increase in plasma volume suppresses renin release from the juxtaglomerular apparatus and these patients usually have low plasma renin levels. Salt restriction and upright posture decrease renal perfusion pressure and therefore increase renin release from the juxtaglomerular apparatus. Secondary aldosteronism is due to elevated renin levels and may be caused by heart failure or renal artery stenosis.

5.42

Answer: E　Potassium-sparing diuretic

Potassium-sparing diuretics act by either antagonising the action of aldosterone (spironolactone) or inhibiting Na^+ reabsorption in the distal tubules (amiloride). Mannitol is freely filtered at the glomerulus, but in contrast to glucose is not reabsorbed and produces an osmotic

renal

diuresis. Clinically it is used to treat cerebral oedema and in prerenal azotaemia to convert oliguric acute renal failure. Thiazides inhibit Na^+ and K^+ reabsorption in the distal tubule and loop diuretics (eg ,furosemide, ethacrynic acid) inhibit the $Na^+-K^+-2Cl^-$ co-transporter in the thick ascending loop of Henlé. Carbonic anhydrase inhibitors reduce H^+ secretion and HCO_3^- reabsorption in the proximal tubules. Since these are coupled to Na^+ reabsorption through the Na^+/H^+ countertransport in the luminal membrane, a decrease in HCO_3^- reabsorption also reduces Na^+ reabsorption, causing these ions to remain in the tubular fluid and act as an osmotic diuretic.

5.43

Answer: D   Proximal tubule

The proximal tubule reabsorbs the majority (about two-thirds) of filtered salt and water. This is done in an essentially iso-osmotic manner. Both the luminal salt concentration and the luminal osmolality remain constant (and equal to plasma values) along the entire length of the proximal tubule. Water and salt are reabsorbed proportionally because the water is dependent on and coupled with the active reabsorption of Na^+. The water permeability of the proximal tubule is high and therefore a significant transepithelial osmotic gradient is not possible (a minute gradient of as little as 1 mOsm/l may exist). Sodium is actively transported, mainly by basolateral sodium pumps, into the lateral intercellular spaces; water follows. The glomerulus is where solutes are filtered from the plasma. The juxtaglomerular apparatus produces renin. The thick ascending limb of the loop of Henlé actively transports Na^+ and Cl^- from lumen to the peritubular space using a $Na^+-K^+-Cl^-$ co-transporter. About 30–35% of filtered salt is reabsorbed here. The collecting duct reabsorbs only a small fraction of filtered Na^+.

5.44

Answer: E   Thick ascending limb of the loop of Henlé

Both the thin and the thick ascending limbs of the loop of Henlé have very low permeability to water. Since there are no regulatory mechanisms to alter its permeability, it remains poorly permeable to

renal

water under all circumstances. Sodium and chloride are transported out of the luminal fluid into the surrounding interstitial spaces, where they are reabsorbed. Water must remain behind because it is not reabsorbed, so the solute concentration becomes less and less (the luminal fluid becomes more dilute). This is one of the principal mechanisms (along with diminution of ADH secretion) for the production of a dilute, hypo-osmotic urine (water diuresis). The glomerulus is completely permeable to water, acting as a filter. The proximal tubule is characterised by high water permeability, preventing the establishment of an osmotic gradient across the proximal tubular epithelium, and reabsorption of any solute here is accompanied by reabsorption of water. The juxtaglomerular apparatus produces renin. Water permeability of the collecting duct is under control of ADH, allowing adjustment of the renal function according to the body's state of hydration.

5.45

Answer: E   Is inhibited by parathyroid hormone

Regulation of phosphate excretion is accomplished primarily by parathyroid hormone (PTH), which inhibits phosphate reabsorption in the proximal tubule. At high parathyroid hormone (PTH) concentration, as much as 40% of filtered phosphate may be excreted. Reabsorption of phosphate by renal tubular cells occurs via a carrier co-transport of phosphate and sodium. This mechanism is similarly to the reabsorption of glucose and amino acids and is driven by the Na^+ gradient built by the Na^+/K^+-ATPase at the basolateral membrane of the tubular epithelium. Co-transport with calcium or chloride does not occur. Reabsorption of phosphate occurs against its electrochemical gradient and therefore cannot be passive. Calcitonin has only minor effects on renal calcium and phosphate handling. It lowers serum calcium by suppressing bone osteoclasts, so shifting the balance in favour of calcium deposition in the bone.

renal

SECTION 6:
GASTROINTESTINAL
PHYSIOLOGY – ANSWERS

6.1

Answer: D   Cholesterol

Bile salts are formed in the hepatic cells from cholesterol and in the process of secreting the bile salts about 1–2 g of cholesterol is also secreted each day. Under abnormal conditions, the cholesterol may precipitate, causing cholesterol gallstones to develop in the gallbladder. Cholesterol gallstones account for about 80% of gallstones. Some of the causes of gallstone formation include too much absorption of water or bile acids from bile, too much cholesterol in bile and inflammation of gallbladder epithelium. Pigment stones are small, dark stones made of bilirubin and calcium salts that are found in bile. They account for the other 20% of gallstones. Risk factors for pigment stones include cirrhosis, biliary tract infections and hereditary blood cell disorders, such as sickle cell anaemia. Stones of mixed origin also occur.

6.2

Answer: B   Hydrolysis

The breakdown of complex foodstuffs, such as carbohydrates, fats and proteins is accomplished by the same basic process of hydrolysis. The only difference is that different enzymes are required to promote the reactions for each type of food.

gastrointestinal

6.3

Answer: A   Pancreas

Pancreatic secretion contains a large quantity of α-amylase, a digestive enzyme that hydrolyses starches, glycogen and most other carbohydrates to form disaccharides and a few trisaccharides.

6.4

Answer: A   Acid pH and pepsin

Pepsin is expressed as a pro-form zymogen, pepsinogen, whose primary structure has an additional 44 amino acids. In other words, pepsinogen is an inactive precursor of the proteolytic enzyme, pepsin. Following secretion from the peptic and mucous cells of the gastric glands, the pepsinogen comes into contact with hydrochloric acid and previously formed pepsin, which split the pepsinogen to form active pepsin.

6.5

Answer: C   Co-transport with the sodium ion

The brush border of the small intestine is equipped with a family of peptidases. Like lactase and maltase, these peptidases are integral membrane proteins rather than soluble enzymes. They function to further the hydrolysis of luminal peptides, converting them to free amino acids and very small peptides. These end-products of digestion, formed on the surface of the enterocyte, are ready for absorption. The mechanism by which amino acids are absorbed is conceptually identical to that of monosaccharides. The luminal plasma membrane of the absorptive cell bears at least four **sodium-dependent amino acid co-transporters** – one each for acidic, basic, neutral and amino acids. These transporters bind amino acids only after binding sodium. The fully loaded transporter then undergoes a conformational change that dumps sodium and the amino acid into the cytoplasm, followed by its reorientation back to the original form. So, absorption of amino acids is also absolutely dependent on the electrochemical gradient of sodium across the epithelium. Further, absorption of amino acids, like that of monosaccharides, contributes to generating the osmotic gradient that drives water absorption. The basolateral membrane of the enterocyte contains additional transporters, which export amino acids from the cell into blood. These are not dependent on sodium gradients.

6.6

Answer: D   Gastric mucosal cells transport hydrogen ions out of the gastric mucosa

Transporting hydrogen ions out of the gastric mucosa decreases the local hydrogen ion concentration and this is believed to offer some protection against autodigestion of the stomach. The gastric mucosa is also protected by a thick layer of mucus. Finally, pepsin is stored as pepsinogen so it will only be released when needed and does not digest the body's own proteins in the stomach's lining.

6.7

Answer: B   Free fatty acids

Fat is transported from one part of the body to another almost entirely in the form of free fatty acids. On leaving the fat cells, the free fatty acids ionise strongly in the plasma and immediately combine with albumin. The concentration of free fatty acid in plasma under resting conditions is about 15 mg/dl and there is only about 0.45 g of fatty acids in the entire circulatory system.

6.8

Answer: E   Must be present in the diet

An essential amino acid or indispensable amino acid, is an amino acid that cannot be synthesised de novo by the organism (usually referring to humans) and therefore must be supplied in the diet. Nutritional essentiality is characteristic of the species, not the nutrient. Nine amino acids are generally regarded as essential for humans. They are: histidine, isoleucine, leucine, lysine, methionine, phenylalanine, threonine, tryptophan and valine. In addition, the amino acids arginine, cysteine, glycine and tyrosine are considered

gastrointestinal

conditionally essential, meaning they are not normally required in the diet, but must be supplied exogenously to specific populations that do not synthesise it in adequate amounts. An example would be with the disease phenylketonuria (PKU). Patients living with PKU must keep their intake of phenylalanine extremely low to prevent mental retardation and other metabolic complications. However, phenylalanine is the precursor for tyrosine synthesis. Without phenylalanine, tyrosine cannot be made and so tyrosine becomes essential in the diet of PKU patients.

6.9

Answer: A   Following total colectomy and ileostomy, the volume and water content of ileal discharge decreases over time.

Following total colectomy and ileostomy, the volume and water content of ileal discharge decreases over time and most patients can lead an essentially normal life. Iron absorption occurs in the upper gastrointestinal (GI) tract, not the colon and the vitamin B_{12}–intrinsic factor complex is absorbed in the ileum. As long as the ileum remains intact, deficiency of these factors essential for erythropoiesis is not expected.

6.10

Answer: E   Lipoprotein lipase

The features presented in this vignette are suggestive of hypertriglyceridaemia secondary to lipoprotein lipase deficiency. Lipoprotein lipase (LPL) is an enzyme that hydrolyses lipids in lipoproteins, like those found in chylomicrons and very-low-density lipoproteins (VLDL), into three fatty acids and one glycerol molecule. It requires Apo-CII as a co-factor. LPL deficiency leads to hypertriglyceridaemia. Lipoprotein lipase is specifically found in endothelial cells lining the capillaries. Insulin is known to enhance LPL synthesis in adipocytes and its placement in the capillary endothelium.

gastrointestinal

6.11

Answer: D   Osmotic

There are at least four types of diarrhoea: secretory diarrhoea, osmotic diarrhoea, motility-related diarrhoea and inflammatory diarrhoea.

- **Secretory diarrhoea** means that there is an increase in the active secretion or there is an inhibition of absorption. There is little to no structural damage. The most common cause of this type of diarrhoea is a cholera toxin that stimulates the secretion of anions, especially chloride ions. Therefore, to maintain a charge balance in the lumen, sodium is carried with it, along with water.

- **Osmotic diarrhoea** occurs when there is a loss of water due to a heavy osmotic load. This can occur when there is maldigestion (eg pancreatic disease or coeliac disease), where the nutrients are left in the lumen, which pulls water into the lumen.

- **Motility-related diarrhoea** occurs when the motility of the gastrointestinal tract is abnormal. If the food moves too quickly, there is not enough contact time between the food and the membrane, meaning that there is not enough time for the nutrients and water to be absorbed. This can follow a vagotomy or diabetic neuropathy.

- **Inflammatory diarrhoea** occurs when there is damage to the mucosal lining or brush border, which leads to a passive loss of protein-rich fluids and a decreased ability to absorb these lost fluids. Features of all three of the other types of diarrhoea can be found in this type of diarrhoea. It can be caused by bacterial infections, viral infections, parasitic infections or autoimmune problems such as inflammatory bowel disease.

gastrointestinal

6.12

Answer: E   Vitamin B$_{12}$ deficiency

The ileum is the final section of the small intestine. It is about 2–4 m long in humans, follows the duodenum and jejunum and is separated from the caecum by the ileocaecal valve. The pH in the ileum is usually between 7 and 8 (neutral or slightly alkaline). The chief function of the ileum is to absorb the products of digestion. The wall itself is made up of folds, each of which has many tiny finger-like projections, known as villi, on its surface. In turn, the epithelial cells that line these villi possess even larger numbers of microvilli. Therefore, the ileum has an extremely large surface area both for the adsorption (attachment) of enzyme molecules and for the absorption of products of digestion. The cells that line the ileum contain the protease and carbohydrase enzymes responsible for the final stages of protein and carbohydrate digestion. These enzymes are present in the cytoplasm of the epithelial cells. The villi contain large numbers of capillaries, which take the amino acids and glucose produced by digestion to the hepatic portal vein and the liver. Lacteals are small lymph vessels and are present in villi. They absorb fatty acid and glycerol, the products of fat digestion. Ileal resection will result in increased fat content of the stool.

Another important function of ileum, which will be lost after ileal resection, is absorption of vitamin B$_{12}$. The jejunum absorbs more water than the ileum, but the colon is the most efficient water-absorbing segment of the gut. Therefore, extracellular fluid volume deficiency is least likely to be seen after ileal resection. Finally, like most mineral nutrients such as calcium, iron from digested food or supplements is almost entirely absorbed in the duodenum by enterocytes of the duodenal lining and the absorption of iron or calcium will not be affected by ileal resection.

6.13

Answer: A   Chylomicron

Chylomicrons are large lipoprotein particles (having a diameter of 75–1200 nm) that are created by the absorptive cells of the small intestine. Chylomicrons transport exogenous lipids to liver, adipose, cardiac and skeletal tissue where they are broken down by lipoprotein lipase. The chylomicrons are released by exocytosis from enterocytes into lacteals – lymphatic vessels originating in the villi of the small intestine – and are then secreted into the bloodstream at the thoracic duct's connection with the left subclavian vein. Nascent chylomicrons are primarily composed of triglycerides (85%) and contain some cholesterol and cholesteryl esters. The main apolipoprotein component is apolipoprotein B-48 (ApoB-48).

6.14

Answer: D   Intrinsic factor

An active transport process has been implicated in the absorption of vitamin B_{12}. Four physiologically important forms of vitamin B_{12} are cyanocobalamin, hydroxycobalamin, methylcobalamin and deoxyadenosylcobalamin. Up to 5 milligrams of vitamin B_{12} is stored in the liver; about 70% of the vitamin B_{12} present in the bile is reabsorbed. This liver storage is thought to be sufficient for 3–6 years. Most cobalamins are bound to proteins and absorbed in the intestine. The low pH of the stomach and pepsin release cobalamins. These cobalamins are bound to R proteins, ie, haptocorrin (HC) secreted from salivary glands and gastric juice. Intrinsic factor (IF) is a cobalamin-binding protein secreted by the gastric parietal cells. Its secretory rate usually parallels that of HCl. Dietary cobalamin bound to food proteins is released in the stomach by pepsin and acid pH and more free cobalamin binds to HC than IF. The cobalamin–HC complex moves to the intestinal lumen, is digested by pancreatic proteases and the liberated cobalamin now complexes with IF. The cobalamin–IF complex moves through the small intestine and binds to a transmembrane receptor (IFCR) in the ileum. After endocytosis of the complex, cobalamin is released intracellularly and transferred to transcobalamin II (TC II). This cobalamin–TC II complex leaves the ileal mucosal cell and enters the circulation.

6.15

Answer: A   Acid secreted by stomach enhances iron absorption

Dietary iron contains both inorganic iron and haem. Both forms are actively absorbed by the duodenum. Iron is released from haem inside the mucosal cell and transferred into the body as inorganic iron. Fe^{2+} is absorbed faster than Fe^{3+} because ferric iron is insoluble above pH 3, whereas ferrous iron remains soluble at pH 8. Dietary constituents such as phosphates, carbonates and oxalates reduce iron absorption because they form insoluble complexes with iron. These iron complexes are more soluble at low pH. Therefore, HCl secreted by the stomach enhances iron absorption and that is why patients with gastrectomy often have iron-deficiency anaemia. Ascorbate also promotes iron absorption. The quantity of iron in the body is maintained by controlled absorption from the duodenum. Iron deficiency enhances erythropoiesis and hypoxia increases intestinal iron absorption. Iron is stored in the mucosal cell as a ferritin complex. When iron absorption is increased, no ferritin complex is formed and the iron is rapidly delivered into the plasma. When iron absorption is depressed, more iron is trapped in the form of a ferritin complex and retained in the mucosal cell. When Fe^{2+} leaves the mucosal cell, transferrin in the circulating blood is the carrier that delivers it to other tissues via transferrin receptors in the plasma membrane.

6.16

Answer: C   Glucose-6-phosphatase

Glycogen storage disease type I or von Gierke's disease is the most common of the glycogen storage diseases. This genetic disease results from deficiency of the enzyme glucose-6-phosphatase. This deficiency impairs the ability of the liver to produce free glucose from glycogen and from gluconeogenesis. Since these are the two principal metabolic mechanisms by which the liver supplies glucose to the rest of the body during periods of fasting, it causes severe hypoglycaemia. Reduced glycogen breakdown results in increased glycogen storage in liver and kidneys, causing enlargement of both. Both organs function normally in childhood but are susceptible to a variety of problems in the adult years. Other metabolic derangements include lactic acidosis and hyperlipidaemia. Frequent or continuous feedings of cornstarch or other carbohydrates are the principal treatment. Other therapeutic measures may be needed for associated problems.

gastrointestinal

6.17

Answer: E   Is facilitated by employing the valsalva manoeuvre

Defecation is a complex, neurally controlled act that includes voluntary and involuntary elements. Mass movements or co-ordinated segmental contractions of the colon deliver faecal matter to the rectum. Stretch receptors in the wall of the rectum and anal canal respond and trigger the rectosphincteric reflex. Afferent signals are sent to the cerebral cortex, where the urge to defecate is recognised, to the autonomic ganglia and to the spinal centres, which provide the efferent innervation of the sphincters. As distension increases, rectal contractions are reflexly induced. When the rectum is distended, the immediate reflex response is relaxation of the internal sphincter and contraction of the external sphincter. If conditions are perceived to be appropriate (ie, socially acceptable) for defecation, the external sphincter is voluntarily relaxed and defecation occurs. If conditions are inappropriate, contraction of the external sphincter is voluntarily maintained, the rectal stretch receptors adapt and the rectum relaxes to accommodate the contained faecal matter. The act of defecation is facilitated by assuming a squatting or seated position to align and dilate the recto–anal junction and by employing the Valsalva manoeuvre to increase intra-abdominal pressure.

6.18

Answer: D   Serum fatty acids

Starvation is a severe reduction in nutrient, vitamin and energy intake and is the most extreme form of malnutrition. In humans, prolonged starvation (in excess of 1–2 months) causes permanent organ damage and will eventually result in death. Starved individuals lose substantial fat and muscle mass as the body breaks down these tissues for energy.

gastrointestinal

6.19

Answer: A   Aganglionosis in the rectum

Hirschsprung's disease or congenital aganglionic megacolon, involves an enlargement of the colon, caused by bowel obstruction resulting from an aganglionic section of bowel that starts at the anus and progresses upwards. The length of bowel that is affected varies but seldom stretches for more than 30 cm or so. The lack of ganglion cells disables the muscular peristalsis needed to move stool through the colon, so creating a blockage. One in 5000 children suffer from Hirschsprung's disease; four times as many men get the disease than women. It develops in the fetus during the early stages of pregnancy. Typical symptoms for infants include not having their first bowel movement (meconium) within 48 hours of birth and repeated vomiting. Some infants may have a swollen abdomen. Two-thirds of the cases of Hirschsprung's disease are diagnosed within 3 months of the birth. Occasionally symptoms do not appear until early adulthood. In some cases, the child may have delayed toilet training. A barium enema is the mainstay of diagnosis of Hirschsprung's disease, though a rectal biopsy showing the lack of ganglion cells is the only certain method of diagnosis. The usual treatment is 'pull-through' surgery, in which the portion of the colon that does have nerve cells is pulled through and sewn over the part that lacks nerve cells.

6.20

Answer: A   Acetylcholine increases gastric acid secretion

Physiological agonists of gastric acid secretion are acetylcholine (ACh), histamine and gastrin, acting through their respective receptors on oxyntic (parietal) cells to stimulate HCl release. These all act by using cAMP as the secondary messenger. They increase the number of H^+/K^+-ATPase molecules and Cl^- channels, thereby increasing H^+ and Cl^- secretion. Endogenous antagonists of HCl secretion are somatostatin, secretin, epidermal growth factor and prostaglandins that act directly on parietal cells. Atropine is an antagonist to ACh and the histamine antagonist cimetidine inhibits HCl secretion.

6.21

Answer: D   Pepsin

Pepsin is a digestive protease released by the chief cells in the stomach that functions to degrade food proteins into peptides. Pepsin is expressed as a pro-form zymogen, pepsinogen, whose primary structure has an additional 44 amino acids. In the stomach, chief cells release pepsinogen. This zymogen is activated by hydrochloric acid (HCl), which is released from parietal cells in the stomach lining. The hormone gastrin and the vagus nerve trigger the release of both pepsinogen and HCl from the stomach lining when food is ingested. HCl creates an acidic environment that allows pepsinogen to unfold and cleave itself in an autocatalytic fashion, thereby generating pepsin (the active form). Pepsin cleaves the 44 amino acids from pepsinogen to create more pepsin. It will digest up to 20% of ingested proteins by cleaving preferentially at carboxylic groups of aromatic amino acids such as phenylalanine and tyrosine. It will not cleave at bonds containing valine, alanine or glycine; peptides may be further digested by other proteases (in the duodenum) and eventually absorbed by the body. Pepsin is stored as pepsinogen so it will be released only when needed and does not digest the body's own proteins in the stomach's lining. Pepsin functions best in acidic environments, particularly those at a pH of 2.

6.22

Answer: A   Achalasia

Achalasia, also known as oesophageal achalasia, achalasia cardia, cardiospasm, dyssynergia oesophagus and oesophageal aperistalsis, is an oesophageal motility disorder. In this disorder, inappropriate contraction of the smooth muscle layer of the oesophagus leads to reduced peristalsis (muscular ability to move food down the oesophagus) and failure of the lower oesophageal sphincter to relax properly in response to swallowing. The most common form is primary achalasia (with no underlying cause), but a small proportion is due to oesophageal cancer or (in South America) Chagas' disease. The classical triad of achalasia is dysphagia (difficulty swallowing) to fluids and (later) solids, regurgitation of undigested food and chest pain. Other symptoms may include difficulty belching, frequent

gastrointestinal

hiccups, cough (especially on reclining) and weight loss (due to inadequate nutrient intake). Because of the similarity of symptoms, achalasia can be misdiagnosed as other disorders, such as gastro-oesophageal reflux disease, hiatus hernia and even psychosomatic disorders.

Investigations for achalasia include:

- X-ray with a barium swallow or oesophagography. This shows narrowing at the level of the gastro-oesophageal junction ('bird/parrot beak' or 'rat tail' presentation of the lower oesophagus) and various degrees of megaoesophagus (oesophageal dilatation) as the oesophagus is gradually stretched by retained food. A 5-minute timed barium swallow is useful to measure the effectiveness of treatment.

- Manometry, the key test for establishing the diagnosis. A probe measures the pressure waves in different parts of the oesophagus and stomach during the act of swallowing. A thin tube is inserted through the nose (this is called a nasogastric intubation) and the patient is instructed to swallow several times.

- Endoscopy, which provides a view inside the oesophagus and stomach.

- CT scan may be used to exclude pseudoachalasia or achalasia symptoms resulting from a different cause, usually oesophageal cancer.

- Pathological examination reveals a defect in the nerves that control the motility of the oesophagus (the myenteric plexus). The oesophagus is dilated and hypertrophied. In Chagas' disease, the ganglion cells are destroyed by *Trypanosoma cruzi*, the causative parasite.

gastrointestinal

418

6.23

Answer: D   Lactase

Lactase, a member of the β-galactosidase family of enzymes, is a glycoside hydrolase involved in the hydrolysis of the disaccharide lactose into constituent galactose and glucose monomers. In humans, lactase is present predominantly along the brush border membrane of the differentiated enterocytes lining the villi of the small intestine. Lactase is essential for digestive hydrolysis of lactose in milk. Deficiency of the enzyme causes lactose intolerance; most humans become lactose intolerant as adults. Lactase has an optimum temperature of about 48 °C (118.4 °F) for its activity and an optimum pH of 6.5.

6.24

Answer: A   Cholecystokinin

The woman in this clinical vignette has symptoms suggestive of gallstones. During the ingestion of a meal, vagal parasympathetic discharges stimulate gallbladder contractions. Intraluminal fats or amino acids in the intestine stimulate cholecystokinin (CCK) cells in the duodenum to release CCK, which causes sustained gallbladder contractions and relaxation of the sphincter of Oddi. In the presence of gallstones, inflammation of the gallbladder occurs and CCK, by causing gallbladder contractions in the presence of gallstones, aggravates the inflammation.

6.25

Answer: E   8.0

There are four major components of saliva:

- mucus that serves as a lubricant

- α-amylase, an enzyme that initiates the digestion of starch

- lingual lipase, an enzyme that begins the digestion of fat

gastrointestinal

- a slightly alkaline electrolyte solution that moistens food.

Human saliva is always hypotonic to plasma. Na^+ and Cl^- concentrations are less than that of plasma, but K^+ and HCO_3^- concentrations are higher in saliva than in plasma. Salivary osmolality increases as the secretion rate increases, reaching about 70% of plasma osmolality at maximal secretion rates. In addition, the pH changes from being slightly acidic (at rest) to basic (pH 8) at ultimate stimulation. This increase in alkalinity is due to the increase of HCO_3^- in the saliva. At low flow rates of saliva secretion, Na^+ is actively absorbed, Cl^- passively absorbed, but K^+ and HCO_3^- are secreted as the saliva moves out of the ducts into the mouth. However, at higher flow rates, salivary ducts are not as efficient in reabsorbing Na^+ and Cl^- because their levels now more closely approach those of the plasma. Therefore, at high flow rates, besides being rich in HCO_3^- and K^+, saliva also has high concentrations of Na^+ and Cl^- and is more basic. Amylase and mucus also increase in concentration after stimulation.

6.26

Answer: D   Pancreatitis

The test for amylase is easier to perform than lipase, making it the primary test used to test for and monitor pancreatitis. Laboratories will usually measure either pancreatic amylase or total amylase. If only pancreatic amylase is measured, an increase will not be noted with mumps or other salivary gland trauma. Unfortunately, because of the small amount present, timing is critical when sampling blood for this measurement. Blood should preferably be taken soon after a bout of pancreatitis pain, as amylase is excreted rapidly by the kidneys. Increased plasma levels in humans are found in:

- salivary trauma (including anaesthetic intubation)
- mumps – due to inflammation of the salivary glands
- pancreatitis – because of damage to the cells that produce amylase
- renal failure – due to reduced excretion.

gastrointestinal

Total amylase readings of over 10 times the upper limit of normal (ULN) are suggestive of pancreatitis; 5–10 times the ULN may indicate ileus or duodenal disease or renal failure. Lower elevations are commonly found in salivary gland disease.

6.27

Answer: E   When acid secretion is stimulated in the stomach, the potential difference between mucosa and serosa falls to −20 mV

The mucosal surface of the stomach is always electrically negative; the serosa, positive. At rest, the potential difference is −60 to −80 mV. When acid secretion is stimulated, the potential difference falls to −20 mV. Cl^- from plasma is transported from the extracellular fluid to the lumen of the gland against a concentration gradient. H^+ moves down an electrical gradient into the lumen against a high chemical concentration gradient. At maximum rates of H^+ secretion, H^+ is pumped against a concentration gradient of one million to one. Energy is required to transport H^+ and Cl^- against their electrochemical gradients. H^+ is transported across the mucosal membrane, using the H^+/K^+-ATPase system. The secretion of H^+ causes the parietal cell to become alkaline. This alkalinity must be dissipated or H^+ secretion would cease. OH^- leaves in exchange for Cl^-, causing alkalinisation of the plasma, referred to as the alkaline tide.

6.28

Answer: B   Calcium is concentrated

The gallbladder concentrates bile by removing sodium, chloride and water. It acidifies the bile by removing Na^+ in exchange for H^+ ions. Bile salts are concentrated fivefold and bilirubin tenfold in the gallbladder bile; cholesterol, fatty acids and lecithin are concentrated as much as tenfold in gallbladder bile. Gallbladder bile contains K^+ and Ca^{2+} several-fold more concentrated than in liver bile. Liver bile contains Cl^- and HCO_3^-, in four- and threefold greater concentration than gallbladder bile. This will be made available to promote digestion after the next meal. Sodium and chloride are pumped into the blood along with some Ca^{2+} ions, but Ca^{2+} concentration remains higher in the gallbladder than in blood.

gastrointestinal

6.29

Answer: D   Bile becomes more acidic in the gall-bladder

Canalicular bile is formed in response to the osmotic filtration of bile acid anions. In the sinusoidal plasma, bile acid anions pass through the fenestrations of endothelial cells and diffuse through the space of Disse. They are taken up across the hepatocyte sinusoidal membrane by a sodium (Na^+/K^+-ATPase) coupled transport system. Bile acids in the hepatocytes are bound to cytosolic proteins, ie glutathione *S*-transferase. Unconjugated bile acids are conjugated to glycine or taurine. The bile acid anions are then actively secreted into the canaliculus. This transport can concentrate bile acids 20–200 times more than their concentration in a hepatocyte. Plasma water and solutes pass through tight junctions that separate the canalicular lumen from the space of Disse and this restores isotonicity in the canaliculus and the canalicular bile is formed. Canalicular bile is estimated to be secreted at the rate 0.15 ml/min. Canalicular bile consists of solutes needed to induce bile formation and secondary solutes, plasma electrolytes, amino acids, monosaccharides and organic acids. As the bile flows down the bile duct, some modifications occur. However, they are not viewed as very important because they do not affect the delivery of bile acid to the small intestine or the excretion of bile acids, bilirubin and cholesterol. Glucose, amino acids and secondary solutes are absorbed by ductular cells. Secretin induces increased water and bicarbonate secretion in the ductal bile. Somatostatin inhibits ductular water and bicarbonate secretion and may even lead to bicarbonate absorption. Ductule secretion of bile is estimated at 0.11 ml/min. The gallbladder concentrates bile by removing sodium, chloride and water. It acidifies the bile by removing Na^+ in exchange for H^+ ions.

After an overnight fast, about half the hepatic bile enters the gall-bladder. The remainder enters the small intestine. Secreted bile acids are absorbed from the terminal ileum and re-secreted into bile. The length of overnight fast determines the amount that is stored. A greater percentage of bile acids will be stored in the gall-bladder after an overnight fast. During the ingestion of a meal, vagal parasympathetic discharges stimulate gallbladder contractions. Intraluminal fats or amino acids in the intestine stimulate CCK cells in the duodenum to release CCK, which causes sustained gallbladder contractions and relaxation of the sphincter of Oddi. The slow contractions of the gallbladder discharge two-thirds of its stored bile within the first hour of digestion. Bile is not stored in the gallbladder during digestion; therefore, during ingestion of a meal, bile stored in the gallbladder is discharged into the small intestine. The total estimated bile output is about 500–600 ml per day. Only bile acids, of all the steroids and lipids in the bile, undergo an enterohepatic circulation. The enterohepatic circulation uses a large mass of previously synthesised bile acids that can pass through hepatocytes to generate a bile flow and these bile acids are now again available to facilitate fat digestion.

6.30

Answer: C   Gastrocolic reflex

The gastrocolic reflex or gastrocolic response is one of a number of physiological reflexes controlling the motility or peristalsis, of the gastrointestinal tract. It involves an increase in motility, of the colon in response to stretch in the stomach and by-products of digestion in the small intestine. The small intestine also shows a similar motility response. The reflex was demonstrated by myoelectric recordings in the colons of animals and humans, which showed an increase in electrical activity as soon as 15 min after eating. The recordings also demonstrated that the gastrocolic reflex is uneven in its distribution throughout the colon. The sigmoid colon is more greatly affected than the right side of the colon in terms of a phasic response; however, the tonic response across the colon is uncertain. A number of neuropeptides have been proposed as mediators of the gastrocolic reflex. These include serotonin, neurotensin, cholecystokinin and gastrin. Clinically, the gastrocolic reflex has been implicated in pathogenesis of irritable bowel syndrome. Also, the serotonin antagonist ondansetron decreases the tonic response to stretch.

gastrointestinal

6.31

Answer: A A decrease in the sodium content of the body

Diarrhoea results mainly from excess faecal water, which can have infectious, drug-induced, food-related, surgical, inflammatory, transit-related or malabsorptive causes. These causes produce diarrhoea by four distinct mechanisms: increased osmotic load, increased secretion, inflammation and decreased absorption time. Paradoxic diarrhoea results from stool oozing around a faecal impaction. Acute diarrhoea (< 4 days) is predominantly caused by self-limited conditions such as food poisoning or infections.

Complications may result from diarrhoea of any aetiology. Fluid loss with consequent dehydration, electrolyte loss (Na^+, K^+, Mg^{2+}, Cl^-) and even vascular collapse sometimes occur. Collapse can develop rapidly in patients who have severe diarrhoea (eg patients with cholera) or are very young, very old or debilitated. HCO_3^- loss can cause metabolic acidosis. Hypokalaemia can occur in severe or chronic diarrhoea or if the stool contains excess mucus. Hypomagnesaemia after prolonged diarrhoea can cause tetany.

6.32

Answer: D Hepatic disease if plasma albumin is low and serum aminotransferase elevations > 500 units

In a patient with jaundice, aminotransferases and alkaline phosphatase levels should be measured. Mild hyperbilirubinaemia (eg, bilirubin < 3 mg/dl [< 51 μmol/l]) with normal aminotransferase and alkaline phosphatase levels is often unconjugated (eg, due to haemolysis or Gilbert's syndrome rather than hepatobiliary disease). Moderate or severe hyperbilirubinaemia, bilirubinuria, high alkaline phosphatase levels or high aminotransferase levels suggest hepatobiliary disease. Unconjugated hyperbilirubinaemia is usually confirmed by bilirubin fractionation. However, because hyperbilirubinaemia produced by any hepatobiliary disease is largely conjugated, bilirubin fractionation is unwarranted if test results reflect hepatobiliary disease.

Other blood tests should be performed selectively. For example, hepatitis serology should be obtained for suspected acute or chronic hepatitis, prothrombin time (PT) or international normalised ratio (INR) for suspected hepatic insufficiency, albumin and globulin levels for suspected chronic liver disease and antimitochondrial antibody levels for suspected primary biliary cirrhosis. In cases of isolated elevation of alkaline phosphatase, γ-glutamyl transpeptidase (GGT) should be obtained; levels are elevated in hepatobiliary disease but not if the high alkaline phosphatase level is due to a bone disorder.

In hepatobiliary disease, neither bilirubin fractionation nor the degree of bilirubin elevation helps differentiate hepatocellular from cholestatic jaundice. Aminotransferase elevations > 500 units suggest a hepatocellular cause such as hepatitis or acute liver hypoxia; disproportionate increases of alkaline phosphatase (eg, alkaline phosphatase > 3 times normal and aminotransferase < 200 units) suggest cholestasis. Liver infiltration can also increase alkaline phosphatase disproportionately to aminotransferases but usually increases bilirubin only slightly or not at all.

Because hepatobiliary disease alone rarely causes bilirubin levels > 30 mg/dl (> 513 μmol/l), higher levels usually reflect a combination of severe hepatobiliary disease and haemolysis or renal dysfunction. Low albumin and high globulin levels suggest chronic rather than acute liver disease. An elevated PT or INR that decreases after giving vitamin K (5–10 mg IM for 2–3 days) favours cholestasis over hepatocellular disease but is not conclusive. Imaging is best for diagnosing infiltrative and cholestatic causes of jaundice. Abdominal ultrasound, CT or MRI is usually performed first. These tests can detect abnormalities within the biliary tree and focal liver lesions, but are less accurate in diagnosing diffuse hepatocellular disorders (eg, hepatitis, cirrhosis). In extrahepatic cholestasis, endoscopic or magnetic resonance cholangiopancreatography (ERCP, MRCP) provides a more accurate assessment of the biliary tree; ERCP also permits treatment of the obstruction (eg, stone removal, stenting of strictures).

Liver biopsy is seldom required for diagnosing jaundice, but can help in intrahepatic cholestasis and in some kinds of hepatitis. Laparoscopy (peritoneoscopy) permits direct inspection of the liver and gallbladder without the trauma of a full laparotomy. Unexplained cholestatic jaundice warrants laparoscopy occasionally and diagnostic laparotomy rarely.

gastrointestinal

6.33

Answer: A   Blockage of the common bile duct

The woman in this clinical vignette has laboratory investigations suggestive of obstructive jaundice. Cholestasis (obstructive jaundice) can cause conjugated hyperbilirubinaemia. Cholestasis results when bile flow is impaired. The term cholestasis is preferred to obstructive jaundice because mechanical obstruction is not always present. Bile flow may be impaired at any point, from the liver cell canaliculus to the ampulla of Vater. Intrahepatic causes include hepatitis, drug toxicity and alcoholic liver disease. Less common causes include primary biliary cirrhosis, cholestasis of pregnancy and metastatic cancer. Extrahepatic causes include a common duct stone and pancreatic cancer. Less common causes include benign stricture of the common duct (usually related to prior surgery), ductal carcinoma, pancreatitis or pancreatic pseudocyst and sclerosing cholangitis.

Mechanisms are complex, even in mechanical obstruction. The pathophysiological effects reflect absence of bile constituents (most importantly, bilirubin, bile salts and lipids) in the intestines and their backup, which causes spillage into the systemic circulation. Stools are often pale because less bilirubin reaches the intestine. Absence of bile salts can produce malabsorption, leading to steatorrhoea and deficiencies of fat-soluble vitamins (particularly A, K and D); vitamin K deficiency can reduce prothrombin levels. In long-standing cholestasis, concomitant vitamin D and Ca^{2+} malabsorption can cause osteoporosis or osteomalacia.

Bilirubin retention produces mixed hyperbilirubinaemia. Some conjugated bilirubin reaches and darkens the urine. High levels of circulating bile salts are associated with, but may not cause, pruritus. Cholesterol and phospholipid retention produces hyperlipidaemia despite fat malabsorption (although increased liver synthesis and decreased plasma esterification of cholesterol also contribute); triglyceride levels are largely unaffected. The lipids circulate as a unique, abnormal, low-density lipoprotein called lipoprotein X.

gastrointestinal

6.34

Answer: D   The pH of the pancreatic juice is alkaline

The pancreas is a mixed gland. The exocrine part elaborates pancreatic juice, while the endocrine part synthesises and secretes insulin, glucagon, pancreatic polypeptide and somatostatin. The exocrine pancreas comprises 98% of the gland. The endocrine pancreas makes up the remaining 2%. The pancreas is characterised by islands of endocrine cells among the exocrine pancreas; therefore, the endocrine part is often called the islets of Langerhans. The 100-g pancreas synthesises and secretes about 1.5 l of pancreatic juice per day. The alkaline juice neutralises the duodenal chyme and contains enzymes for digesting proteins, fats and carbohydrates.

The secretions of the acinar cells that synthesise and secrete pancreatic juice leave the cells via exocytosis. They drain into intercalated ducts, which in turn drain into intralobular ducts and ultimately drain into the extralobular duct that empties into the duodenum along with the common bile duct. The exocrine pancreas is supplied by blood from the coeliac and superior mesenteric arteries.

The pancreas is innervated by preganglionic parasympathetic branches of the vagus that synapse with cholinergic neurones within the pancreas. Sympathetic nerves from the coeliac and superior mesenteric plexuses innervate the blood vessels of the pancreas. Sympathetic nerve impulses inhibit and parasympathetic nerve impulses stimulate pancreatic juice secretion.

6.35

Answer: B HCO_3^- content is greater in response to secretin

The columnar epithelial cells of the pancreatic ducts secrete most of the aqueous component of the pancreatic juice. Na^+ and K^+ concentrations are similar to those in the plasma. HCO_3^- increases threefold above basal levels during high secretory rates. HCO_3^- and Cl^- concentrations usually vary reciprocally. After initial secretion, the aqueous component contains a high concentration of HCO_3^- and is slightly hypertonic. Water equilibrates with the aqueous component rich in HCO_3^-, causing it to be isotonic, and some Cl^- is exchanged

gastrointestinal

for HCO_3^- at rest. Most of the aqueous component is synthesised by cells of the intercalated ducts. When secretin strongly stimulates the aqueous component, it is secreted mostly by extralobular ducts. CCK stimulates secretion of small quantities of isotonic aqueous component, but the secretin-stimulated component is of greater quantity and has a greater concentration of bicarbonate.

6.36

Answer: D   Will result after vagotomy

The cephalic phase of pancreatic secretion is triggered by the central nervous system through recognition and integration of the sight, smell and taste of food. When human subjects see, smell and chew food without swallowing, HCO_3^- and pancreatic enzyme secretion increases. The degree of enzyme secretion in the cephalic phase is about 50% of the maximal response elicited with exogenous CCK and secretin. The vagus nerve modulates secretion by means of cholinergic fibres, which innervate pancreatic acinar cells. The vagus also modulates peptidergic nerve fibres, which innervate duct cells.

6.37

Answer: E   Results in increased passage of maltose in stool

Maltase is one enzyme produced by the cells lining the small intestine to break down disaccharides. It comes under the enzyme category carbohydrase (which is a subcategory of hydrolase) and the disaccharide it hydrolyses is maltose. Maltase is secreted by the surface cells of the villi, which are thin projections on the mucosa. These are found throughout the small intestine, but differ in shape in the duodenal and ileal sections. Maltase works like any other enzyme, with the substrate (maltose) binding with the active site. When the maltose binds with maltase, the former is hydrolysed, that is to say it is split into its component parts, ie two molecules of α-glucose. This is done by breaking the glycosidic bond between the 'first' carbon of one glucose and the 'fourth' carbon of the other (a 1–4 bond). Maltase deficiency will result in increased passage of maltose in the stool.

gastrointestinal

6.38

Answer: D   Is accompanied by hypochloraemic metabolic alkalosis

Vomiting is a reflex controlled by a centre in the medulla that receives afferent input from the gastrointestinal (GI) tract, the labyrinth receptors of the inner ear, gag receptors in the throat and pain receptors. It also receives afferents from a medullary chemoreceptor trigger zone that responds to certain circulating chemicals, such as apomorphine. Higher centres may also influence the medullary centre.

The most common stimulus for vomiting is irritation of the upper GI tract, but it can also be induced by motion sickness, olfactory, visual and painful stimuli. The act of vomiting is usually preceded by the sensation of nausea. Initially there is a diffuse sympathetic discharge with tachycardia, tachypnoea, sweating and inhibited gastric motility. This is followed by parasympathetic activation with relaxation of upper and lower oesophageal sphincters (although not always simultaneously), increased salivation and a transient increase in gastric motility. A deep inspiration that follows moves the stomach and diaphragm down into the abdomen. The anterior abdominal muscles then contract forcefully, compressing the flaccid stomach and expelling the gastric contents into the oesophagus. If the upper oesophageal sphincter is not relaxed, secondary peristalsis returns the contents to the stomach. This phase of the process is termed retching and may be repeated many times. If the upper oesophageal sphincter is relaxed, the act of vomiting is completed with the expulsion of the gastric contents through the mouth.

The consequences of vomiting relate to the composition of gastric juice, which is characteristically acidic, high in chloride and relatively high in potassium. The major effects of vomiting are dehydration (due to volume loss), hypokalaemia (due to potassium loss) and hypochloraemic metabolic alkalosis due to loss of hydrogen ion and chloride.

gastrointestinal

6.39

Answer: B   Gastric emptying

Although both neural and hormonal components control gastric emptying, brainstem co-ordination is not required for gastric emptying. The former components influence the motor activity of the stomach, the gastroduodenal junction and the duodenum. Receptive relaxation and low-intensity tonic contraction of the orad stomach accommodate ingested food. The more intense peristaltic activity in the distal stomach provides the force for propelling gastric contents through the gastroduodenal junction. Resistance to flow across the junction can be further regulated by the diameter of the pylorus. An additional resistance to flow across the gastroduodenal junction is provided by duodenal pressure, which is determined by duodenal motility, particularly segmentation. Increased motility of the orad stomach (decreased distensibility) or of the distal stomach (increased peristalsis), decreased pyloric tone, decreased duodenal motility or a combination of these will increase the rate of gastric emptying.

The major control mechanism for gastric emptying involves duodenal gastric feedback. The duodenum has receptors that respond to the presence of acid, carbohydrate, fat and protein digestion products, to osmolarity different from that of plasma, and to distension. Activating these receptors decreases the rate of emptying. Neural mechanisms involve both enteric and vagal pathways and vagotomy impairs the regulation of gastric emptying. CCK, which is released primarily by fat and protein digestion products, slows gastric emptying at physiological levels of the hormone. Gastrin, secretin and glucose-1-phosphate (GIP) also slow gastric emptying, but require higher doses to demonstrate the effect and their physiolological significance is questionable. CCK, which increases both gastric and duodenal motility, may exert its effect by causing a relatively greater increase in pyloric contraction and/or duodenal segmentation rather than increasing the motility of the distal stomach.

gastrointestinal

6.40

Answer: D   Segmentation

Segmentation and peristalsis are the two major types of contractions observed in the intestine. Segmentation, primarily a function of circular muscle, is observed most frequently. It consists of a 2- or 3-cm segment that contracts while the muscle on either side of it relaxes. Chyme in the segment is displaced in both orad and aborad directions from the site of contraction. As the contracted segment relaxes, the previously relaxed segments on either side may contract.

Segmentation cycling efficiently mixes the chyme with the digestive secretions and maximally exposes the mucosal absorptive surface to the luminal contents.

Segmentation also serves a propulsive function. This is in part related to the characteristics of the slow wave. Because slow-wave frequency decreases along the intestine, contraction occurs more frequently in the orad portions. Also, the relatively greater muscle mass of the orad portions allow them to develop greater force. These factors are responsible for establishing a pressure gradient along the intestine, which allows segmentation to contribute to the aborad movement of chyme.

Peristalsis is a propulsive wave of contraction that is initiated by distension of the intestine. The peristaltic wave in the intestine is short lived and travels only a few centimetres before dying out. Long segments of the small intestine do not normally undergo peristalsis. The combined effects of intestinal peristalsis and segmentation provide for both adequate mixing of the intestinal contents and slow, steady movement of chyme. This allows adequate time for digestive processing and absorption.

6.41

Answer: D   Obstructive jaundice due to carcinoma of common bile duct

Bilirubin is a tetrapyrrole created by the normal breakdown of haem. Most bilirubin is produced during the breakdown of haemoglobin

gastrointestinal

and other haemoproteins. Accumulation of bilirubin or its conjugates in body tissues produces jaundice, which is characterised by high plasma bilirubin levels and deposition of yellow bilirubin pigments in skin, sclerae, mucous membranes and other less visible tissues. Because bilirubin is highly insoluble in water, it must be converted into a soluble conjugate before elimination from the body. In the liver, uridine diphosphate (UDP)–glucuronyl transferase converts bilirubin to a mixture of monoglucuronides and diglucuronides, referred to as conjugated (direct) bilirubin, which is then secreted into the bile by an ATP-dependent transporter. This process is highly efficient under normal conditions, so plasma unconjugated bilirubin concentrations remain low. Normal serum values of total bilirubin typically are 0.2–1 mg/dl (3.4–17.1 mmol/l), of which no more than 0.2 mg/dl (3.4 mmol/l) is directly reacting. Conjugated hyperbilirubinaemia results from reduced secretion of conjugated bilirubin into the bile, such as occurs in patients with hepatitis, or it results from impaired flow of bile into the intestine, such as occurs in patients with biliary obstruction due to tumours in the head of pancreas or common bile duct. Bile formation is very sensitive to a variety of hepatic insults, including high levels of inflammatory cytokines such as may occur in patients with septic shock. Diseases that increase the rate of bilirubin formation, such as haemolysis, or diseases that reduce the rate of bilirubin conjugation, such as Gilbert's syndrome, produce unconjugated hyperbilirubinaemia (*see also* answer to 6.33).

6.42

Answer: C H^+/K^+ ATPase

The key player in acid secretion is an H^+/K^+-ATPase or 'proton pump' located in the canalicular membrane. This ATPase is magnesium-dependent and not inhibitable by ouabain. Parietal cells secrete an essentially isotonic solution of pure hydrochloric acid (HCl) containing 150 mmol/l Cl^- and 150 mmol/l H^+ (pH < 1). Intracellular H^+ of parietal cells is 10^{-4} meg/l(pH = 7.0) and active transport is necessary to transport H^+ against this gradient. This is achieved by H^+/K^+-ATPase in the apical membrane that exchanges H^+ for K^+. Omeprazole is a proton pump inhibitor and blocks H^+/K^+-ATPase.

gastrointestinal

6.43

Answer: D   Vasoactive intestinal peptide

A number of agents released into the circulation may affect gastrointestinal (GI) blood flow. Important vasoconstrictors include noradrenaline, adrenaline and dopamine released from the adrenal medulla, angiotensin II generated as a consequence of renal renin release and vasopressin released from the posterior pituitary. Important vasodilators include vasoactive intestinal peptide and the hormones gastrin, cholecystokinin and glucagon.

6.44

Answer: E   Vasopressin

Gastric blood flow is influenced by both neural and humoral factors. Vagal stimulation, gastrin, histamine and acetylcholine stimulate gastric secretion and the production of vasodilator metabolites, which, in turn, cause increased gastric blood flow. Acetylcholine and histamine also have direct vasodilator effects on the gastric arterioles. Inhibitors of secretion, such as catecholamines and secretin, inhibit gastric acid secretion and decrease gastric blood flow by reducing the concentration of local vasodilator metabolites. Sympathetic stimulation mediated by noradrenaline causes vasoconstriction, as does circulating vasopressin. The gastric circulation shows the autoregulatory escape phenomenon with sustained sympathetic stimulation. Maintaining the integrity of gastric mucosal blood flow is important for protecting against damage from the high acidity of stomach contents.

6.45

Answer: A   Decrease in body temperature

Among the factors affecting BMR are weight and body surface area. The latter provides the best relationship to use to normalise the BMR data. Age affects the BMR. The rate is 30 kcal/m² per hour at birth; at age 2, the rate is 57 kcal/m² per hour; and at age 20, 41 kcal/m² per hour. Thereafter it declines by about 10% between ages 20 and 60 years. Women have a 10% lower BMR than men

gastrointestinal

because of their greater fat content. A one-degree increase in body temperature leads to a 10% increase in metabolic rate; a one-degree decrease in body temperature leads to a 10% decrease in metabolic rate, but shivering increases metabolic rate. An increase in ambient temperature in a hot climate causes an increase in BMR, especially if body temperature is elevated. Hyperthyroid individuals have an increased BMR. Stress must be avoided because an increase in adrenal catecholamines increases BMR, as do caffeine and theophylline. Diet-induced thermogenesis accounts for an increased metabolic rate and heat production during food assimilation. It accounts for 30% of the caloric value of protein and 5% of the caloric value of carbohydrate and fat. This is why BMR is measured after an overnight fast. Physical activity affects the metabolic rate; the metabolic rate varies with the activity level. The total caloric expenditure is the sum of basal caloric expenditure plus that which can be attributed to physical activity.

gastrointestinal

SECTION 7: NEUROPHYSIOLOGY – ANSWERS

7.1

Answer: B   Confusion

Lesions of the orbitofrontal cortex in non-human primates attenuate behavioral expression of anger and frustration following incorrect choices on delayed-response problems. During the late 1930s, such findings suggested the treatment of prefrontal leukotomy in mentally disturbed humans. Prefrontal leukotomy severs connections between the prefrontal cortical association area and the thalamus and so functionally isolates vast areas of the prefrontal and orbitofrontal association cortex. The effects of such surgical resections affect both frontal granular areas involved with motor and spatial planning and the orbitofrontal cortex, which is involved with control of autonomic and limbic functions. Therefore, in addition to the desired reduction of expressed anger and frustration, there are also other undesirable changes in mood and affect, as well of symptoms of confusion following leukotomy. Prefrontal leukotomy is no longer prevalent as a treatment for psychiatric disorders, because of undesirable and permanent side-effects and because of improved pharmacological treatment of mental disorders.

7.2

Answer: A   Alpha

Electroencephalography is the neurophysiological measurement of the electrical activity of the brain by recording from electrodes placed on the scalp or, in special cases, subdurally or in the cerebral cortex. The resulting traces are known as an electroencephalogram (EEG) and represent an electrical signal (postsynaptic potentials) from a large number of neurones. These are sometimes called brainwaves, though this use is discouraged. The EEG is a brain function test, but in clinical use it is a 'gross correlate of brain activity'. Electrical currents are not measured, but rather voltage differences between different parts of the brain.

Historically, four major types of continuous rhythmic sinusoidal EEG activity are recognised (alpha, beta, delta and theta). There is no precise agreement on the frequency ranges for each type. Alpha (Berger's wave) is the frequency range from 8 Hz to 12 Hz. It is characteristic of a relaxed, alert state of consciousness. Alpha rhythms are best detected with the eyes closed. Alpha attenuates with drowsiness and open eyes and is best seen over the occipital (visual) cortex. An alpha-like normal variant called mu is sometimes seen over the motor cortex (central scalp) and attenuates with movement or, rather, with the intention to move.

7.3

Answer: A   Cerebellar diseases

The patient in this vignette has cerebellar tremor as suggested by the signs and symptoms. Cerebellar tremor is a slow, broad tremor of the extremities that occurs at the end of a purposeful movement, such as trying to press a button or touching a finger to the tip of one's nose. Cerebellar tremor is caused by lesions in or damage to the cerebellum resulting from stroke, tumour or disease such as multiple sclerosis or some inherited degenerative disorder. It can also result from chronic alcoholism or overuse of some medicines. In classic cerebellar tremor, a lesion on one side of the brain produces a tremor in that same side of the body that worsens with directed movement. Cerebellar damage can also produce a 'wing-beating' type of tremor called rubral or Holmes' tremor – a combination of rest, action and postural tremors. The tremor is often most prominent when the affected person is active or is maintaining a particular posture. Cerebellar tremor may be accompanied by dysarthria (speech problems), nystagmus (rapid, involuntary rolling of the eyes), gait problems and postural tremor of the trunk and neck.

7.4

Answer: E Spasticity

An upper motor neurone lesion is a lesion of the neural pathway above the anterior horn cell or motor nuclei of the cranial nerves. This is in contrast to a lower motor neurone lesion, which affects nerve fibres travelling from the anterior horn of the spinal cord to the relevant muscle(s). The features of an upper motor neurone lesion include:

- 'spastic' increase in tone in the extensor muscles (lower limbs) or flexor muscles (upper limbs)

- 'clasp-knife' response where initial resistance to movement is followed by relaxation

- weakness in the flexors (lower limbs) or extensors (upper limbs), but no muscle wasting

- brisk tendon jerk reflexes

- Babinski sign positive, where the big toe is raised rather than curled downwards on stimulation of the sole of the foot.

7.5

Answer: E Substantia nigra

Parkinson's disease is a degenerative disorder of the central nervous system that often impairs the sufferer's motor skills and speech. Parkinson's disease belongs to a group of conditions called movement disorders. It is characterised by muscle rigidity, tremor, a slowing of physical movement (bradykinesia) and, in extreme cases, a loss of physical movement (akinesia). The primary symptoms are the results of excessive muscle contraction, normally caused by the insufficient formation and action of dopamine, which is produced in the dopaminergic neurones of the brain. Secondary symptoms may include high-level cognitive dysfunction and subtle language problems. Parkinson's disease is both chronic and progressive.

Parkinson's disease is the most common cause of Parkinsonism, a group of similar symptoms. Parkinson's disease is also called 'primary

Parkinsonism' or 'idiopathic Parkinson's disease ('idiopathic' meaning of no known cause). While most forms of Parkinsonism are idiopathic, there are some cases where the symptoms may result from toxicity, drugs, genetic mutation, head trauma or other medical disorders.

The symptoms of Parkinson's disease result from the loss of pigmented dopamine-secreting (dopaminergic) cells and subsequent loss of melanin, secreted by the same cells, in the pars compacta region of the substantia nigra (literally 'black substance'). These neurones project to the striatum and their loss leads to alterations in the activity of the neural circuits within the basal ganglia that regulate movement, in essence an inhibition of the direct pathway and excitation of the indirect pathway.

The direct pathway facilitates movement and the indirect pathway inhibits movement, so the loss of these cells leads to a hypokinetic movement disorder. The lack of dopamine results in increased inhibition of the ventral lateral nucleus of the thalamus, which sends excitatory projections to the motor cortex, so leading to hypokinesia. There are four major dopamine pathways in the brain: the nigrostriatal pathway, referred to above, mediates movement and is the most conspicuously affected in early Parkinson's disease. The other pathways are the mesiocortical, the mesiolimbic and the tuberoinfundibular. These pathways are associated with, respectively: volition and emotional responsiveness; desire, initiative and reward; sensory processes and maternal behaviour. Disruption of dopamine along the non-striatal pathways probably explains much of the neuropsychiatric pathology associated with Parkinson's disease.

7.6

Answer: A   Dopamine

Dopamine is a chemical naturally produced in the body. In the brain, dopamine functions as a neurotransmitter, activating dopamine receptors. Dopamine is also a neurohormone released by the hypothalamus. It has many functions in the brain. Most importantly, it is central to the reward system. Dopamine neurones are activated when an unexpected reward is presented. In nature, we learn to repeat behaviours that lead to unexpected rewards. Dopamine is therefore believed by many to provide a teaching signal to parts of the brain responsible for acquiring new motor sequences, ie behaviours. Dopamine affects the basal ganglia motor loop that in turn affects the way the brain controls our movements. Shortage of dopamine, particularly the death of dopamine neurones in the nigrostriatal pathway, causes Parkinson's disease, in which a person loses the ability to execute smooth, controlled movements. The phasic, dopaminergic activation seems to be crucial with respect to a lasting internal encoding of motor skills.

In the frontal lobes, dopamine controls the flow of information from other areas of the brain. Dopamine disorders in this region of the brain can cause a decline in neurocognitive functions, especially memory, attention and problem solving. Reduced dopamine concentrations in the prefrontal cortex are thought to contribute to attention-deficit disorder and some symptoms of schizophrenia. Conversely, antipsychotic medications rely on their inhibition of dopamine uptake and are used in the treatment of positive symptoms in schizophrenia.

Dopamine is the primary neuroendocrine regulator of the secretion of prolactin from the anterior pituitary gland. Dopamine produced by neurones in the arcuate nucleus of the hypothalamus is secreted into the hypothalamo–hypophysial blood vessels of the median eminence, which supply the pituitary gland. The lactotrophic cells that produce prolactin, in the absence of dopamine, secrete prolactin continuously; dopamine inhibits this secretion. Dopamine is also commonly associated with the pleasure system of the brain, providing feelings of enjoyment and re-inforcement to motivate a person proactively to perform certain activities. Dopamine is released (particularly in areas such as the nuclei accumbens and striatum) by naturally rewarding experiences such as food, sex, use of certain drugs and the neural stimuli that become associated with them. This theory is often discussed in terms of drugs (such as cocaine and the amphetamines), which seem to be directly or indirectly related to the increase of dopamine in these areas and in relation to neurobiological theories of chemical addiction, arguing that these dopamine pathways are pathologically altered in addicted people.

7.7

Answer: E   Vision

The lateral geniculate nucleus (LGN) of the thalamus is a part of the brain, which is the primary processor of visual information, received from the retina, in the central nervous system. The LGN receives information directly from the retina and sends projections directly to the primary visual cortex. In addition, it receives many strong feedback connections from the primary visual cortex. Although the function of the LGN is unknown, it has been shown that it introduces coding efficiencies by cancelling out redundant information from the retina, but there is almost certainly much more going on. Like other areas of the thalamus, particularly other relay nuclei, the LGN probably helps the visual system focus its attention on the most important information. That is, if you hear a sound slightly to your left, the auditory system probably 'tells' the visual system, through the LGN, to direct visual attention to that part of space. The LGN is also a station that refines certain receptive fields.

7.8

Answer: B   Regulation of circadian rhythm

The suprachiasmatic nucleus (SCN) is a region of the brain, located in the hypothalamus, that is responsible for controlling endogenous circadian rhythms. The SCN receives inputs from specialised photoreceptive retinal ganglion cells, via the retinohypothalamic tract. Destruction of the SCN leads to a complete loss of circadian rhythm. The SCN also controls 'slave oscillators' in the peripheral tissues, which exhibit their own 24-hour rhythms, but are crucially synchronised by the SCN. The importance of entraining our bodies to an exogenous cue, such as light, is reflected by several circadian rhythm sleep disorders, in which this process does not function normally.

7.9

Answer: D Pons

Rapid eye movement (REM) sleep is the stage of sleep characterised by rapid movements of the eyes. During this stage, the summed activity of the brain's neurones is quite similar to that during waking hours; for this reason, the phenomenon is often called paradoxical sleep. Most of the vividly recalled dreams occur during REM sleep. REM sleep is so physiologically different from the other phases of sleep that the others are collectively referred to as non-REM sleep.

During a night of sleep, a person usually has about four or five periods of REM sleep, which are quite short at the beginning of the night and longer at the end. It is common to wake for a short time at the end of a REM phase. The total time of REM sleep per night is about 90–120 min for an adult. However, the relative amount of REM sleep varies considerably with age: a newborn baby spends more than 80% of total sleep time in REM, while people over 70 years old spend less than 10%. The average is 20%.

Physiologically, certain neurones in the brainstem, known as REM sleep-on cells (located in the pontine tegmentum), are particularly active during REM sleep and are probably responsible for its occurrence. The release of certain neurotransmitters, the monoamines (noradrenaline, serotonin and histamine), is completely shut down during REM. This causes REM atonia, a state in which the motor neurones are not stimulated and so the body's muscles do not move. Lack of such REM atonia causes REM behaviour disorder; sufferers act out the movements occurring in their dreams.

Heart rate and breathing rate are irregular during REM sleep, again similar to the waking hours. Body temperature is not well regulated during REM. Erections of the penis (nocturnal penile tumescence) is an established accompaniment of REM sleep and is used diagnostically to determine if male erectile dysfunction is of organic or psychological origin. Clitoral enlargement, with accompanying vaginal blood flow and transudation (ie lubrication) is also present during REM. The eye movements associated with REM are generated by the pontine nucleus with projections to the superior colliculus and are associated with PGO (pons, geniculate, occipital) waves.

7.10

Answer: D   Gracile nucleus

The gracile nucleus, located in the medulla oblongata, is one of the dorsal column nuclei that participates in the sensation of fine touch and proprioception. It contains second-order neurones of the dorsal column–medial lemniscus system that receive inputs from sensory neurones of the dorsal root ganglia and send axons that synapse in the thalamus. The neurones contained within the nucleus form a visible bump called the gracile tubercle on the posterior side of the closed medulla at the floor of the 4th ventricle. The gracile nucleus and fasciculus carry epicritic, kinaesthetic and conscious proprioceptive information from the lower part of the body (below the level of T6 in the spinal cord). The counterpart to the gracile nucleus and fasciculus is the cuneate nucleus and fasciculus, which carries the same type of information, but from the upper body (above T6, excepting the face and ear – the information from the face and ear is carried by the primary sensory trigeminal nucleus).

7.11

Answer: E   Right lateral spinothalamic tract

The spinothalamic tract is a sensory pathway originating in the spinal cord that transmits information about pain, temperature, itch and crude touch to the thalamus. The pathway decussates at the level of the spinal cord, rather than in the brainstem like the posterior column–medial lemniscus pathway and corticospinal tract.

The neurones that make up the spinothalamic tract are located principally within the dorsal horn of the spinal cord. These neurones receive synaptic inputs from sensory fibres, which innervate the skin and internal organs.

There are two main parts of the spinothalamic tract:

- the lateral spinothalamic tract transmits pain and temperature
- the anterior spinothalamic tract transmits touch (crude touch).

The types of sensory information transmitted via the spinothalamic tract are described as affective sensation. This means that the sensation is accompanied by a compulsion to act. For instance, an itch is accompanied by a need to scratch and a painful stimulus makes us want to withdraw from the pain. Unilateral lesion of the lateral spinothalamic tract usually causes contralateral anaesthesia (loss of pain) and temperature. Anaesthesia will normally begin one to two segments below the level of lesion, affecting all caudal body areas. This is clinically tested by using pinpricks. So in this clinical vignette the patient has a lesion of right lateral spinothalamic tract.

7.12

Answer: A   Fine touch

The posterior column–medial lemniscus pathway is the sensory pathway responsible for transmitting fine touch and conscious proprioceptive information from the body to the cerebral cortex. The name comes from the two structures that the sensation travels up: the posterior (or dorsal) columns of the spinal cord and the medial lemniscus in the brainstem. Because the posterior columns are also called dorsal columns, the pathway is often called the dorsal column–medial lemniscus system or DCML for short. (Also called posterior column–medial lemniscus or PCML pathway).

Discriminative sensation is well developed in the fingers of humans and allows us to feel fine textures and determine what an unknown object in our hands is without looking at it. This fine sensation is detected by Meissner's corpuscles that lie in the dermis of the skin close to the epidermis. When these structures are stimulated by slight pressure, an action potential is started. The action potential travels up an axon (the cell body of the neurone will be in a dorsal root ganglion). (The neurones are classified as *unipolar,* so they are regarded as having just one long process, an axon.) Therefore, the sensation travels from the skin, along the axon, past the neuronal cell body and into the dorsal column of the spinal cord. The axons continue inside the spinal cord, running up the posterior (dorsal) column. Axons from the lower body are most medial (closer to the midline) and run in the *gracile tract* of the spinal column. Sensory axons from the upper body enter the spinal cord later, so are more lateral and travel up the *cuneate tract.*

At the level of the closed medulla oblongata, these axons synapse with neurones in the *gracile* and *cuneate nuclei*. The secondary neurones (that start in the nuclei) cross over to the other side of the medulla (as *internal arcuate fibres*) to form the medial lemniscus. At the medulla, the medial lemniscus is orientated perpendicular to the way the fibres travelled in the posterior columns. For example, in the columns, lower limb is medial, upper limb is more lateral. At the medial lemniscus, axons from the leg are more ventral, arm fibres more dorsal. Fibres from the trigeminal nerve (supplying the head) come in dorsal to the arm fibres and travel up the lemniscus too. The medial lemniscus rotates 90 degrees at the pons. The secondary axons from neurones giving sensation to the head stay at around the same place, while the leg axons move outwards. The axons travel up the rest of the brainstem and synapse at the thalamus (at the *ventral posterolateral nucleus*). Neurones starting in the thalamus travel up the posterior limb of the internal capsule, and again, head and leg swap relative positions. The axons synapse in the primary sensory cortex, with lower body sensation most medial (eg, the paracentral lobule) and upper body more lateral.

7.13

Answer: E   Substance P

Substance P is a neuropeptide: a short-chain polypeptide that functions as a neurotransmitter and as a neuromodulator. It belongs to the tachykinin neuropeptide family. Substance P is an 11-amino acid polypeptide with the sequence: Arg–Pro–Lys–Pro–Gln–Gln–Phe–Phe–Gly–Leu–Met–NH_2. In the central nervous system, substance P has been associated in the regulation of pain, mood disorders, anxiety, stress, re-inforcement, neurogenesis, respiratory rhythm, neurotoxicity, nausea and emesis. It also has effects as a potent vasodilator. This is caused by the release of nitric oxide from the endothelium. Its release can cause hypotension. The endogenous receptor for substance P is neurokinin 1 receptor (NK1-receptor, NK1R). It belongs to the tachykinin receptor subfamily of G-protein-coupled receptors.

7.14

Answer: B   Cerebellum

The cerebellum (Latin: 'little brain') is a region of the brain that plays an important role in the integration of sensory perception and motor output. Many neural pathways link the cerebellum with the motor cortex – which sends information to the muscles, causing them to move – and the spinocerebellar tract – which provides feedback on the position of the body in space (proprioception). The cerebellum integrates these pathways, using the constant feedback on body position to fine-tune motor movements. Because of this 'updating' function of the cerebellum, lesions within it are not so debilitating as to cause paralysis, but rather present as feedback deficits resulting in disorders in fine movement, equilibrium, posture and motor learning. The patient in this vignette has cerebellar tremor as suggested by the signs and symptoms. Cerebellar tremor is a slow, broad tremor of the extremities that occurs at the end of a purposeful movement, such as reaching for coffee cup or touching a finger to the tip of one's nose (*see also* answer to 7.3).

7.15

Answer: E   Meningitis

Although diagnosis of meningitis as well as its specific aetiology are important, laboratory testing takes time. Because bacterial meningitis is such an urgent issue, treatment is usually instituted before a definite diagnosis is made. When a patient is suspected of meningitis, blood should be drawn for culture and empiric antibiotics started immediately. Diagnosis of meningitis can then be carried out with examination of cerebrospinal fluid (CSF) with a lumbar puncture (LP). However, if the patient has had recent head trauma, is immunocompromised, has known malignancy or central nervous system neoplasm or focal neurological deficits such as papilloedema or altered consciousness, computed tomography (CT) or MRI should be performed before the LP to avoid a potentially fatal brain herniation during the procedure. Otherwise, the CT or MRI should be performed after the LP, with MRI preferred over CT due to its superiority in demonstrating areas of cerebral oedema, ischaemia and meningeal enhancement. Antibiotics started within 4 hours of lumbar puncture will not significantly affect lab results. The opening pressure is noted during the LP and the CSF sent for examination of white and red blood cell counts, glucose, protein, Gram stain, culture and possibly latex agglutination test, litmus, lysates or polymerase chain reaction (PCR) for bacterial or viral DNA. If the patient is immunocompromised, the doctor may also consider testing the CSF for toxoplasmosis, Epstein–Barr virus, cytomegalovirus, JC virus and fungal infection. CSF analysis in bacterial meningitis will show:

- opening pressure: > 180 mmH$_2$O

- white blood cell count: 10–10 000/µl with neutrophil predominance

- glucose: < 40 mg/dl

- CSF glucose to serum glucose ratio: < 0.4

- protein: > 4.5 mg/dl

- Gram stain: positive in > 60%

- culture: positive in > 80%

- latex agglutination: may be positive in meningitis due to *Streptococcus pneumoniae*, *Neisseria meningitidis*, *Haemophilus influenzae*, *Escherichia coli*, group B streptococci

- Limulus, lysates: positive in Gram-negative meningitis.

CSF cultures are usually positive in 30–70% of patients with viral meningitis and those with negative cultures will usually have a positive CSF PCR test.

7.16

Answer: C   Muscle wasting

Lower motor neurones (LMNs) are the motoneurones connecting the brainstem and spinal cord to muscle fibres, bringing the nerve impulses from the upper motor neurones out to the muscles. Lower motor neurones are classified based on the type of muscle fibres they innervate. Alpha motor neurones (α-MNs) innervate extrafusal muscle fibres, the most numerous type of muscle fibre and the one most involved in contraction of a muscle. Gamma motor neurones (γ-MNs) innervate intrafusal muscle fibres, which are involved with muscle spindles and the sense of body position. Damage to lower motor neurones is indicated by abnormal electromyographic potentials, fasciculations, paralysis, weakening muscles and neurogenic atrophy (wasting) of skeletal muscle(s).

7.17

Answer: B   Guillain–Barré syndrome

Guillain–Barré syndrome (GBS) is an acute, autoimmune, polyradiculoneuropathy affecting the peripheral nervous system, usually triggered by an acute infectious process. There are several types of GBS, but unless otherwise stated, GBS refers to the most common form, acute inflammatory demyelinating polyneuropathy. It is frequently severe and usually exhibits as an ascending paralysis noted by weakness in the legs that spreads to the upper limbs and the face along with complete loss of deep tendon reflexes. About 75% of patients with GBS have a history of acute infection within the past 1–4 weeks, usually respiratory or gastrointestinal. 20–30% of these cases are due to *Campylobacter jejuni* and a similar proportion due to cytomegalovirus or Epstein–Barr virus. The risk of developing Guillain–Barré syndrome following campylobacter infection is less than two per 10 000 in the following 2 months. Less common infectious agents include *Mycoplasma pneumoniae*, HIV and herpes simplex virus. Immunisations have also been implicated in GBS. With prompt treatment with immunoglobulins and supportive care, the majority of patients will regain full functional capacity. However, death may occur if severe pulmonary complications and dysautonomia are present.

7.18

Answer: C   Ipsilateral spastic paralysis, ipsilateral loss of vibration and proprioception (position sense) and contralateral loss of pain and temperature sensation beginning one or two segments below the lesion

Brown–Séquard syndrome, also known as Brown–Séquard's hemiplegia and Brown–Séquard's paralysis, is a loss of motricity (paralysis and ataxia) and sensation caused by the lateral hemisection of the spinal cord. Other synonyms are crossed hemiplegia, hemiparaplegic syndrome, hemiplegia and hemiparaplegia spinalis and spinal hemiparaplegia. The hemisection of the cord results in a lesion of each of the three main neural systems: the principal upper motor neurone pathway of the corticospinal tract, one or both dorsal columns and the spinothalamic tract. Because of the injury to these three main brain pathways the patient will present with three lesions. The corticospinal lesion produces spastic paralysis on the same side of the body (the loss of moderation by the upper motor neurones). The lesion to fasciculus gracilis or fasciculus cuneatus results in ipsilateral loss of vibration and proprioception (position sense). The loss of the spinothalamic tract leads to pain and temperature sensation being lost from the contralateral side beginning one or two segments below the lesion. At the lesion site, all sensory modalities are lost on the same side, and an ipsilateral flaccid paralysis.

7.19

Answer: B   Impaired two-point discrimination and vibratory sensibility on the left side of body below the lesion

The hemisection of the cord results in a lesion of each of the three main neural systems: the principal upper motor neurone pathway of the corticospinal tract, one or both dorsal columns and the spinothalamic tract. As a result of the injury to these three main brain pathways the patient will present with three lesions. The corticospinal lesion produces spastic paralysis on the same side of the body (the loss of moderation by the upper motor neurones). The lesion to fasciculus gracilis or fasciculus cuneatus results in ipsilateral loss of vibration and proprioception (position sense). The loss of the spinothalamic tract leads to pain and temperature sensation being lost from the contralateral side beginning one or two segments below the lesion. At the lesion site, all sensory modalities are lost on the same side, and an ipsilateral flaccid paralysis. So in this vignette B is the correct option.

neurophysiology

7.20

Answer: C   Pacinian corpuscle

Pacinian corpuscles are one of the four major types of mechanoreceptor, responsible for sensitivity to deep pressure, touch and high-frequency vibration. These corpuscles are found in mesenteries, especially the pancreas, and are often found near joints. Like Ruffini endings, they are found in deep subcutaneous tissue and are considered rapidly adapting receptors. Similar in physiology to the Meissner's corpuscle, Pacinian corpuscles are larger and fewer in number than both Merkel cells and Meissner's corpuscles. The Pacinian corpuscle is ovoid and approximately 1 mm in length. The entire corpuscle is wrapped by a layer of connective tissue. It has 20–60 concentric lamellae composed of fibrous connective tissue and fibroblasts, separated by gelatinous material. The lamellae are very thin, flat, modified Schwann cells. In the centre of the corpuscle is the inner bulb, a fluid-filled cavity with a single afferent unmyelinated nerve ending. Pacinian corpuscles detect gross pressure changes and vibrations. Any deformation in the corpuscle causes action potentials to be generated, by opening pressure-sensitive sodium ion channels in the axon membrane. This allows sodium ions to influx, creating a receptor potential (independent of potassium channels). These corpuscles are especially susceptible to vibrations, which they can sense even centimetres away. Pacinian corpuscles cause action potentials when the skin is rapidly indented but not when the pressure is steady, due to the layers of connective tissue that cover the nerve ending. It is thought that they respond to high velocity changes in joint position. Pacinian corpuscles have a large receptive field on the skin's surface, with an especially sensitive centre. They only sense stimuli that occur within this field.

7.21

Answer: D   In upper motor neurone lesion

A stretch reflex is a muscle contraction in response to stretching within that muscle. It is a monosynaptic reflex that provides automatic regulation of skeletal muscle length. Muscle spindles are sensory apparatus sensitive to stretch of the muscle in which they lie. Suppose a person standing in the upright position begins to lean to one side.

The postural muscles that are closely connected to the vertebral column on the side will stretch. Because of this, stretch receptors in those muscles contract to correct posture. The patellar (knee jerk) reflex is an example. Another example is the group 1a fibres in the calf muscle, which synapse with motor neurones supplying muscle fibres in the same muscle. A sudden stretch, such as tapping the Achilles' tendon, causes a reflex contraction in the muscle as the spindles sense the stretch and send an action potential to the motor neurones, which then cause the muscle to contract; this particular reflex causes a contraction in the soleus–gastrocnemius group of muscles. This reflex can be enhanced by the Jendrassik manoeuvre. In upper motor neurone lesion the stretch reflexes are brisk, due to loss of inhibitory signals on gamma neurones through the lateral reticulospinal tract.

7.22

Answer: B   Level of wakefulness

The reticular activating system is the name given to part of the brain (the reticular formation and its connections) believed to be the centre of arousal and motivation in animals (including humans). The activity of this system is crucial for maintaining the state of consciousness. It is situated at the core of the brainstem between the myelencephalon (medulla oblongata) and mesencephalon (midbrain).

It is involved with the circadian rhythm; damage can lead to permanent coma. It is thought to be the area affected by many psychotropic drugs. General anaesthetics work through their effect on the reticular formation. Fibres from the reticular formation are also vital in controlling respiration, cardiac rhythms and other essential functions. The reticular activating system has received attention from neuroscientists interested in various pathological conditions affecting behaviour, such as Alzheimer's disease. More recently, results of research on the area has prompted extrapolations from the data into various areas such as motivational programmes and attention-deficit hyperactivity disorder (ADHD). The reticular activating system is believed to cause ADHD due to an unbalance of noradrenaline in the cells. This leads to the over-arousal and lack of motivation associated with these disorders. Although the functioning of this system is a prerequisite for consciousness to occur, it is generally assumed that this system's role is indirect and it does not, by itself, generate consciousness. Instead, its unique anatomical and physiological characteristics ensure that the thalamocortical system fires in such a way that is compatible with conscious experience.

7.23

Answer: D   Loss of satiety

The ventromedial nucleus of the hypothalamus (sometimes referred to as the ventromedial hypothalamus) has two parts: superior and anterior. The *superior part* is responsible for satiety. This means if it is taken out of an animal, the animal will overeat because there is nothing telling the body that the animal is satisfied. The *anterior part* is responsible for the female sexual drive.

7.24

Answer: C   Hyperaesthesia

Cerebrovascular accidents can cause thalamic syndrome, which results in contralateral hemianaesthesia, burning or aching sensation in one half of a body (hyperaesthesia), often accompanied by mood swings. Ischaemia of the territory of the paramedian artery, if bilateral, causes serious troubles, including akinetic mutism accompanied or not by oculomotor troubles.

7.25

Answer: C   It only occurs during voluntary movements

The cerebellum is generally considered to play an important role in the co-ordination and smoothing out of voluntary movements. Intention tremor, which may be observed in cerebellar disease, is absent at rest but appears at the onset of voluntary movements. This aspect of the tremor readily differentiates it from tremor observed with degeneration of the nigrostriatal dopaminergic tracts in Parkinson's disease, which produces tremor that is present at rest. Frequency of tremor is a less reliable means to distinguish these types of tremor and the amplitude of oscillations is not generally constant throughout a voluntary movement (*see also* answer to 7.3).

7.26

Answer: E   Phentolamine causes pupil constriction

Pupil diameter is determined by the balance between sympathetic tone to the radial fibres of the iris and parasympathetic tone to the pupillary sphincter muscle. Phentolamine is a blocker of α-adrenergic receptors, which causes pupil constriction. Pupil dilatation occurs during increased sympathetic activity, eg emotional excitement, decreased parasympathetic activity during darkness or block of muscarinic receptors by atropine.

7.27

Answer: A   Convection currents in endolymph

Water that is either higher or lower than body temperature when introduced into the external auditory meatus may set up convection currents within the endolymph of the inner ear. These currents may result in the stimulation of the semicircular canals by causing movements of the ampullar cristae. Conflicting information from the right and left sides may in turn result in vertigo and nausea. Decreased movement or immobilisation of the otoliths or the ampullar cristae is not caused by such changes in temperature. Furthermore, changes in the discharge rate of vestibular afferents, which must occur with caloric stimulation, are most likely to be caused by the changes in the activity of the receptors, rather than being a direct response of the afferents to changes in temperature.

7.28

Answer: D   The location of maximal basilar membrane displacement moves toward the base of the cochlea

The primary change in the cochlea due to an increase in the frequency of a sound wave is a change in the position of maximal displacement of the basilar membrane. A sound of low pitch produces the greatest displacement toward the apex of the cochlea and produces the greatest activation of hair cells at that location. As the pitch is increased, the position of greatest displacement moves closer to the base of the cochlea. Increased amplitude of basilar membrane displacement and increases in the number of hair cells that are activated and in the frequency of discharge of units in the auditory nerve fibres, together with an increase in range of frequencies to which such units respond, are all more likely to be observed in response to increases in the intensity or a sound stimulus rather than to increases in pitch. In the auditory cortex, sound frequencies are organised topographically so that a change in pitch may be represented by a change in the location of activated cortical units.

7.29

Answer: D   Response of skeletal muscle to nerve stimulation is weakened

Myasthenia gravis is an autoimmune disease characterised by progressive muscle weakness due to formation of antibodies against the nicotinic acetylcholine (ACh) receptor of the motor endplate. Impairment of neuromuscular transmission results in a weakened response of the muscle to nerve stimulation, but a normal response to direct electrical stimulation. Improvement of muscle weakness by small doses of acetylcholinesterase inhibitors, physostigmine or edrophonium, are diagnostic for this disease. A large dose of physostigmine worsens muscle weakness because of desensitisation of the endplate to persistent ACh. Radiolabelled snake venom α-bungarotoxin is a useful investigative tool to quantify the number of ACh receptors at the motor endplate; the test should be performed in vitro on a muscle biopsy specimen.

7.30

Answer: E   Penile erections

Normal sleep occurs in alternating cycles between slow-wave sleep (non-REM sleep) and REM sleep, the latter characterised by high metabolic brain activity and desynchronisation of the EEG. Somnambulism (sleepwalking), enuresis (bedwetting) and night terrors occur during slow-wave sleep or arousal from slow-wave sleep. During REM sleep, there is hypotonia of all major muscle groups except the ocular muscles, due to a generalised spinal inhibition that prevents acting out of dreams. Dreams, nightmares and penile erections in

neurophysiology

the male all occur during REM sleep. Sleep spindles in the EEG are characteristic for the early sleep stages (*see also* answer to 7.9).

7.31

Answer: D   Ptosis (hanging of the upper eyelid) on the left side

The patient in question has Horner's syndrome. Unilateral loss of sympathetic innervation of the face results in ptosis and pupil constriction, not dilatation. Vasodilatation of the skin vessels and loss of sweating results in dry and red skin, not pale or sweaty skin. Lateral deviation of the eye would suggest damage to the third cranial nerve.

7.32

Answer: D   This patient's condition can be corrected with convex glasses

Hyperopia or farsightedness, is due either to an insufficient refractive power of the lens or too short an eyeball. This condition can be corrected using glasses with convex lenses. Myopia or nearsightedness, is due to either unusually large refractive power of the lens or too long an eyeball. This condition can be corrected using glasses with concave lenses. Presbyopia is a condition of decreased accommodation range of the lens due to a decline of lens elasticity with age. Like hyperopia, this condition can also be corrected with convex glasses (reading glasses).

7.33

Answer: C   Lower motor neurone lesions

Muscle tone is determined by the firing rate of the α-motor neurones and damage to these so-called lower motor neurones will result in flaccid paralysis. In contrast, damage to the corticospinal tract (ie upper motor neurone lesions) results in spastic paralysis because of hyperactive stretch reflexes. Activation of γ-efferent fibres to muscle spindles also increase muscle tone due to reflex activation of the motor neurones (stretch reflex). Pathological increased γ-efferent discharge results in muscle clonus. Parkinson's disease is characterised by muscle rigidity and tremor. Anxiety is also associated with increased muscle tension.

7.34

Answer: B   Non-selective cation channels

The photoreceptor cell membrane is relatively depolarised in darkness due to Na^+ entry through non-selective cation channels. Openings of these channels are maintained by the high intracellular cGMP levels in photoreceptors during darkness and the Na^+ inward current through these channels is usually called 'dark current'. Illumination by light causes a conformational change in the photosensitive pigment rhodopsin, which is linked via a G protein to a cGMP-specific phosphodiesterase. Activation of phosphodiesterase lowers cGMP levels and, since cGMP is required to maintain openings of the non-selective cation channels, results in membrane hyperpolarisation with light exposure. Cl^- channels or non-selective anion channels do not contribute to the dark current of photoreceptors. Ryanodine receptors are located on the sarcoplasmic reticulum (SR) and when opened release stored Ca^{2+} from the SR. These channels are locked into the open state by the plant alkaloid, ryanodine (hence the name). Like in most other cells, the Na^+/K^+ pump is responsible for the high intracellular K^+ concentration in photoreceptor cells.

7.35

Answer: E   Right posterior parietal cortex

Large injury to the non-dominant parietal cortex may cause the patient to ignore the serious nature of his illness and to neglect or even deny the presence of the paralysis affecting the side of the body opposite to the lesion. Occasionally this neglect may involve not only the patient's body but also the perception of the external world. Smaller injuries to the non-dominant parietal cortex involving the precentral gyrus (primary motor cortex) or postcentral gyrus (primary sensory cortex) result in contralateral spastic paralysis or contralateral loss of tactile sensation, respectively. Injury to the dominant hemisphere involving the posterior inferior gyrus of the frontal lobe (Broca's area) produces an expressive or motor aphasia in which the patient's comprehension of language, involving the posterior superior gyrus of the temporal lobe (Wernicke's area), produces a sensory aphasia in which words are spoken fluently but without meaning. The patient does not understand his own word 'salad', either.

7.36

Answer: C   Fibrosis causing fixation of the ossicles

Because the cochlea is embedded in bone, vibrations in the bone can be transmitted directly to the cochlear fluid. For this reason, damage to the ossicles or tympanic membrane would not be detected from a bone conduction test.

7.37

Answer: D   There is a latent period before the attenuation reflex can occur

When a loud sound is transmitted into the central nervous system, an attenuation reflex occurs after a latent period of 40–80 ms. The reflex involves the contraction of two muscles that pull the malleus and stapes toward each other, thereby causing the entire ossicular system to develop a high degree of rigidity. In turn, the ossicular conduction of low-frequency sounds to the cochlea can be reduced by as much as 30–40 decibels. Since loud sounds are usually low-frequency sounds, the attenuation reflex can protect the cochlea from damage caused by loud sounds when they develop slowly.

7.38

Answer: A   The ciliary muscles are relaxed

This patient probably suffers from myopia (nearsightedness). Myopia is due to either eyeballs that are too long or a lens that is too strong. To focus a distant object onto the retina (far accommodation) the lens has to decrease its refractive power, ie, increase its focal length. This is accomplished through relaxation of the ciliary muscles that oppose the pull of the sclera, resulting in a tightening of the zonular fibres and a flattening of the lens. Relaxation of the zonular fibres, rounding of the lens and shortening of the focal length, all occur during near accommodation. The pupils also constrict during near accommodation, perhaps to increase depth of field.

7.39

Answer: C   Glaucoma is a rare cause of blindness in the UK

This patient suffers from an acute glaucoma attack. The aqueous humour leaves the eye in the anterior chamber, passes through a meshwork of trabeculae and enters the canal of Schlemm, which empties into extraocular veins. Pupil dilatation tends to open the canal of Schlemm and enhance outflow because of the proximity of the pupillary dilator muscle insertion at the sclera to the canal and trabeculae. Normal ocular pressure is around 15 mmHg and remains constant in a normal eye throughout the day, usually within about ± 2 mmHg. The production rate of aqueous humour is approximately 2–3 µl/min and intraocular pressure is mainly determined by the balance of rate of production and outflow. Closure of the ocular angle (canal of Schlemm) leads to an acute glaucoma attack. Because of the high risk of permanent damage to the retina and optic nerve, this medical emergency should be treated with drugs that dilate the pupils. Drugs of choice are antimuscarinics (pilocarpine) or β-blockers (timolol). In addition, carbonic anhydrase inhibitors reduce the rate of production of aqueous humour during acute attacks, but are not useful for long-term treatment. Corticosteroids play no role in the emergency management of acute glaucoma. Glaucoma is not a rare cause of blindness in the United Kingdom, but rather one of the most common causes of acquired blindness.

7.40

Answer: E   Supplementary motor area

Monitoring regional cerebral blood flow (rCBF) is a method of measuring the dynamics of the physiological substrate of speech. The physiological assumption is that active areas command increased blood flow. In fact, blood flow to the speech areas increases during various types of linguistic function. During periods of silent counting, rCBF increases within the superior speech cortex (supplementary motor area). Speaking aloud increase rCBF in the motor cortex and medial temporal lobe, in addition to the superior speech cortex. Both silent reading and reading aloud increases rCBF within the region of Broca's anterior speech cortex, in addition to the areas increased by speaking aloud.

7.41

Answer: E   Vibratory sensations from the ipsilateral arm

At this level, the lateral portion of the dorsal columns (dorsal funiculus) is composed of the fasciculus cuneatus. Axons carrying tactile, proprioceptive and vibratory information from the ipsilateral arm enter the spinal cord via the dorsal root, ascend the cord in the fasciculus cuneatus and synapse in the nucleus cuneatus of the caudal medulla. Secondary neurones from this nucleus give rise to internal arcuate fibres, which decussate and ascend to the thalamus (ventral posterolateral nucleus, VPL) as the medial lemniscus. Tertiary neurones from the VPL project to the ipsilateral somatosensory cortex. Therefore, damage to the fasciculus cuneatus would result in a deficit in tactile, proprioceptive and vibratory sensations in the ipsilateral arm, because the fibres that carry this information do not cross until they reach the medulla.

Fine motor control of the fingers is principally carried by the ipsilateral lateral corticospinal tract in the lateral funiculus of the cord. Motor control of the contralateral foot is carried by the ipsilateral corticospinal tract in the lateral funiculus of the cord. Hemi-anhidrosis (lack of sweating) of the face could be produced by interruption of sympathetic innervation to the face. The hypothalamospinal tract projects from the hypothalamus to the intermediolateral cell column at levels T1 to T2. It descends the cord in the lateral funiculus. Interruption of this tract results in Horner's syndrome (miosis, ptosis, hemi-anhidrosis). Proprioception from the ipsilateral leg is carried by the fasciculus gracilis in the medial part of the dorsal columns.

7.42

Answer: B   Intercollicular brainstem transection

Decerebrate 'rigidity' is a condition of increased muscle tone and stretch reflexes, particularly in extensor muscles. It is produced by intercollicular brainstem transection. This disconnects certain reticulospinal neurones from their most important source of excitatory synaptic drive, eliminates rubrospinal inhibition and leads to the appearance of the positive neurological signs of increased muscle tone and stretch reflexes. Disinhibition of extensor motor neurones is the major culprit, but ongoing excitation from the vestibulospinal tract is also important. Decerebrate rigidity comes about through the following interactions:

- The pontine reticular formation (N. reticularis pontis oralis and caudalis) facilitates alpha and gamma motor neurones of extensor muscles. Pontine reticulospinal neurones receive excitatory drive from somato-sensory receptors as well as from the cerebral cortex (forebrain). These reticulospinal neurones continue to fire even when they are disconnected from the forebrain.

- The medullary reticular formation (N. reticularis gigantocellularis) facilitates flexor LMNs (not shown) and inhibits, via inhibitory inter-neurones, alpha and gamma motor neurones of extensor muscles. Medullary reticulospinal neurones do not receive much excitatory drive from somatosensory receptors and so depend on excitatory drive from the cerebral cortex for maintaining their normal rate of firing. Medullary reticulospinal neurones cease firing when disconnected from the forebrain, so inhibitory synaptic drive onto extensor motor neurones is decreased.

- Tonic reciprocal inhibition of extensor motor neurones from rubrospinal tract axons is eliminated by brainstem transection. This further inhibits the extensor LMNs.

- The net result of the transection is to cause an imbalance in descending influences onto alpha and gamma extensor motor neurones: excitation out-weighs inhibition. This occurs because inhibitory action from the medullary reticular formation and the red nucleus is much reduced while excitatory action from the pontine reticular formation and the lateral vestibular nucleus persists.

- Because gamma motor neurones are most excitable (recall the 'size principle'), the stretch reflex arc becomes spontaneously active. This causes a large, tonic increase in extensor muscle tone (hypertonia) with increased stretch reflexes (decreased threshold and increased amplitude, referred to as hyper-reflexia).

An interesting feature of decerebrate hypertonia is that section of the dorsal roots to a limb 'melts' (abolishes) the rigidity in that limb. The explanation for this effect is as follows. The small, highly excitable gamma motor neurones are powerfully excited in the decerebrate preparation. They cause the stretch reflex arc to be hyperactive, which means that the group Ia afferent fibres from the muscle spindles are hyperactive. Cutting the dorsal roots knocks out the afferent limb of the stretch reflex arc. This diminishes the excessive excitatory synaptic drive to alpha motor neurones enough to stop them from firing. This type of hypertonia, which is sensitive to dorsal root section, is called 'gamma rigidity'.

Another noteworthy feature of decerebrate rigidity is that ablation (destruction) of the anterior lobe of the cerebellum enhances the hypertonia. This effect is due to disinhibition of the spontaneously active vestibulospinal tract cells. Disinhibition arises due to the loss of the inhibitory action of Purkinje cells, which project from the anterior lobe of the cerebellum to the lateral vestibular nucleus.

7.43

Answer: A   Areflexia

Complete spinal cord transection produces the following:

- Spinal shock: immediately following the transection, spinal reflexes below the level of cord transection are lost (areflexia). This is a classic negative sign due to profound disfacilitation of LMNs, as well as interneurones in reflex circuits. These cells are disfacilitated due to transection of all motor pathways.

- Mass reflex: with time, somatic and autonomic reflexes return and may become hyperactive. Flexion reflexes return before stretch reflexes. Light tactile stimulation may produce bilateral flexion of legs and trunk accompanied by bladder and bowel evacuation. Hyperactive reflexes probably arise due to two reasons: development of denervation supersensitivity in spinal cord neurones; and sprouting of the central terminals of primary afferent fibres.

7.44

Answer: D   Postcentral gyrus

The primary somatic sensory (S1) cortex in the postcentral gyrus is the first and largest cortical receiving area for the analysis of information from somatosensory receptors. It receives and analyses information from the ventrobasal (VPL + VPM) nucleus of the thalamus. S1 cortex is necessary for the conscious awareness: (1) that a stimulus has occurred; (2) of stimulus quality; (3) of stimulus location; (4) of stimulus amplitude; and (5) of stimulus duration. The S1 cortex is not, however, the 'end station' in the somatic sensory pathway. S1 cortex sends information, via corticocortical fibres, to other areas of the neocortex. Further important analysis of somatosensory information occurs in the posterior parietal association cortex.

7.45

Answer: C Precentral gyrus

The primary motor cortex (or M1) works in association with premotor areas to plan and execute movements. M1 contains large neurones known as Betz cells, which send long axons down the spinal cord to synapse onto alpha motor neurones, which connect to the muscles. Premotor areas are involved in planning actions (in concert with the basal ganglia) and refining movements based upon sensory input (this requires the cerebellum). The human primary motor cortex is located in the dorsal part of the precentral gyrus and the anterior bank of the central sulcus. The precentral gyrus is in front of the postcentral gyrus, from which it is separated by the central sulcus. Its anterior border is the precentral sulcus, while inferiorly it borders to the lateral fissure (Sylvian fissure). Medially, it is contiguous with the paracentral lobule.

SECTION 8:
ENDOCRINE PHYSIOLOGY –
ANSWERS

8.1

Answer: E   Water intake is appropriately adjusted

In diabetes insipidus, appropriate water intake from thirst will adequately compensate for the potential excess volume loss. Only if access to appropriate intake is prevented will a large volume loss occur. All of the other changes listed would tend to maintain blood volume, but all are either short-term effects or the result of extreme stimuli, such as haemorrhage or intense sympathetic activity.

8.2

Answer: C   Low serum concentration of glucose

Hypoglycaemia is the most potent stimulus for glucagon secretion. High serum levels of amino acids (especially alanine and arginine) will also induce glucagon release. Hyperglycaemia is a potent stimulus for insulin release from pancreatic β-cells. Somatostatin inhibits glucagon secretion. While parasympathetic stimulation to the pancreas stimulates acinar secretion, it does not stimulate α-cells to secrete glucagon.

8.3

Answer: A   Angiotensin II

Secondary hyperaldosteronism in hypertensive states either is secondary to a primary overproduction of renin by the kidneys or is caused by an overproduction of renin secondary to a decrease in renal blood flow or perfusion pressure (eg, malignant hypertension). Principal stimuli for aldosterone release are circulating adrenocorticotrophic hormone (ACTH) from the pituitary gland, angiotensin II and high plasma K$^+$ levels. In addition, low plasma Na$^+$ may also have a direct stimulatory effect on the adrenal cortex. Hypokalaemia and hypernatraemia reduce aldosterone secretion. Volume depletion, eg, haemorrhage, increases aldosterone release through activation of the renin–angiotensin system. Overhydration has the opposite effect: atrial natriuretic peptide is secreted from atrial myocytes under conditions of expanded extracellular volume and acts on renal mesangial cells and ductal epithelium to decrease Na$^+$ reabsorption.

8.4

Answer: C   Low serum sodium due to the dilutional effect of ADH-induced water retention in the collecting tubules

Antidiuretic hormone (ADH) acts on the collecting tubules in the kidney to induce water retention. Inappropriately high levels of ADH, as an achieved in SIADH, result in the renal retention of free water, which consequently exercise a dilutional effect on serum ion concentrations. So, serum sodium can fall dramatically in SIADH. While ADH also increases Na$^+$ reabsorption in the papillary collecting ducts, this effect is not enough to overcome the dilution of plasma caused by the increased renal water reabsorption in the presence of ADH. High sodium levels might be expected with decreased ADH levels, decreased renal responsiveness to ADH or in patients dehydrated from any other cause.

8.5

Answer: D   Increased plasma osmolarity

Increased plasma osmolarity is the most potent stimulus for ADH release. An increase in plasma osmolarity of only 1% is sufficient to increase ADH levels. Decreased plasma volume also stimulates ADH release but is a less potent stimulus. Plasma ADH levels are not affected until blood volume is reduced by about 10%. Nevertheless the decreased blood volume and arterial pressure in patients with severe haemorrhage result in ADH secretion, causing increased water reabsorption by the kidneys that helps to restore blood pressure and volume. Hypothalamic releasing factors control release of anterior pituitary hormones TSH, ACTH, FSH, LH, GH and prolactin, but not the release of posterior pituitary hormones ADH and oxytocin.

8.6

Answer: E   Patient has significantly reduced glomerular filtration rate

Glucose excretion by the kidneys depends on the glomerular filtration and tubular reabsorption rates. Glucose first appears in the urine when the capacity of the glucose transporters in the proximal tubuli cells is exceeded. This usually occurs at plasma glucose levels higher than 180 mg/dl. Patients with long-standing diabetes mellitus often have decreased renal function and reduced glomerular filtration rate. Under these circumstances the threshold (ie plasma level) for excretion of glucose will be higher than in a healthy person. Patients with diabetes insipidus have a large urine output due to absence of ADH or defective renal ADH receptors, but should not have a plasma glucose level of 200 mg/dl. Antidiuresis increases the concentration of solutes in the urine and increases the sensitivity to detect urine glucose. Reabsorption of filtered glucose occurs in the proximal tubule by active transport. A defect in glucose transporters would result in glucosuria even at normal plasma glucose concentration. Urine dipsticks nowadays are both sensitive and specific for glucose, detecting as little as 100 mg/dl. Earlier dipstick tests were sensitive but not specific, ie they detected other reducing sugars in addition to glucose.

8.7

Answer: C   Decreased   Increased   Decreased

Glycogen synthesis and breakdown depend on the balance of glycogen synthase activity (glycogen synthesis) and glycogen phosphorylase activity (glycogen breakdown). These enzymes are under the control of cAMP-dependent protein kinases. Phosphorylation of glycogen phosphorylase activates this enzyme

endocrine

and promotes glycogen degradation. This phosphorylation is carried out by an enzyme called glycogen phosphorylase kinase, which itself is activated by a cAMP-dependent protein kinase. Therefore, hormones that increase liver cell cAMP promote glycogen breakdown, while hormones that decrease liver cell cAMP promote glycogen synthesis. Adrenaline and glucagon stimulate the mobilisation of glycogen by triggering the cAMP cascade. Cortisol, the main glucocorticoid, regulates the metabolism of proteins, fats and carbohydrates. On most organs cortisol acts catabolically, however on the liver it has anabolic effects, increasing glycogen synthesis and accumulation in the liver.

8.8

Answer: D   Periorbital swelling and lethargy

An increased TSH combined with a low T_3 resin uptake (and low free T_4) are characteristic of hypothyroidism. Clinical signs and symptoms of hypothyroidism include dull facial expression, puffiness and periorbital swelling caused by infiltration with mucopolysaccharides, decreased adrenergic drive, lethargy, bradycardia and cold intolerance. The periorbital swelling must be distinguished from exophthalmus due to increased retro-orbital tissue, which is a specific sign for hyperthyroidism caused by Graves' disease. Tachycardia, fever, palpitations and anxiety are all seen in hyperthyroidism. Additional clinical signs seen with hyperthyroidism may include heat intolerance, tremor, sweating and sleeplessness.

8.9

Answer: B   Osteomalacia due to secondary hyperparathyroidism

Osteomalacia in chronic renal failure is caused by decreased production of vitamin D and phosphate retention by the kidneys. The rise in serum phosphate causes increased binding of calcium, resulting in a decrease in ionised calcium concentration, which stimulates parathyroid hormone (PTH) secretion by the parathyroid glands (secondary hyperparathyroidism). PTH stimulates release of calcium from the bones, leading to demineralisation. Osteoporosis is a reduction in bone mass, particularly a decrease in cortical thickness.

In contrast to osteomalacia, the ratio of mineral to organic phase is normal in osteoporosis. Bone loss occurs with age in both men and women at a rate of about 0.5% per year. Osteoporosis predominantly involves the spine, hip and distal radius. In postmenopausal women, an accelerated loss of bone mass is superimposed on the age-related loss due to declining oestrogen levels. In men, bone modelling is less dependent on sex steroids. Osteomalacia occurs with both primary and secondary hyperparathyroidism. In patients with chronic renal failure, hyperparathyroidism is secondary to reduced ionised calcium concentration in the serum. Lack of active vitamin D also contributes to osteomalacia in this patient. In chronic renal failure the conversion of 25-hydroxycholecalciferol to the active 1,25-dihydroxycholecalciferol by the kidneys is impaired. Lack of dietary vitamin D is less likely in this patient.

8.10

Answer: D   Prolactin

The hypophyseal portal system is the system of blood vessels that links the hypothalamus and the anterior pituitary. It allows endocrine communication between the two structures. The anterior pituitary receives releasing and inhibitory hormones in the blood. Using these the anterior pituitary is able to fulfil its function of regulating the other endocrine glands. It is one of only a few portal systems of circulation in the body; that is, it involves two capillary beds connected by venules rather than arterioles. The hypothalamic–hypophyseal venous portal system carries prolactin-inhibitory hormone from the hypothalamus to the anterior pituitary gland. In the absence of this hormone, prolactin secretion increases to about three times normal levels.

8.11

Answer: C   Hypoglycaemia between meals

Addison's disease results from failure of the adrenal cortices to produce adrenocortical hormones. Addison's disease usually develops slowly (over several months) and symptoms may not be present or be noticed until some stressful illness or situation occurs.

endocrine

Common symptoms are:

- chronic fatigue that gradually worsens

- muscle weakness

- weight loss and loss of appetite

- nausea, diarrhoea or vomiting

- hypotension, abnormally low blood pressure that falls further when standing (orthostatic hypotension)

- areas of hyperpigmentation (darkened skin), known as melasma suprarenalis caused by increases in pro-opiomelanocortin. Although cutaneous pigmentation will most probably disappear following therapy, pigmentation of the oral mucosa tends to persist

- irritability

- depression

- craving for salt and salty foods

- for women, menstrual periods become irregular or cease

- tetany (particularly after drinking milk) due to phosphate excess

- numbness of the extremities, sometimes with paralysis, due to potassium excess

- increased number of eosinophils

- polyuria

- hypovolaemia

- dehydration

- tremors

- tachycardia

- restlessness

- diaphoresis (excessive sweating)

- dysphagia (difficulty swallowing)

- hyponatraemia (low blood sodium levels), possibly worsened by loss of production of the hormone aldosterone, but it occurs in secondary (pituitary) adrenal insufficiency as well. This underscores the point that the hyponatraemia is primarily due to cortisol deficiency per se. Such deficiency causes poor vascular tone and decreased cardiac output, thereby leading to an (effective) decrease in blood volume, so stimulating ADH secretion

- hyperkalaemia (raised blood potassium levels), due to loss of production of the hormone aldosterone

- axillary or pubic hypotrichosis

- hypoglycaemia (worse in children).

Loss of cortisol secretion makes it impossible to maintain normal blood glucose concentration between meals because glucose cannot be synthesised in significant quantities by gluconeogenesis.

8.12

Answer: D   Increased thyroid-stimulating hormone (TSH) secretion

Graves' disease is a thyroid disorder that may manifest several different conditions, including goitre and hyperthyroidism (over-activity of thyroid hormone production), infiltrative exophthalmos (protuberance of one or both eyes and associated problems) and infiltrative dermopathy (a skin condition usually of the lower extremities). This disorder is the most common cause of hyperthyroidism. It is known to be related to an antibody-mediated type of autoimmunity, but the trigger for the reaction is unknown. Most individuals with Graves' disease have an enlarged thyroid gland with each cell secreting more than normal amounts of thyroid hormone; however, the plasma levels of thyroid-stimulating hormone (TSH) are found to be less than normal and often zero. Instead, thyroid-stimulating antibodies, designated as TSAb, which bind to the same membrane receptors as TSH, are found in the plasma and the high levels of thyroid hormone in turn suppress anterior pituitary formation of TSH.

endocrine

469

8.13

Answer: B   Increase blood glucose concentration

Glucagon increases blood glucose concentration, mainly by causing glycogenolysis and gluconeogenesis in the liver. Growth hormone increases blood glucose concentration by decreasing glucose utilisation and uptake by the cells. In addition, growth hormone increases the mobilisation of fatty acids from adipose tissue and increases the use of fatty acids for energy.

8.14

Answer: B   Glucagon

Glucagon is a 29-amino acid polypeptide acting as an important hormone in carbohydrate metabolism. The polypeptide has a molecular mass of 3485 Da and was discovered in 1923 by Kimball and Murlin. Glucagon helps maintain the level of glucose in the blood by binding to glucagon receptors on hepatocytes, causing the liver to release glucose – stored in the form of glycogen – through a process known as glycogenolysis. As these stores become depleted, glucagon then encourages the liver to synthesise additional glucose by gluconeogenesis. This glucose is released into the bloodstream. Both of these mechanisms lead to glucose release by the liver, preventing the development of hypoglycaemia.

8.15

Answer: E   Insulin

Hormone-sensitive lipase is a protein found in the cytosol of adipocytes. It functions to hydrolyse triacylglycerols from the lipid droplet, freeing fatty acids and glycerols. It may be activated by two mechanisms. In the first, it is phosphorylated by perilipin A, causing it to move to the surface of the lipid droplet, where it may begin hydrolysing the lipid droplet. Alternatively, it may be activated by a cAMP-dependent protein kinase. This pathway is significantly less effective than the first, which is necessary to lipid mobilisation in response to cAMP. In lipid metabolism, high levels of the hormone glucagon favour an increase in plasma levels of fatty acids and glycerol through activation of hormone-sensitive lipase. Insulin inhibits the action of hormone-sensitive lipase.

8.16

Answer: B   High plasma levels of thyroid-stimulating hormone (TSH)

Lack of iodine in the diet prevents the production of both thyroxine and tri-iodothyronine but does not stop the formation of thyroglobulin. Thus no hormone is available to inhibit secretion of TSH, allowing the anterior pituitary to secrete large quantities of TSH. The TSH causes the thyroid cells to secrete excessive amounts of thyroglobulin into the follicles and the gland then grows larger and larger.

8.17

Answer: C   Deplete fat stores

Exophthalmos occurs in many individuals with hyperthyroidism, but the condition is not caused by the high levels of thyroxine in the plasma. Instead, exophthalmos is thought to result from an autoimmune process in which antibodies directed against the extraocular muscles cause the muscles to weaken and the eyeball to protrude. Excess thyroxine mobilises lipids from fat tissue, depleting fat stores. Other effects include weight loss (often accompanied by a ravenous appetite), intolerance to heat, fatigue, weakness, hyperactivity, irritability, apathy, depression, polyuria and sweating. Additionally, patients may present with a variety of symptoms such as palpitations and arrhythmias (notably atrial fibrillation), shortness of breath (dyspnoea), loss of libido, nausea, vomiting and diarrhoea. In the elderly, these classical symptoms may not be present and they may present only with fatigue and weight loss leading to apathetic hyperthyroidism.

endocrine

8.18

Answer: A   1,25-Dihydroxycholecalciferol

Vitamin D$_3$ is cholecalciferol. Vitamin D$_3$ is converted to 25-hydroxycholecalciferol in the liver and this, in turn, is converted in the kidney to the active form, 1,25-dihydroxycholecalciferol.

8.19

Answer: D   Increased formation of 1,25-dihydroxycholecalciferol

Parathyroid hormone increases tubular reabsorption of calcium in the ascending limbs of the loops of Henlé, distal tubules and collecting ducts and at the same time it decreases reabsorption of phosphate in the proximal tubules. Parathyroid hormone also enhances calcium and phosphate absorption from the intestines by increasing the formation of 1,25-dihydroxycholecalciferol from vitamin D in the kidneys and increases absorption of calcium and phosphate from the bone by stimulating both the proliferation and activity of the osteoclasts.

8.20

Answer: D   Extracellular ionised calcium

Parathyroid hormone (PTH) is secreted by the parathyroid glands as a polypeptide containing 84 amino acids. It acts to increase the concentration of calcium in the blood, whereas calcitonin (a hormone produced by the thyroid gland) acts to decrease calcium concentration. Increased ionised calcium concentration in the blood acts (via feedback inhibition) to decrease parathyroid hormone (PTH) secretion by the parathyroid glands. This is achieved by the activation of calcium-sensing receptors located on parathyroid cells.

endocrine

8.21

Answer: E   Vasopressin

Only vasopressin (also called antidiuretic hormone) and oxytocin are secreted by the posterior pituitary. The table below summarises these two hormones:

Hormone	Target	Effect	Source
Oxytocin	Uterus, mammary glands	Uterine contractions, lactation	Paraventricular nuclei
Vasopressin (antidiuretic hormone; ADH)	Kidneys, arterioles	Stimulates water retention and raises blood pressure by contracting arterioles	Supraoptic nucleus

8.22

Answer: C   Low plasma concentration of 1,25-dihydroxycholecalciferol

In vitamin D deficiency, extra amounts of parathyroid hormone are released, which maintain the plasma calcium concentration at a value only slightly lower than normal. However, plasma phosphate concentration falls to extremely low levels because the increased parathyroid activity increases the excretion of phosphates in the urine.

8.23

Answer: D   Increased skin pigmentation

The clinical condition in this vignette is Addison's disease. This patient will have:

- hypoglycaemia
- chronic fatigue that gradually worsens
- muscle weakness
- weight loss and loss of appetite
- nausea, diarrhoea or vomiting

endocrine

- hypotension, abnormally low blood pressure that falls further when standing (orthostatic hypotension)

- areas of hyperpigmentation (darkened skin), known as melasma suprarenalis caused by increases in pro-opiomelanocortin. Although cutaneous pigmentation will most probably disappear following therapy, pigmentation of the oral mucosa tends to persist

- irritability

- depression

- craving for salt and salty foods

- for women, menstrual periods become irregular or cease

- tetany (particularly after drinking milk) due to phosphate excess

- numbness of the extremities, sometimes with paralysis, due to potassium excess

- increased number of eosinophils

- polyuria

- hypovolaemia

- dehydration

- tremors

- tachycardia

- restlessness

- diaphoresis (excessive sweating)

- dysphagia (difficulty swallowing)

- hyponatraemia (low blood sodium levels), possibly worsened by loss of production of the hormone aldosterone, but it occurs in secondary (pituitary) adrenal insufficiency as well. This underscores the point that the hyponatraemia is primarily due to cortisol deficiency per se. Such deficiency causes poor vascular tone and decreased cardiac output, thereby leading to an (effective) decrease in blood volume, so stimulating ADH secretion

- hyperkalaemia (raised blood potassium levels), due to loss of production of the hormone aldosterone

- axillary or pubic hypotrichosis

- decreased daily excretion of 17-ketosteroids and 17-hydroxysteroids.

See also answer to 8.11.

8.24

Answer: A   Addisonian crisis

In some cases, Addison's symptoms may present rapidly. This 'acute adrenal failure' is known as an Addisonian crisis and is a severe medical emergency. An illness or accident can aggravate the adrenal problems causing the Addisonian crisis (most common in untreated sufferers), although the most common cause (for those already diagnosed) is abrupt discontinuation of corticosteroid therapy without tapering the dose. Untreated, an Addisonian crisis can be fatal. It is a medical emergency, usually requiring admission to hospital. Symptoms that may occur include:

- sudden penetrating pain in the legs, lower back or abdomen

- severe vomiting and diarrhoea, resulting in dehydration

- hypotension

- loss of consciousness/syncope

- hypoglycaemia

- confusion, psychosis.

endocrine

8.25

Answer: B   Decreased serum free fatty acid levels

Growth hormone (GH or somatotrophin) is a 191-amino acid, single chain polypeptide hormone that is synthesised, stored and secreted by the somatotroph cells within the lateral wings of the anterior pituitary gland, which stimulates growth and cell reproduction in humans. Height growth in childhood is the best known effect of GH action and appears to be stimulated by at least two mechanisms:

- GH directly stimulates division and multiplication of the chondrocytes of cartilage. These are the primary cells in the growing ends (epiphyses) of children's long bones (arms, legs, digits).

- GH also stimulates production of insulin-like growth factor-1 (IGF-1, formerly known as somatomedin C), a hormone homologous to pro-insulin. The liver is a major target organ of GH for this process and is the principal site of IGF-1 production. IGF-1 has growth-stimulating effects on a wide variety of tissues. Additional IGF-1 is generated within target tissues, making it apparently both an endocrine and an autocrine/paracrine hormone. IGF-1 will also have stimulatory effects on osteoblast and chondrocyte activity to promote bone growth.

Although height growth is the best known effect of GH, it serves many other metabolic functions as well:

- it increases calcium retention and strengthens and increases the mineralisation of bone, as suggested by increased alkaline phosphatase activity

- it increases muscle mass through the creation of new muscle cells (which differs from hypertrophy)

- it promotes lipolysis, which results in the reduction of adipose tissue (body fat) and increased serum free fatty acid levels

- it increases protein synthesis and stimulates the growth of all internal organs excluding the brain, resulting in decreased BUN

- it plays a role in fuel homeostasis

- it reduces liver uptake of glucose, an effect that opposes that of insulin

- it also contributes to the maintenance and function of pancreatic islets

- it stimulates the immune system.

8.26

Answer: E   Increased plasma aldosterone levels

Severe dehydration as experienced by the student in this clinical vignette will result in increased plasma angiotensin II levels, increased urine osmolarity, decreased glomerular filtration rate and increased plasma aldosterone levels – all attempts on the part of the body to conserve fluid. Severe diarrhoea will lead to decreased extracellular fluid volume.

8.27

Answer: D   Increased renin

Hyperaldosteronism is a medical condition in which too much aldosterone is produced by the adrenal glands, which can lead to lowered levels of potassium. Primary hyperaldosteronism, often caused by a tumour, is also known as Conn's syndrome. Secondary hyperaldosteronism is due to overactivity of the renin–angiotensin system.

8.28

Answer: D   Sheehan's syndrome

Sheehan's syndrome, also known as post-partum hypopituitarism or post-partum pituitary necrosis, is hypopituitarism (decreased functioning of the pituitary gland), caused by necrosis due to blood loss and hypovolaemic shock during and after childbirth. It is a rare complication of pregnancy, usually occurring after excessive

endocrine

blood loss; the presence of disseminated intravascular coagulation also appears to be a factor in its development. Hypertrophy and hyperplasia of lactotrophs during pregnancy results in the enlargement of the anterior pituitary, without a corresponding increase in blood supply. Secondly, the anterior pituitary is supplied by a low-pressure portal venous system. These vulnerabilities, when affected by major haemorrhage or hypotension during the peripartum period, can result in ischaemia of the affected pituitary regions, leading to necrosis. The posterior pituitary is usually not affected due to its direct arterial supply.

8.29

Answer: E   Tyrosine kinase

The insulin receptor is a transmembrane receptor that is activated by insulin. It belongs to the large class of tyrosine kinase receptors. Two alpha subunits and two beta subunits make up the insulin receptor. The beta subunits pass through the cellular membrane and are linked by disulphide bonds. Tyrosine kinase receptors, including the insulin receptor, mediate their activity by causing the addition of a phosphate group to particular tyrosines on certain proteins within a cell. The 'substrate' proteins, which are phosphorylated by the insulin receptor, include a protein called IRS-1 (insulin receptor substrate 1). IRS-1 binding and phosphorylation eventually leads to an increase in glucose transporter (GLUT4) molecules on the outer membrane of insulin-responsive tissues, including muscle cells, liver and adipose tissue and therefore to an increase in the uptake of glucose from blood into these tissues. Briefly, the glucose transporter (GLUT4), is transported from cellular vesicles to the cell surface, where it then can mediate the transport of glucose into the cell.

8.30

Answer: C   Noradrenaline

A phaeochromocytoma is a neuroendocrine tumour of the medulla of the adrenal glands originating in the chromaffin cells, which secretes excessive amounts of catecholamines, usually adrenaline and noradrenaline. Extra-adrenal paragangliomas (often described as extra-adrenal phaeochromocytomas) are closely related, though less common, tumours that originate in the ganglia of the sympathetic nervous system and are named based upon the primary anatomical site of origin. Traditionally it is known as the 10% tumour, since bilateral disease is present in approximately 10% of patients, approximately 10% of tumours are malignant and approximately 10% are located in chromaffin tissue outside the adrenal gland.

8.31

Answer: B Exercise

Peptides released by neurosecretory nuclei of the hypothalamus into the portal venous blood surrounding the pituitary are the major controllers of growth hormone (GH) secretion by the somatotrophs. Growth hormone releasing hormone (GHRH) from the arcuate nucleus and ghrelin promote GH secretion; somatostatin from the periventricular nuclei inhibits it. GH secretion is also affected by negative feedback from circulating concentrations of GH and insulin-like growth factor-1. Although the balance of these stimulating and inhibiting peptides determines GH release, this balance is affected by many physiological stimulators and inhibitors of GH secretion. Stimulators of GH secretion include (among others) sleep, exercise, hypoglycaemia, dietary protein and oestradiol. Inhibitors of GH secretion include dietary carbohydrate and glucocorticoids.

8.32

Answer: D Gene transcription

As steroids are lipid soluble, they can diffuse freely from the blood through the cell membrane and into the cytoplasm of target cells. In the cytoplasm, the steroid may or may not undergo an enzyme-mediated alteration such as reduction, hydroxylation or aromatisation. In the cytoplasm, the steroid binds to the specific receptor, a large metalloprotein. Upon steroid binding, many kinds of steroid receptor dimerize: two receptor subunits join together to form one functional DNA-binding unit that can enter the cell nucleus. In some of the hormone systems known, the receptor is associated with a heat-shock protein, which is released on the binding of the

endocrine

ligand, the hormone. Once in the nucleus, the steroid–receptor–ligand complex binds to specific DNA sequences and induces transcription of its target genes.

8.33

Answer: C Hyperthyroidism

Hyperthyroidism (or 'overactive thyroid gland') is the clinical syndrome caused by an excess of circulating free thyroxine (T_4) or free tri-iodothyronine (T_3) or both. Major clinical features include weight loss (often accompanied by a ravenous appetite), intolerance to heat, fatigue, weakness, hyperactivity, irritability, apathy, depression, polyuria and sweating. Additionally, patients may present with a variety of symptoms such as palpitations and arrhythmias (notably atrial fibrillation), shortness of breath (dyspnoea), loss of libido, nausea, vomiting and diarrhoea. In the elderly, these classical symptoms may not be present and they may present only with fatigue and weight loss leading to apathetic hyperthyroidism. Neurological manifestations are tremor, chorea, myopathy and periodic paralysis. Stroke of cardioembolic origin due to co-existing atrial fibrillation may be mentioned as one of the most serious complications of hyperthyroidism. A diagnosis is suspected through blood tests, by measuring the level of thyroid-stimulating hormone (TSH) in the blood. A low TSH (the job of TSH taken over by thyroid-stimulating immunoglobulin [TSI] that acts like TSH) indicates increased production of T_4 and/or T_3. Measuring specific antibodies, such as anti-TSH-receptor antibodies in Graves' disease, may contribute to the diagnosis. In all patients with hyperthyroxinaemia, scintigraphy is required to distinguish true hyperthyroidism from thyroiditis.

8.34

Answer: E Hypothalamic failure

Hypothyroidism is the disease state in humans caused by insufficient production of thyroid hormones by the thyroid gland. There are several distinct causes for chronic hypothyroidism in human beings, the most common being Hashimoto's thyroiditis (an autoimmune disease) and radioiodine therapy for hyperthyroidism. Historically,

endocrine

iodine deficiency was the most common cause of hypothyroidism world-wide. The disease may also be caused by a lack of thyroid gland or a deficiency of hormones from either the hypothalamus or the pituitary.

Secondary hypothyroidism occurs if the pituitary gland does not create enough thyroid-stimulating hormone (TSH) to induce the thyroid gland to create a sufficient quantity of thyroxine. Although not every case of secondary hypothyroidism has a clear-cut cause, it is usually caused when the pituitary is damaged by a tumour, radiation or surgery so that it is no longer able to instruct the thyroid to make enough hormone.

Tertiary hypothyroidism, also called hypothalamic–pituitary axis hypothyroidism, results when the hypothalamus fails to instruct the pituitary to produce sufficient TSH.

8.35

Answer: D   Elevated thyroid-stimulating hormone (TSH)

Total thyroidectomy results in removal of thyroid gland, with a fall in the production of T_3 and T_4 hormones. The synthesis and secretion of thyroid hormones is under control of TSH from the anterior pituitary gland, through its secondary messenger, cAMP. TSH secretion in turn is controlled by negative feedback from the thyroid hormones. A fall in T_3 and T_4 levels will result in increased secretion of TSH and elevated TSH levels after total thyroidectomy. Serum calcium level can occasionally fall after total thyroidectomy due to iatrogenic removal of parathyroid glands.

8.36

Answer: A   Anxiety

The signs and symptoms of a phaeochromocytoma are those of sympathetic nervous system hyperactivity, which can generally be described as those of 'impending doom', including:

- elevated heart rate
- elevated blood pressure; a clue to the presence of

phaeochromocytoma is orthostatic hypotension, a fall in systolic blood pressure greater than 10 mmHg on making the patient stand

- palpitations

- anxiety often resembling that of a panic attack

- diaphoresis

- headaches

- pallor.

A phaeochromocytoma can also cause resistant arterial hypertension. A phaeochromocytoma can be fatal if it causes malignant hypertension.

8.37

Answer: D   Increased calcitriol

Patients who are hyperparathyroid usually suffer from a tumour (adenoma) of one of the parathyroid glands. An increase in parathyroid hormone (PTH) level leads to hypercalcaemia, which is usually due to the demineralisation of bone. This could lead to osteoporosis or osteomalacia. With the influence of calcitriol, high PTH also results in the increased intestinal absorption of calcium and initially increased reabsorption of calcium from the kidneys. Although calcium and phosphate are absorbed in the intestine by active and passive diffusion, most of the calcium is absorbed by facilitated diffusion. PTH stimulates the 1-α hydroxylation of 25-hydroxycholecalciferol to 1,25-dihydroxycholecalciferol (calcitriol) in the kidney. Calcitriol increases the synthesis of calcium-binding protein, which results in higher levels of calcium being absorbed from the intestine. Therefore, calcitriol is the hormone responsible for increased calcium absorption from the gut. The action of PTH is indirect; it stimulates increased production of calcitriol. If there is less PTH, as in hypoparathyroidism, there is less calcium absorbed; in hyperparathyroidism, significantly greater amounts of calcium are absorbed. With time, hypercalciuria and phosphaturia lead to kidney stones and calcium-phosphate deposits on soft tissue. In addition, muscle weakness increases due to decreased muscle excitability.

PTH assays, calcium and phosphorus determinations and X-ray of selected bones are used to diagnose this condition (*see also* answer to 8.19).

8.38

Answer: A   Congenital adrenal hyperplasia

Congenital adrenal hyperplasia (CAH) due to 21-hydroxylase deficiency, in all its forms, accounts for about 95% of diagnosed cases of congenital adrenal hyperplasia and 'CAH' in most contexts refers to 21-hydroxylase deficiency.

Severe 21-hydroxylase deficiency causes *salt-wasting CAH,* with life-threatening vomiting and dehydration occurring within the first weeks of life. Severe 21-hydroxylase deficiency is also the most common cause of ambiguous genitalia due to prenatal virilisation of genetically female (XX) infants. Moderate 21-hydroxylase deficiency is referred to as *simple virilising CAH;* and typically is recognised by causing virilisation of prepubertal children. Still milder forms of 21-hydroxylase deficiency are referred to as *non-classical CAH* and can cause androgen effects and infertility in adolescent and adult women.

The defective enzyme 21-hydroxylase is embedded in the smooth endoplasmic reticulum of the cells of the adrenal cortex. It catalyses hydroxylation of 17-hydroxyprogesterone to 11-deoxycortisol in the glucocorticoid pathway from pregnenolone to cortisol. It also catalyses hydroxylation of progesterone to 11-deoxycorticosterone in the mineralocorticoid pathway from pregnenolone to aldosterone. Deficient activity of this enzyme reduces the efficiency of cortisol synthesis, with consequent elevation of ACTH levels and hyperplasia of the adrenal cortex. ACTH stimulates uptake of cholesterol and synthesis of pregnenolone. Steroid precursors up to and including progesterone, 17-hydroxypregnenolone and especially 17-hydroxyprogesterone (17OHP) accumulate in the adrenal cortex and in circulating blood. Blood levels of 17OHP can reach 10–1000 times the normal concentration.

Since 21-hydroxylase activity is not involved in synthesis of androgens, a substantial fraction of the large amounts

endocrine

of 17-hydroxypregnenolone is diverted to synthesis of dehydroepiandrosterone androstenedione and testosterone, beginning in the third month of fetal life in both sexes. Synthesis of aldosterone is also dependent on 21-hydroxylase activity. Although fetal production is impaired, it causes no prenatal effects, as the placental connection allows maternal blood to 'dialyse' the fetus and maintain both electrolyte balance and blood volume.

8.39

Answer: C   Cholesterol to pregnenolone

Adrenocorticotrophic hormone (ACTH) is the hormone of the adenohypophysis that controls the function of the adrenal cortex. The precursor molecule of ACTH is a glycoprotein of about 31 kDa, pro-opiomelanocortin (POMC). This large molecule is produced by corticotrophes in the anterior lobe, intermediate lobe and in the brain. POMC is processed in the anterior pituitary to ACTH and β-lipotropin. The latter compound is in turn cleaved to γ-lipotrophin and β-endorphin. In the rudimentary intermediate lobe, POMC is cleaved to α-MSH, corticotrophin-like intermediate lobe peptide (CLIP), γ-lipotrophin and β-endorphin. In the brain, the main products are ACTH and β-endorphin. ACTH consists of 39 amino acids, the first 13 of which (counting from the N-terminus) may be cleaved to form α-MSH. (This common structure is one reason that patients with hypercortisolism, in which ACTH levels are elevated, often present with excessively tanned skin.) The half-life of ACTH in human blood is about 10 min.

ACTH secretion is controlled by hypothalamic corticotropin-releasing hormone, augmented by antidiuretic hormone (ADH). ACTH acts to stimulate the growth and maintenance of the adrenal cortex. Specifically, it acts on cells of the zona fasciculata to stimulate the synthesis and secretion of the glucocorticoid, cortisol. It also acts on the zona reticularis cells to stimulate the production of weak androgens such as dehydroepiandrosterone (DHEA). Specifically, it stimulates new hormone synthesis, which facilitates the transport of the cholesterol into the inner membrane of the mitochondria where the cholesterol side-chain cleavage enzyme is located. It also regulates enzymes involved in steroidogenesis. It promotes production of cortisol by converting cholesterol to pregnenolone. It also stimulates the pentose shunt that yields NADPH$^+$ H$^+$ and ribose-5-phosphate, necessary in steroidogenesis and mRNA synthesis, respectively. (Cells of the outermost zone of the adrenal cortex, the zona glomerulosa, are under control of angiotensin II.) The pituitary–adrenocortical axis is stimulated by stress and sympathetic nervous system activation. High circulating levels of cortisol, after the stressful stimulation is no longer operative, feed back to the pituitary to stop the production of ACTH; this is known as negative feedback.

Because ACTH has a partial amino acid sequence similar to that of MSH, it is not surprising that in Addison's disease (primary adrenal insufficiency), elevated ACTH levels cause skin darkening. ACTH-secreting tumours are the third most prevalent human pituitary tumour.

8.40

Answer: C   Decreased gluconeogenesis

The actions of insulin on human metabolism include:

- Increased glycogen synthesis – insulin forces storage of glucose in liver (and muscle) cells in the form of glycogen; lowered levels of insulin cause liver cells to convert glycogen to glucose and excrete it into the blood. This is the clinical action of insulin, which is directly useful in reducing high blood glucose levels as in diabetes.

- Increased fatty acid synthesis – insulin forces fat cells to take in blood lipids, which are converted to triglycerides; lack of insulin causes the reverse.

- Increased esterification of fatty acids – forces adipose tissue to make fats (ie triglycerides) from fatty acid esters; lack of insulin causes the reverse.

- Decreased proteolysis – forces reduction of protein degradation; lack of insulin increases protein degradation.

- Decreased lipolysis – forces reduction in conversion of fat cell lipid stores into blood fatty acids; lack of insulin causes the reverse.

endocrine

- Decreased gluconeogenesis – decreases production of glucose from various substrates in liver; lack of insulin causes glucose production from assorted substrates in the liver and elsewhere.

- Increased amino acid uptake – forces cells to absorb circulating amino acids; lack of insulin inhibits absorption.

- Increased potassium uptake – forces cells to absorb serum potassium; lack of insulin inhibits absorption.

8.41

Answer: E   Hypothyroidism

To diagnose primary hypothyroidism, occasionally the amount of thyroid-stimulating hormone (TSH) being produced is measured. High levels of TSH indicate that the thyroid is not producing sufficient levels of thyroid hormones (mainly as thyroxine [T_4] and smaller amounts of tri-iodothyronine [T_3]). However, measuring just TSH fails to diagnose secondary and tertiary forms of hypothyroidism, so leading to the following suggested minimum blood testing:

- thyroid-stimulating hormone (TSH)
- free tri-iodothyronine (fT_3)
- free levothyroxine (fT_4)
- total T_3
- total T_4.

Additionally, the following measurements may be needed:

- antithyroid antibodies – for evidence of autoimmune diseases that may be damaging the thyroid gland

- serum cholesterol – which may be elevated in hypothyroidism

- prolactin – as a widely available test of pituitary function.

8.42

Answer: A   Adrenocorticotrophic hormone (ACTH)

Pro-opiomelanocortin (POMC) is a precursor polypeptide with 241 amino acid residues. It is synthesised by corticotroph cells of the anterior pituitary gland, melanotroph cells of the intermediate lobe of the pituitary gland, about 3000 neurones in the arcuate nucleus of the hypothalamus and smaller populations of neurones in the dorsomedial hypothalamus and brainstem.

The large molecule of POMC is the source of several important biologically active substances. POMC can be cleaved enzymatically into the following peptides:

- adrenocorticotrophic hormone (ACTH) and beta-lipotrophin (β-LPH) in the anterior pituitary gland

- corticotrophin-like intermediate peptide (CLIP), gamma-lipotropin (γ-LPH), alpha-melanocyte-stimulating hormone (α-MSH) and β-endorphin in the intermediate lobe

- gamma-melanocyte-stimulating hormone (γ-MSH)

- met-encephalin

- beta-melanocyte-stimulating hormone (β-MSH).

Each of these peptides is packaged in large dense-core vesicles that are released from the cells by exocytosis in response to appropriate stimulation. Alpha-melanocyte-stimulating hormone produced by neurones in the arcuate nucleus has important roles in the regulation of appetite and sexual behaviour, while α-MSH secreted from the intermediate lobe of the pituitary regulates the production of melanin. ACTH is a peptide hormone that regulates the secretion of glucocorticoids from the adrenal cortex. Beta-endorphin and met-encephalin are endogenous opioid peptides with widespread actions in the brain.

endocrine

8.43

Answer: D   Pregnenolone

Pregnenolone is an intermediary involved in the steroidogenesis of progesterone, mineralocorticoids, glucocorticoids, androgens and oestrogens. As such, it is a prohormone. Like other steroids, pregnenolone consists of four interconnected cyclic hydrocarbons. It contains ketone and hydroxyl functional groups, two methyl branches and a double bond at C5, in the B cyclic hydrocarbon ring. Like all steroid hormones, it is hydrophobic. Its esterised version, pregnenolone sulphate, is water-soluble. Pregnenolone is synthesised from cholesterol. This conversion involves hydroxylation at the side chain at C20 and C22 positions, with cleavage of the side chain. The enzyme performing this task is cytochrome P450, located in the mitochondria and controlled by pituitary trophic hormones, such as ACTH, FSH, and LH. Pregnenolone undergoes further steroid metabolism in one of two ways:

- Pregnenolone can be converted to progesterone. The critical enzyme step is twofold using a 3β-hydroxysteroid dehydrogenase and a δ4–5-isomerase. The latter transfers the double bond from C5 to C4 on the A ring. Progesterone is the entry into the δ4 pathway resulting in production of 17-hydroxyprogesterone and androstenedione, precursor to testosterone and oestrone. Aldosterone and corticosteroids are also derived from progesterone or its derivatives.

- Pregnenolone can be converted to 17-hydroxypregnenolone by the enzyme 17α-hydroxylase. Using this pathway, termed δ5 pathway, the next step is conversion to dehydroepiandrosterone (DHEA) using a desmolase. DHEA is the precursor of androstenedione.

8.44

Answer: C Hypothyroidism due to a primary abnormality in the hypothalamus

Tertiary hypothyroidism, also called hypothalamic–pituitary axis hypothyroidism, results when the hypothalamus fails to instruct the pituitary to produce sufficient TSH. This young woman's hypothyroidism improves with TRH administration, confirming the diagnosis of tertiary hypothyroidism.

8.45

Answer: E Stimulates the synthesis of androgen binding protein

In men, FSH helps to maintain Sertoli cells (large cells in the seminiferous tubules that nourish the developing sperm). FSH and testosterone synergise to stimulate the synthesis of androgen-binding protein (ABP). ABP keeps the levels of testosterone high in the tubular fluid. Sertoli cells cannot synthesise androgens but rely on the diffusion of androgens from interstitial cells of Leydig. FSH is necessary for spermatids to mature into sperm. Oestrogen and testosterone feedback do not completely suppress FSH secretion; inhibin, produced by ovarian granulosa cells and testicular Sertoli cells, is necessary for complete suppression.

8.46

Answer: E Short QT interval on ECG

Hypercalcaemia is an elevated calcium level in the blood. (Normal range: 9–10.5 mg/dl or 2.2–2.6 mmol/l.) It can be an asymptomatic laboratory finding, but because an elevated calcium level is often indicative of other diseases, a diagnosis should be undertaken if it persists. It can be due to excessive skeletal calcium release, increased intestinal calcium absorption or decreased renal calcium excretion. Hypercalcaemia per se can result in fatigue, depression, confusion, anorexia, nausea, vomiting, constipation, pancreatitis or increased urination; if it is chronic, it can result in urinary calculi (renal stones or bladder stones). Abnormal heart rhythms can result and an electrocardiogram (ECG) finding of a short QT interval suggests

endocrine

hypercalcaemia. Symptoms are more common at high calcium levels (12.0 mg/dl or 3 mmol/l). Severe hypercalcaemia (above 15–16 mg/dl or 3.75–4 mmol/l) is considered a medical emergency: at these levels, coma and cardiac arrest can result. Hyperparathyroidism and malignancy account for ~90% of cases.

8.47

Answer: E Increases normal sensitivity of vascular smooth muscle to the vasoconstrictor effects of catecholamines

Cortisol is needed to maintain normal vascular integrity and responsiveness and normal volume of body fluids. In the absence of cortisol, exaggerated vasodilatation occurs: normal sensitivity of vascular smooth muscle to the vasoconstrictor effects of adrenaline and noradrenaline is lost and abnormal vasodilatation results, with loss of vascular tone. The filling of the vascular bed is reduced and blood pressure falls. Intercellular 'cement' between capillary epithelial cells is not maintained and allows blood leakage. Normal renal function requires cortisol. In its absence, glomerular filtration falls and water cannot be excreted as rapidly. Cortisol also has some mineralocorticoid effect that is responsible for part of normal sodium retention and potassium excretion. Although aldosterone is some 300–600 times more potent a mineralocorticoid than cortisol, usually 200 times more cortisol than aldosterone is secreted. Therefore, cortisol has an important overall influence on sodium retention. In fact, cortisol insufficiency is diagnosed clinically by using a water-load challenge. A subject is given 1 l of water to drink. In a normal individual, this load will be cleared in 1–2 hours, but not for at least 12 hours in cortisol insufficiency. This effect is not reversed by aldosterone.

8.48

Answer: B Reabsorption of Na^+

Although aldosterone's primary action is to increase sodium reabsorption in the distal tubules, it also increases the reabsorption of sodium in other places – saliva, sweat and stool.

8.49

Answer: B   Aldosterone

The arrangement of blood flow from the outer cortex into the medulla is thought to account for the differentiation of secretions from the various zones. Subcapsular cells are capable of generating all three cortical zones. One theory holds that the youngest cells differentiate just beneath the capsule, forming the zona glomerulosa and over time the cells migrate downward. The inner zona reticularis cells being the oldest and showing signs of progressive loss of functional activity.

A critical distinction of the cells within each zone is that they contain different sets of enzymes and therefore have different steroid hormone biosynthetic capabilities. The zona glomerulosa lacks 17α-hydroxylase, but exhibits 18-hydroxylase activity. Therefore, these cells can produce the mineralocorticoid, aldosterone (50–200 µg/day), but not the glucocorticoid, cortisol. Hence, destruction of zona glomerulosa cells will result in lack of aldosterone secretion. The zona fasciculata cells exhibit 17α-hydroxylase but no 18-hydroxylase activity, so, cortisol is synthesised (15–30 mg/day), but not aldosterone. The cells of the innermost zona reticularis have lost their ability to produce cortisol and the primary secretion is the weak androgen, dehydroepiandrosterone. Additionally, the zona glomerulosa is under the control of angiotensin II, which binds to membrane-bound receptors and enhances the rate-limiting step of cholesterol side-chain cleavage, leading to increased synthesis of aldosterone. The fasciculata and reticularis, on the other hand, are regulated by ACTH from the pituitary.

8.50

Answer: C   Hyponatraemia

Addison's disease (also known as chronic adrenal insufficiency or hypocortisolism) is a rare endocrine disorder, which results in the body not producing sufficient amounts of certain adrenal hormones. The symptoms of Addison's disease are caused by the failure of the adrenal glands to produce enough of the hormone cortisol in both primary and secondary adrenal insufficiency. In primary adrenal insufficiency (classic Addison's disease), the hormone aldosterone

endocrine

is also deficient. Many of the symptoms of Addison's disease arise due to the hyposecretion of aldosterone leading to hyperkalaemia and metabolic acidosis. Often the production of adrenaline is also diminished or eliminated. Primary Addison's disease is caused by damaged adrenal glands where the damage causes the insufficient production of the above-mentioned hormones. Most often, the damage is caused by autoimmune disease, where the body creates antibodies that attack the glands (as if it were a disease) in the same way the immune system fights infection. Hence, it is not surprising that this form of adrenal gland damage is associated with other autoimmune diseases such as hypothyroidism (Hashimoto's thyroiditis), rheumatoid arthritis, type I diabetes, etc. Other causes of failure of the adrenal glands may include the following:

- tuberculosis

- infections of the adrenal glands

- spread of cancer to the adrenal glands

- bleeding into the adrenal glands (seen in patients using anticoagulants such as heparin or warfarin)

- Addison's disease usually develops slowly (over several months) and symptoms may not be present or be noticed until some stressful illness or situation occurs.

Common symptoms are:

- chronic fatigue that gradually worsens

- muscle weakness

- weight loss and loss of appetite

- nausea, diarrhoea or vomiting

- hypotension that aggravates further when standing (orthostatic hypotension)

- hyperpigmentation (darkened skin), known as melasma suprarenalis caused by increases in pro-opiomelanocortin. Although cutaneous pigmentation will most probably disappear following therapy, pigmentation of the oral mucosa tends to persist

- irritability

- depression

- craving for salt

- hypoglycaemia (worse in children)

- for women, menstrual periods become irregular or cease

- tetany (particularly after drinking milk) due to hyperphosphataemia

- numbness of the extremities, sometimes with paralysis, due to potassium excess

- increased umber of eosinophils

- polyuria

- hypovolaemia (decreased blood volume)

- dehydration

- tremors

- tachycardia

- restlessness

- diaphoresis (excessive sweating)

- dysphagia (difficulty swallowing)

- hyponatraemia (low blood sodium levels), possibly worsened by loss of production of the hormone aldosterone, but occurs in secondary (pituitary) adrenal insufficiency as well. This underscores the point that the hyponatraemia is primarily due to cortisol deficiency per se. Such deficiency causes poor vascular tone and decreased cardiac output, thereby leading to an (effective) decrease in blood volume, so stimulating ADH secretion.

- hyperkalaemia due to loss of production of the hormone aldosterone

- axillary or pubic hypotrichosis.

See also answer to 8.11.

8.51

Answer: E   Insulin deficiency

Diabetic ketoacidosis (DKA) is one consequence of untreated diabetes mellitus and is linked to an impaired glucose cycle. In a diabetic patient, DKA begins with deficiency in insulin. This is most commonly due to undiagnosed diabetes mellitus or, in patients who have been diagnosed with diabetes, failure to take prescribed insulin. DKA has a 100% mortality rate if left untreated. A key component of DKA is that there is no or very little circulating insulin, so it occurs mainly (but not exclusively) in type 1 diabetes (because type 1 diabetes is characterised by a lack of insulin production in the pancreas). It is much less common in type 2 diabetes because that is closely related to cell insensitivity to insulin, not shortage or absence of insulin. Some type 2 diabetics have lost their own insulin production and must take external insulin; they have some susceptibility to DKA. Although glucagon plays a role as a hormone antagonistic to insulin when there are low blood glucose levels, mainly by stimulating the process of glycogenolysis in hepatocytes (liver cells), insulin is the much more important hormone, with more widespread effects throughout the body. Its presence or absence can by itself regulate most of DKA's pathological effects; notably, it has a short half-life in the blood of only a few minutes (typically about 6 min), so little time is needed between cessation of insulin release internally and the reduction of insulin levels in the blood.

Despite possibly high circulating levels of plasma glucose, the liver will act as though the body is starving if insulin levels are low. In starvation situations, the liver produces another form of fuel: ketone bodies. Ketogenesis, which is a fat metabolic process (beginning with lipolysis), makes ketone bodies as intermediate products in the metabolic sequence when fatty acids (formerly attached to a glycerol backbone in triglycerides) are processed. The ketone bodies β-hydroxybutyrate and acetoacetate enter the bloodstream and are usable as fuel for some organs such as the brain, though the brain still requires a substantial proportion of glucose to function. If large quantities of ketone bodies are produced, the metabolic imbalance known as ketosis may develop, though this condition is not necessary harmful. The negative charge of ketone bodies causes decreased blood pH. An extreme excess of ketones can cause ketoacidosis.

8.52

Answer: D   PTH secretion is increased by increased plasma
phosphate level

Parathyroid hormone (PTH) is rapidly released from the parathyroid gland in response to decreased plasma calcium ion concentration. A negative feedback system exists between plasma calcium levels and PTH levels. When plasma calcium levels are low, PTH secretion increases and PTH mobilises calcium from bones, increases calcium reabsorption from the kidney or indirectly stimulates increased calcium absorption from the small intestine (this will be explained in detail in the next section). Conversely, if calcium is high, PTH secretion is inhibited and calcium is deposited in bones. Intracellular calcium and the phosphoinositol–diacyl glycerol system appear to be the mediators in the regulation of PTH secretion by extracellular calcium. Calcium is the major regulator of PTH secretion.

Activated vitamin D, 1,25-dihydroxycholecalciferol, diffuses into chief cells and inhibits prepro-PTH mRNA, so inhibiting PTH synthesis. A decrease in plasma magnesium, like decreased calcium, stimulates PTH secretion; an increase in magnesium inhibits PTH. It appears that magnesium is acting directly on the parathyroid gland, but the exact mechanism has not been elucidated. Phosphate action on the parathyroid gland is different; an increase in plasma phosphate stimulates PTH secretion by lowering plasma calcium levels and inhibiting the formation of 1,25-dihydroxycholecalciferol (*see also* answer to 8.20).

8.53

Answer: C   Increased blood level of glucose due to
glycogenolysis in liver and muscle cells

Composed mainly of hormone-producing chromaffin cells, the adrenal medulla is the principal site of the conversion of the amino acid tyrosine into the catecholamines adrenaline and noradrenalin. In response to stresses such as exercise or imminent danger, adrenal medullary cells release catecholamines into the blood in an 85 : 15 ratio of adrenaline to noradrenaline. Notable effects of adrenaline and noradrenaline include increased heart rate, blood vessel constriction including cutaneous, splanchnic and muscle, bronchial dilatation and increased glycogenolysis and lipolysis, all of which are characteristic of the fight-or-flight response. Although these effects appear extraordinarily diverse, they constitute a marvellous set of integrated responses. Catecholamines co-ordinate adjustments in all bodily functions to promote survival in the face of extreme challenges. On the whole, cardiovascular effects maximise cardiac output and ensure perfusion of the brain and skeletal muscles. Metabolic effects ensure an adequate supply of glucose for the central nervous system (CNS) and offer alternative substrates for other tissues by mobilizing fat. Effects on skeletal muscle and transmitter release from motor neurones increase muscular performance and quiescence of the gut permits diversion of blood flow, oxygen and energy substrates to re-inforce these effects.

8.54

Answer: C   Increased protein breakdown

Metabolic effects of insulin include: stimulation of the formation of glycogen from glucose and inhibition of glycogenolysis; stimulation of fatty acid (FA) production from stored lipids and inhibition of FA release into the blood; stimulation of FA uptake and storage; inhibition of protein catabolism and of gluconeogenesis, in which glucose is synthesised (mostly from some amino acid, released by protein catabolism). A lack of insulin or inadequately controlled diabetes will result in reversal of all these effects of insulin, all of which contribute to increasing blood glucose levels, increased fat metabolism and protein degradation.

8.55

Answer: A   Activates adenylate cyclase

Biochemical mechanisms of signal transduction follow the pharmacological subdivisions of the adrenergic receptors. Stimulation of either β_1- or β_2-receptors activates adenylate cyclase. Beta-adrenergic responses typically result from increased production of cAMP. The only salient difference between β_1- and β_2-

receptors is the low sensitivity of the β_2 receptors to noradrenaline. Stimulation of the α_2-receptors inhibits adenylate cyclase and may block the increase in cAMP produced by other agents. For β effects, the recognition subunit of the adrenergic receptor communicates with adenylate cyclase through the stimulatory guanosine binding subunit of the receptor complex (G protein).

8.56

Answer: A   Adrenocorticotrophic hormone (ACTH)

Upon stimulation with adrenocorticotrophic hormone (ACTH), the adrenal cortex secretes cortisol, which inhibits further secretion of ACTH in a typical negative feedback pattern. Cortisol exerts its inhibitory effects on corticotrophin-releasing hormone (CRH) neurones in the hypothalamus and corticotrophs. Superimposed on this system is a diurnal rhythm in the release of ACTH and hence oscillation in plasma levels of cortisol. Hormone levels are highest in the early morning hours, rising in anticipation of arousal and becoming lowest in the evening. The rhythmic secretion can be explained in terms of the negative feedback model by considering a set-point element within the feedback system that monitors existing levels of plasma cortisol. The set point oscillates throughout the day (the diurnal rhythm). In this negative feedback system, the set-point element compares its set point with the existing plasma concentration of cortisol. If the concentration is below the set point, a positive signal is sent to the CRH hypothalamic neurones that, in turn, release CRH into the portal capillaries and stimulate release of ACTH. ACTH then reaches the adrenal cortex in the circulation and stimulates cortisol synthesis. Plasma cortisol rises and when it reaches a concentration equal to the set point, no signal is sent to the CRH neurones and stimulation for further release of cortisol is withdrawn. As plasma cortisol levels gradually fall below the set point, the cycle repeats. The anatomy and biochemical equivalent of the 'set-point' element is not known. However, it has been suggested that changes in sensitivity of CRH-secreting cells to cortisol may account for this behaviour. Decreased sensitivity to inhibitory effects of cortisol in the early morning results in increased output of CRH, ACTH and cortisol. As the day progresses, sensitivity

endocrine

to cortisol increases and there is a decrease in the output of CRH and hence ACTH and cortisol. The exact mechanisms regulating these changes are not understood. However, the important points are: (1) secretion of ACTH is driven by changes in CRH secretion; and (2) although cortisol concentrations change with time of day, they are controlled precisely.

8.57

Answer: C   Purple striae on the trunk

Cushing's syndrome or hypercortisolism or hyperadrenocorticism is an endocrine disorder caused by excessive levels of the endogenous corticosteroid hormone cortisol. It may also be induced iatrogenically by treatment with exogenous corticosteroids for other medical conditions. Clinical features include rapid weight gain, particularly of the trunk and face with sparing of the limbs (central obesity), 'moon face', excess sweating, telangiectasia (dilatation of capillaries), atrophy of the skin (which gets thin and bruises easily) and other mucous membranes, purple or red striae on the trunk, buttocks, arms, legs or breasts, proximal muscle weakness (hips, shoulders) and hirsutism (facial male-pattern hair growth). A common sign is the growth of fat pads along the collarbone and on the back of the neck (known as a buffalo hump). The excess cortisol may also affect other endocrine systems and cause, for example, reduced libido, impotence, amenorrhoea and infertility. Patients frequently suffer various psychological disturbances, ranging from euphoria to frank psychosis. Depression and anxiety, including panic attacks, are common. Other signs include persistent hypertension (due to the aldosterone-like effects) and insulin resistance, leading to hyperglycaemia, which can lead to diabetes mellitus. Untreated Cushing's syndrome can lead to heart disease and increased mortality. Cushing's syndrome due to excess ACTH may also result in hyperpigmentation of the skin, due to its ability to stimulate melanocyte receptors.

8.58

Answer: A   Angiotensin II

Aldosterone is the primary mineralocorticoid. It arises from the outer zona glomerulosa and is primarily under the control of angiotensin and of serum potassium and ACTH to a lesser degree. Since the major function of aldosterone is to control body fluid volume by increasing the reabsorption of sodium by the kidneys, it is appropriate that the major stimulus for aldosterone synthesis and secretion arises in the kidneys. The juxtaglomerular apparatus consists of modified myoepithelial cells in the renal afferent arterioles, contiguous to the macula densa of the distal tubule. These cells synthesise and secrete the proteolytic enzyme, renin. Renin is released into the blood, where it comes in contact with its substrate, angiotensinogen, a 14 amino acid alpha-globulin synthesised by the liver. Renin catalyses the cleavage of 4 amino acids, giving rise to the 10 amino acid peptide angiotensin I. Angiotensin I is inactive, but is rapidly converted to the very active 8 amino acid peptide, angiotensin II, by the action of converting enzyme found especially abundantly in the lungs, arising from the plasma membrane of vascular endothelial cells.

Angiotensin II exerts two major actions: (1) as a direct arteriolar vasoconstrictor; and (2) as a stimulus to aldosterone secretion. It binds to specific membrane receptors in the zona glomerulosa to stimulate aldosterone synthesis directly. These two actions, working in concert, maintain the volume and pressure of the arterial circulation. They provide the major support to the circulation in times of fluid loss or fall in blood pressure. Angiotensin II has a half-life of 1–3 min in the circulation. It is inactivated by blood, kidney and liver. All of the actions of renin are mediated through its generation of angiotensin II, which serves as the primary stimulus to aldosterone synthesis.

Plasma potassium concentration and ACTH also stimulate aldosterone. The potassium effect appears appropriate, as a major effect of aldosterone is to increase renal excretion of potassium. The physiological effects of ACTH on release are not pronounced. For example, clinical suppression of ACTH by exogenous glucocorticoids for, say, a pituitary function test, will drastically decrease cortisol synthesis but will not influence aldosterone secretion. ACTH most probably plays a supportive role. When ACTH is deficient, the zona

endocrine

glomerulosa may be less able to respond to other stimuli. However, very large doses of ACTH, as such are released during stress, cause transient stimulation of aldosterone.

8.59

Answer: C　Decreased phagocytosis by white blood cells

Cortisol not only increases the supply of glucose through gluconeogenesis, but also decreases the utilisation of glucose by cells. The supply of glucose is enhanced by increasing the activity and amounts of enzymes involved in conversion of amino acids into glucose and glycogen. Decreased utilisation of glucose by cells involves direct inhibition of glucose transport into cells. Cortisol tends to increase the mobilisation of fatty acids and glycerol from adipose tissue, increasing their concentration in the blood and making more glycerol available for gluconeogenesis. Not only is fat broken down but also less is formed.

Cortisol reduces the utilisation of amino acids for the formation of protein everywhere except the liver. Extrahepatic protein stores are reduced and amino acid levels in the blood increase. Extrahepatic utilisation is decreased because amino acids are not transported into muscle cells, thereby reducing protein synthesis. Breakdown of cellular proteins continues, so that plasma amino acids are further increased. The high levels of blood amino acids are transported more avidly into hepatic cells where they are utilised for gluconeogenesis, glycogen formation and protein synthesis.

Cortisol tempers the inflammatory response through mechanisms not entirely understood. Some of the beneficial effects of cortisol include stabilisation of lysosomal membranes so that proteolytic enzymes are not released, decrease in permeability of capillaries so that less plasma and fewer cells enter the inflamed area, depression of phagocytosis by white blood cells and suppression of thymus-derived lymphocytes. Cortisol also suppresses synthesis of several key proteins that promote the inflammatory process, such as interleukin-1, and inhibits generation of pro-inflammatory prostaglandins.

8.60

Answer: D   Somatostatin and growth hormone-releasing
hormone (GHRH)

This clinical vignette describes the condition 'acromegaly', which
is a hormonal disorder that results when the pituitary gland
produces excess growth hormone (GH). Most commonly, it is a
benign GH-producing tumour derived from a distinct type of cells
(somatotrophs) and called a pituitary adenoma. Acromegaly most
commonly affects middle-aged adults and can result in serious
illness and premature death. Because of its insidious onset and slow
progression, the disease is hard to diagnose in the early stages and
is frequently missed for many years. Features that result from high
levels of GH or expanding tumour include:

- soft-tissue swelling of the hands and feet
- brow and lower jaw protrusion
- enlarging hands
- enlarging feet
- arthritis and carpal tunnel syndrome
- teeth spacing increases
- macroglossia (enlarged tongue)
- heart failure
- compression of the optic chiasm, leading to loss of
  vision in the outer visual fields
- diabetes mellitus
- hypertension
- increased palmar sweating and sebum production over
  the face (seborrhoea).

All these features are clinical indicators of active growth hormone
(GH)-producing pituitary tumours. These symptoms can also be
used to monitor the activity of the tumour after surgery, although
biochemical monitoring is confirmatory.

endocrine

GH is the most abundant hormone in the anterior pituitary and its acidophilic cell type is the most common. It acts on cells of non-classical endocrine target tissue. About half of GH in the general circulation is bound to an α-macroglobulin. Because it lacks a classical negative feedback hormone, GH secretion is controlled by a hypothalamic growth hormone-releasing hormone (GHRH) and a growth hormone inhibitory hormone (somatostatin). After puberty, somatostatin is most abundant in the hypothalamus.

endocrine

SECTION 9:
REPRODUCTIVE
PHYSIOLOGY – ANSWERS

9.1

Answer: D   Ovulation

17β-Oestradiol is a sex hormone. Labelled the 'female' hormone but also present in men, it represents the major oestrogen in humans. Oestradiol has not only a critical impact on reproductive and sexual functioning, but also affects other organs including bone structure. In the normal menstrual cycle oestradiol levels measure typically < 50 ng/ml at menstruation, rise with follicular development reaching a peak before ovulation, drop briefly at ovulation and rise again during the luteal phase for a second peak. At the end of the luteal phase, oestradiol levels drop to their menstrual levels unless there is a pregnancy. During pregnancy, oestrogen levels, including oestradiol, rise steadily towards term. The source of these oestrogens is the placenta that aromatises prehormones produced in the fetal adrenal gland. Serum oestradiol measurement in women reflects primarily the activity of the ovaries. As such, serum oestradiol measurement is useful to detect baseline oestrogen in women with amenorrhoea or menstrual dysfunction and to detect states of hypo-oestrogenicity and menopause. Furthermore, oestrogen monitoring during fertility therapy assesses follicular growth and is useful to monitor the treatment. Oestrogen-producing tumours will demonstrate persistent high levels of oestradiol and other oestrogens. In precocious puberty, oestradiol levels are inappropriately increased.

9.2

Answer: B   The genotype of the mole is 46,XX and is completely paternal in origin

A hydatidiform mole is a disease of trophoblastic proliferation. It can mimic pregnancy, causes high human chorionic gonadotrophin

reproductive

(HCG) levels and therefore gives false positive readings of pregnancy tests. The cause is not completely understood. Potential causes may include defects in the egg, abnormalities within the uterus or nutritional deficiencies. Women under 20 or over 40 years of age have a higher risk. Other risk factors include diets low in protein, folic acid and carotene. The hydatidiform mole is characterised by a conceptus of hyperplastic trophoblastic tissue attached to the placenta; it does not contain the inner cell mass. The hydatidiform mole can be of two types: complete or partial. Complete moles are diploid in nature and are purely paternal. 99% are 46,XX and 10% are 46,XY. They occur when an empty ovum is fertilised by two sperms. The process is called androgenesis. There are no fetal parts. The condition carries risk of malignancy to choriocarcinoma. Partial moles are triploid (69,XXX, 69,XXY) in nature and result from fertilisation of a haploid ovum and duplication of the paternal haploid chromosomes or from dispermy. Some cases are tetraploid. Fetal parts are often seen. Partial mole also carries risk of malignancy to choriocarcinoma, but the risk is lower than with the complete mole.

9.3

Answer: A   Death of the embryo and its subsequent expulsion

Human chorionic gonadotrophin (hCG) is a glycoprotein hormone, produced in pregnancy, which is made by the embryo soon after conception and later by the syncytiotrophoblast (part of the placenta). Its role is to prevent the disintegration of the corpus luteum of the ovary and thereby maintain progesterone production that is critical for a pregnancy in humans. hCG may have additional functions, for instance it is thought that it affects the immune tolerance of the pregnancy. Early pregnancy testing generally is based on the detection or measurement of hCG. Neutralisation of hCG activity will result in disintegration of the corpus luteum, with subsequent death and expulsion of embryo.

9.4

Answer: E   Secretory

The secretory phase of the menstrual cycle begins soon after ovulation occurs. Under the influence of progesterone produced by the corpus luteum in the ovary, the endometrium continues to grow to reach a maximum thickness of 5–7 mm as measured from the muscle wall to the endometrial cavity. The stromal cells continue to increase in size and number. Blood supply to the endometrium increases. The important change in this phase occurs in the endometrial glands. The glands increase in size and become actively secretory, hence the name – 'secretory phase'. In the early stage, the secretions collect in the cells of the glands. However, by the 19th to the 22nd day of the cycle, the secretions are pushed out of the cells and collect in the endometrial cavity. This secretion is rich in glycogen, fructose and glucose. Its main function is to supply nutrition to any fertilised ovum reaching the uterus.

9.5

Answer: B   Atony of uterus

Uterine atony is a loss of tone in the uterine musculature. Normally, contraction of the uterine arteries compresses the vessels and reduces flow. This increases the likelihood of coagulation and prevents bleeds. So, lack of uterine muscle contraction can cause an acute haemorrhage. Clinically, 75–80% of post-partum haemorrhages are due to uterine atony. Many factors can contribute to the loss of uterine muscle tone, including:

- overdistension of the uterus
- multiple gestations
- polyhydramnios
- fetal macrosomia
- prolonged labour
- oxytocin augmentation of labour
- grand multiparity (having given birth five or more times)

reproductive

- precipitous labour (labour lasting less than 3 hours)
- magnesium sulphate treatment of pre-eclampsia
- chorioamnionitis
- halogenated anaesthetics
- uterine leiomyomata.

9.6

Answer: E   Progesterone

Habitual abortion or recurrent pregnancy loss (RPL) is the occurrence of repeated pregnancies that end in miscarriage of the fetus, usually before 20 weeks of gestation. RPL affects about 0.34% of women who conceive. Habitual abortion is the occurrence of three consecutive spontaneous miscarriages (spontaneous abortions). The majority (85%) of women who have had two miscarriages will conceive and carry normally afterwards, so statistically the occurrence of three abortions at 0.34% is regarded as 'habitual'. There are various causes for habitual abortions and some are treatable. Some couples never have a cause identified, often after extensive investigations. One of the causes for habitual abortion is luteal phase defect. The theory behind the concept suggests that an inadequate amount of progesterone is produced by the corpus luteum to maintain the early pregnancy.

9.7

Answer: C   Androgens

The three major naturally occurring oestrogens in women are oestradiol, oestriol and oestrone. From menarche to menopause, the primary oestrogen is 17β-estradiol. In the body, these are all produced from androgens through actions of enzymes. Oestradiol is produced from testosterone and estrone from androstenedione. Oestrone is weaker than oestradiol and in postmenopausal women more oestrone is present than oestradiol.

9.8

Answer: C   Cardiac output increases

The mean arterial pressure (one-third pulse pressure added to the diastolic pressure) reaches its lowest point in the middle trimester, and then rises slowly until term. Mean pressures greater than 90 mmHg during the middle 3 months are associated with gestational hypertension. Similarly, mean arterial pressures exceeding 105 mmHg in the third trimester are regarded as hypertension.

By the end of the first trimester, cardiac output (CO) has increased by 25–50%. Thereafter, an additional 10% increase occurs in the middle trimester. The basal heart rate increases by about 10 beats per minute, which accounts for a small part of the increased output. The major part is due to increases in stroke volume (remember CO [ml/min] = stroke volume [ml] × beats/min). Normal CO is about 4.5–5.0 l/min, but during pregnancy it increases to as much as 6.2–8.1 l/min. Since there is actually a fall in mean arterial pressure (MAP), especially during the middle trimester, there is obviously a significant fall in total peripheral resistance (TPR). In the second half of pregnancy, the uteroplacental circulation constitutes a low resistance shunt, which accounts for a major part of the reduced peripheral resistance. [Remember: CO = MAP/TPR.]

Total plasma volume also increases in early pregnancy and continues to increase throughout pregnancy. The magnitude of the increase varies greatly between individuals, ranging between 40 and 90%. Average increases amount to 1250–1800 ml. Red cell volume also increases, but frequently lags behind the plasma volume, resulting in a reduced haematocrit and haemoglobin concentration. This has sometimes been referred to as the physiological anaemia of pregnancy. However, the total amount of haemoglobin is greater during pregnancy and the oxygen-carrying capacity of the blood more than matches the increase in oxygen consumption. Leukocyte concentration also increases. However, plasma protein concentration falls dramatically in early pregnancy due to expansion in blood volume. Serum albumin concentration falls from a non-pregnant value of 4 g/100 ml to 2.5–3.0 g/100 ml. As a result, oncotic pressure falls, which favours filtration at the capillary, often leading to a general oedema, especially in lower limbs.

reproductive

The uterus is the major target of increased blood flow during pregnancy. The flow rate to the uterus/placenta is about 200 ml/min at mid-pregnancy and at term it is approximately 500 ml/min. The kidneys are the second major site, where renal blood flow rises from about 600 ml/min to 1200 ml/min by 10 weeks of pregnancy and is maintained at this level until term. Vasodilatation in skin occurs in the first weeks of pregnancy, which result in a fivefold increase in flow to the extremities. Other areas such as liver and brain show no increase in blood flow.

Several explanations have been advanced for changes in haemodynamic alterations in pregnancy and the fall in peripheral resistance. Hormonal changes are probably the major influence. Progesterone decreases intrinsic vascular tone by rendering the vessel walls less responsive to angiotensin II, noradrenaline and adrenaline. In addition, endothelial cells increase production of vasodilatory prostaglandins (eg PGI_2), which decreases sensitivity of arterioles to angiotensin II and noradrenaline. By mid-pregnancy, the utero-placental circulation constitutes a low-resistance shunt, which contributes greatly to the increased blood volume. In the final analysis, there is a larger vascular space, and whether this space is physiologically underfilled or overfilled in pregnancy is an interesting theoretical question. Many changes observed in pregnancy appear to be compensatory adjustments to maintain perfusion pressure in the face of an expanded, highly compliant vascular space (represented by the placenta). For example, consider: increased plasma renin activity; increased plasma angiotensinogen; increased angiotensin II; and increased aldosterone. These adjustments serve to increase sodium retention and increase blood volume, which, in turn, increases stroke volume and hence, cardiac output. Even with these changes, there is observed to be a fall in mean arterial pressure and a marked tendency to hypotension in pregnant individuals. This suggests that the vascular space is not sufficiently filled.

9.9

Answer: A   Alveolar ventilation is increased

Although there is no change in the basal respiratory rate or vital capacity during pregnancy, there is a considerable increase in tidal volume. The residual volume and total lung volume are reduced, but the inspiratory capacity is increased.

There is increased alveolar ventilation (60%), so that the distribution and mixing of gas are more efficient during late pregnancy. Total oxygen consumption increases by 20% in late pregnancy, yet alveolar ventilation increases 60%, so there is relative hyperventilation, which results in a lowered $p(CO_2)$. The high circulating levels of progesterone that occur during pregnancy increase the sensitivity of the hypothalamic respiratory centres to small increases in $p(CO_2)$ and also lower the 'set-point'. A rise of 1 mmHg $p(CO_2)$ results in an increased ventilation of 6 l per min, which is several times the change noted in non-pregnant individuals. During pregnancy, normal $p(CO_2)$ values fall from about 40 to 32 mmHg. With this fall in $p(CO_2)$ one might predict a rise in $p(O_2)$. $p(O_2)$ does increase from a non-pregnant value of 95 mmHg to a mean of 106 mmHg. Presumably, the reduced $p(CO_2)$ makes the elimination of CO_2 by the fetus easier. However, if such a fall occurred without other adjustments, pH of maternal blood would increase. To compensate, plasma bicarbonate is reduced through renal excretion, necessarily accompanied by a reduction in plasma sodium concentration. Compensation is complete and pH of the blood is not altered. You may think of this as a physiological chronic respiratory alkalosis fully compensated by chronic metabolic acidosis. The loss of sodium, which must accompany bicarbonate excretion, leads to a drop in plasma osmolality from about 290 to 280 mOsm/kg plasma water. This is more than enough of a drop to turn off ADH (antidiuretic hormone) secretion from the neurohypophysis. This in turn leads to polyuria, to periods of increased thirst and to exaggerated diuresis following water loads.

9.10

Answer: D   Renal plasma flow is increased

Renal plasma flow increases during pregnancy from 600 ml/min to 1200 ml/min in the first trimester, and then returns to the non-gravid flow at term. The glomerular filtration rate (GFR) is normally about 120 ml/min and in pregnancy increases about 60% to 150–180 ml/min. Since the water filtered by the glomeruli is increased some

60%, so are all of the solutes contained in the plasma water and this increases the load of substances presented to the renal tubules for reabsorption. As a result, more solutes are lost in the urine. Clinical glycosuria occurs more often in pregnancy and some individuals become frank diabetics during pregnancy. After parturition blood glucose returns to normal. Also, during pregnancy, there is considerable amino aciduria attributable to the increased GFR.

To prevent sodium wastage in the face of a 60% increase in GFR, the kidney tubule must retain an additional 10 000 mEq of Na$^+$ each day. This it is able to do. However, the interacting forces regulating sodium reabsorption and excretion during pregnancy are so numerous and complex that net sodium flux is difficult to predict. Knowledge of minute changes in the rate of sodium reabsorption is important for management of patients because they can produce profound effects. For example, if the percentage of filtered sodium reabsorbed by the kidneys increased from 99.4% to 99.5% in pregnancy, this would lead to a positive balance of 34 mEq per day and result in an increase in body weight of approximately 0.5 pounds daily.

Those factors that tend to retain sodium during pregnancy include: (1) increase in oestrogen; (2) increase in cortisol; (3) increase in renin activity and angiotensin II concentration; and (4) increase in aldosterone production. Factors favouring sodium excretion in pregnancy include: (1) increase in GFR; (2) increase in progesterone levels, which is natriuretic by antagonising the action of aldosterone at the renal tubule; and (3) excretion of bicarbonate to compensate for respiratory alkalosis.

9.11

Answer: D   Is similar in structure and function to growth hormone

Human placental lactogen (hPL), also called human chorionic somatomammotrophin, is a polypeptide placental hormone. Its structure and function are similar to those of human growth hormone. It modifies the metabolic state of the mother during pregnancy to facilitate the energy supply of the fetus. hPL is an anti-insulin hormone. It consists of 190 amino acids that are linked by two disulphite bonds and is secreted by the syncytiotrophoblast during pregnancy. Its molecular weight is 22 125. Like human growth hormone, hPL is encoded by genes on chromosome 17q22–24. Its biological half-life is 15 min. hPL is only present during pregnancy, with maternal serum levels rising in relation to the growth of the fetus and placenta. Maximum levels are reached near term, typically to 5–7 mg/ml. Higher levels are noted in patients with multiple gestation. Little hPL enters the fetal circulation. In bioassays, hPL mimics the action of prolactin, yet it is unclear if hPL has any role in human lactation. hPL affects the metabolic system of the mother. It increases production of insulin and IGF-1 and increases insulin resistance and carbohydrate intolerance. Chronic hypoglycaemia leads to a rise in hPL. hPL induces lipolysis with the release of free fatty acids, increase in insulin secretion and insulin resistance. With fasting and release of hPL, free fatty acids become available for the mother as fuel, so that relatively more glucose can be utilised by the fetus. In addition, ketones formed from free fatty acids can cross the placenta and be used by the fetus. These events support the energy supply to the fetus in states of starvation.

9.12

Answer: D $p(CO_2)$

During pregnancy, normal $p(CO_2)$ values fall from about 40 to 32 mmHg. Presumably, the reduced $p(CO_2)$ makes the elimination of CO_2 by the fetus easier.

9.13

Answer: E Placental syncytiotrophoblast

Progesterone is an absolute requirement for maintenance of pregnancy. During the first two weeks of pregnancy the corpus luteum produces large amounts under stimulation of luteinising hormone (LH). However, LH levels begin to fall and human chorionic gonadotrophin must be increasing to rescue the corpus luteum from regression. Between the 6th and 9th weeks of pregnancy, the syncytiotrophoblast tissue of the fetal placenta is fully capable of progesterone synthesis and the luteal source becomes a minor contributor.

9.14

Answer: B   Acute fatty liver

Acute fatty liver of pregnancy is a rare life-threatening complication of pregnancy that occurs in the third trimester or the immediate period after delivery. It is thought to be caused by a disordered metabolism of fatty acids by mitochondria in the fetus, caused by deficiency in the LCHAD (long-chain 3-hydroxyacyl-coenzyme A dehydrogenase) enzyme. The condition was previously thought to be universally fatal, but aggressive treatment by stabilising the mother with intravenous fluids and blood products in anticipation of early delivery has improved prognosis. Acute fatty liver of pregnancy (or hepatic lipidosis of pregnancy) usually manifests in the third trimester of pregnancy, but may occur any time in the second half of pregnancy or in the puerperium, the period immediately after delivery. On average, the disease presents during the 35th or 36th week of pregnancy. The usual symptoms in the mother are non-specific, including nausea, vomiting, anorexia (or lack of desire to eat) and abdominal pain; however, jaundice and fever may occur in as many as 70% of patients.

Many laboratory abnormalities are seen in acute fatty liver of pregnancy. Liver enzymes are elevated, with the aspartate aminotransferase (AST) and alanine aminotransferase (ALT) enzymes ranging from minimal elevation to 1000 IU/l, but usually staying in the 300–500 range. Bilirubin is almost universally elevated. Alkaline phosphatase is often elevated in pregnancy due to production from the placenta, but may be additionally elevated. Other abnormalities may include an elevated white blood cell count, hypoglycaemia, elevated coagulation parameters, including the international normalised ratio (INR) and decreased fibrinogen. Frank disseminated intravascular coagulation or DIC, may occur in as many as 70% of patients.

Abdominal ultrasound may show fat deposition in the liver, but, as the hallmark of this condition is microvesicular steatosis, this may not be seen on ultrasound. Rarely, the condition can be complicated by rupture or necrosis of the liver, which may be identified by ultrasound.

HELLP syndrome is a life-threatening obstetric complication considered by many to be a variant of pre-eclampsia. Both conditions occur during the latter stages of pregnancy or sometimes after childbirth. HELLP is an abbreviation of the main findings:

- **H**aemolytic anaemia
- **E**levated **L**iver enzymes and
- **L**ow **P**latelet count.

9.15

Answer: B   Pituitary basophils

In men, luteinising hormone (LH) acts upon the interstitial (Leydig) cells in the testes and is responsible for testosterone production that exerts intratesticular activity in terms of the spermatogenesis and endocrine activity as the 'male hormone'. LH is produced by gonadotrophs, which are basophilic cells in the anterior pituitary gland.

9.16

Answer: E   Progesterone

The high circulating levels of progesterone that occur during pregnancy increase the sensitivity of the hypothalamic respiratory centres to small increases in $p(CO_2)$, and lower the 'set-point'. A rise of 1 mmHg $p(CO_2)$ results in an increased ventilation of 6 l/min, which is several times the change noted in non-pregnant individuals. During pregnancy normal $p(CO_2)$ values fall from about 40 to 32 mmHg (*see also* answer to 9.9).

9.17

Answer: D   Oestrogen

Oestrogen increases circulating level of factors II, VII, IX, X, antithrombin III and plasminogen, as well as increasing platelet adhesiveness.

reproductive

9.18

Answer: D Reduced fat deposition

Bilateral oophorectomy will result in loss of oestrogen synthesis and secretion as oestrogen is produced primarily by developing follicles in the ovaries. Oestrogen has the following effects:

Structural:

- development of female secondary sex characteristics
- stimulation of endometrial growth
- increased uterine growth
- maintenance of vessels and skin
- reduced bone resorption, increased bone formation.

Protein metabolism:

- increased hepatic production of binding proteins.

Coagulation:

- increased circulating level of factors II, VII, IX, X, antithrombin III and plasminogen
- increase platelet adhesiveness.

Lipid metabolism:

- increased HDL, triglycerides, fat deposition
- decreased LDL.

Fluid balance:

- salt and water retention.

Gastrointestinal tract:

- reduced bowel motility
- increased cholesterol in bile.

Bilateral oophorectomy will result in reversal of the effects of oestrogens.

reproductive

9.19

Answer: C   Luteinising hormone (LH)

Luteinizing hormone (LH) is a hormone synthesised and secreted by gonadotrophs in the anterior lobe of the pituitary gland. In concert with the other pituitary gonadotrophin follicle-stimulating hormone, it is necessary for proper reproductive function. In the female, an acute rise of LH – the LH surge – triggers ovulation. In the male, where LH has also been called interstitial cell-stimulating hormone, it stimulates Leydig cell production of testosterone. LH is a glycoprotein. Each monomeric unit is a protein molecule with a sugar attached to it; two of these make the full, functional protein. Its structure is similar to the other glycoproteins, FSH, TSH and hCG. The protein dimer contains two polypeptide units, labelled alpha and beta subunits, which are connected by two disulphide bridges. The alpha subunits of LH, FSH, TSH and hCG are identical and contain 92 amino acids; the beta subunits vary. LH has a beta subunit of 121 amino acids that confers its specific biological action and is responsible for interaction with the LH receptor. This beta subunit contains the same amino acids in sequence as the beta subunit of hCG and both stimulate the same receptor; however, the hCG beta subunit contains an additional 24 amino acids and both hormones differ in the composition of their sugar moieties. The different composition of these oligosaccharides affects bioactivity and speed of degradation: the biological half-life of LH is 20 min, shorter than that of FSH (3–4 h) or hCG (24 h).

9.20

Answer: C   Decreased sperm count

Follicle-stimulating hormone (FSH) is a hormone synthesised and secreted by gonadotrophs in the anterior pituitary gland. In men, FSH enhances the production of androgen-binding protein by the Sertoli cells of the testes and is critical for spermatogenesis. Diminished secretion of FSH can result in failure of gonadal function (hypogonadism). This condition is typically manifest in men as failure in production of normal numbers of sperm.

reproductive

9.21

Answer: B Kallman's syndrome

Kallmann's syndrome is an example of hypogonadism caused by a deficiency of gonadotrophin-releasing hormone (GnRH), which is created by the hypothalamus. Kallmann's syndrome is also known as hypothalamic hypogonadism, familial hypogonadism with anosmia or hypogonadotrophic hypogonadism, reflecting its disease mechanism. It is a form of secondary hypogonadism, reflecting the fact the primary cause of the defect in sex hormone production lies within the pituitary and hypothalamus, rather than a physical defect of the testes or ovaries themselves.

9.22

Answer: B Inhibin

Inhibin is a peptide that is an inhibitor of FSH synthesis and secretion. It contains an alpha and beta subunit linked by disulphide bonds. Two forms of inhibin differ in their beta subunits (A or B), while their alpha subunits are identical. Inhibin belongs to the transforming growth factor-β (TGF-β) family.

9.23

Answer: E Is regulated by FSH

Androgen-binding protein (ABP) is a glycoprotein (β-globulin) produced by the Sertoli cells in the seminiferous tubules of the testis that binds specifically to testosterone, dihydrotestosterone and 17β-oestradiol. By its binding to testosterone and dihydrotestosterone, these hormones are made less lipophilic and become concentrated within the luminal fluid of the seminal vesicles. The higher levels of these hormones enable spermatogenesis in the seminiferous tubules and sperm maturation in epididymis. ABP has the same amino acid sequence as sex-hormone-binding globulin; the difference is the site of production and the addition of different sugar moieties. ABP contains 403 amino acids, resulting in a molecular weight of 44 533. Its gene is located on chromosome 17. ABP's production is regulated under influence of FSH on Sertoli cell, enhanced by insulin, retinol and testosterone.

9.24

Answer: D   Increased gonadotrophin-releasing hormone
secretion

Actions of testosterone produced by Leydig cells in the testes include:

- Negative feedback influence at the hypothalamus is to inhibit GnRH secretion. Decreases responsiveness of pituitary to GnRH. All of which results in preferential inhibition of LH release.

- Facilitates spermatogenesis. Essential for maintenance of sperm production.

- Stimulates development and maintenance of male genitalia and accessory sex glands.

- Stimulates appearance of secondary sex characteristics: (1) pubic hair, beard; (2) deepening of voice; (3) muscular growth – rapidly increases RNA, DNA and protein synthesis.

- Increases calcium retention and synthesis of bone matrix. Stimulates closure of epiphyseal plates.

- Protein anabolism – increases nitrogen retention and metabolic rate. Positive nitrogen balance in tissues throughout the body. Some tissues more influenced than others.

Removal of testes will result in loss of testosterone production with reversal of all the above-mentioned actions of testosterone.

9.25

Answer: C   Large amounts of ascorbic acid

Once thought to store sperm but now known as the most important source of seminal fluid, seminal vesicles provide 50–60% of the normal ejaculate volume (2–5 ml). The secretions contain large amounts of ascorbic acid, inositol, amino acids, phosphorylcholine (used in one of the older tests for the presence of semen in forensic medicine) and large amounts of prostaglandins in man. The fluid is rich in HCO_3^- and alkaline in nature, which serves to neutralise the

reproductive

high acidity conditions normally encountered in the vagina.

9.26

Answer: C   Fructose

The ampulla is an enlargement of the vas. It produces fructose on which sperm depend for an anaerobic source of energy.

9.27

Answer: C   Choriocarcinoma

Choriocarcinoma is a malignant and aggressive cancer of the placenta. It is characterised by early haematogenous spread to the lungs. It belongs to the far end of the spectrum of gestational trophoblastic diseases (GTD). It is preceded by:

- hydatidiform mole (50% of cases)
- abortion of ectopic pregnancy (20% of cases)
- normal term pregnancy (20–30% of cases).

Clinical features include:

- increased quantitative β-hCG levels
- vaginal bleeding
- shortness of breath
- haemoptysis (coughing up blood)
- chest pain
- multiple infiltrates of various shapes in both lungs on chest X-ray.

9.28

Answer: A   Is a calcium-dependent event

Once capacitation has been completed, activation of spermatozoa can proceed. Activation is a calcium-dependent event, which

reproductive

involves extensive changes in the sperm. First, the surface membrane of the front of the sperm fuses at many points with the underlying acrosomal membrane (the acrosomal reaction) creating a vesiculated appearance and exposing the enzymatic contents of the acrosomal vesicle and the inner acrosomal membrane to the exterior. Second, the tail beat changes from regular wave-like flagella beats to 'whip lashing beats' that push the sperm forward in vigorous lurches. Third, the surface membrane of the middle and posterior half of the sperm head becomes able to fuse to the surface membrane of the ovum. The molecular basis of activation is not yet established. However, a destabilisation of the surface membranes may be critical. Activation of spermatozoa takes place in the female reproductive tract.

9.29

Answer: D   Progesterone

Progesterone inhibits lactation during pregnancy. The fall in serum progesterone with passage of the placenta seems to be the important event in establishment of lactogenesis. Furthermore, progesterone administration inhibits casein and α-lactalbumin synthesis in vitro. Once lactogenesis is initiated, prolactin appears to be the key hormone in maintenance of milk synthesis (galactopoiesis) and secretion. Oestrogen and progesterone or even ovariectomy have no effect on lactation once it has been initiated.

9.30

Answer: C   Oxytocin

The suckling stimulus provided by the feeding infant at the nipple sends afferent fibres to the hypothalamic paraventricular and supraoptic nuclei, with subsequent release of oxytocin from the posterior pituitary. Oxytocin stimulates contraction of the smooth muscle cells underlying the milk-producing alveolar cells. The contractions express milk from the alveolar areas into the duct system leading to the surface at the nipple. Without this 'milk letdown' reflex, milk remains unavailable to the infant in spite of adequate production.

reproductive

9.31

Answer: E   Prolactin

The high levels of prolactin that occur during lactation suppress release of gonadotrophins, which in turn prevents a normal menstrual cycle. Because of this, lactation has been exploited as a means of birth control. However, after about 40 days post partum, prolactin sensitivity to suckling decreases markedly, and so loses its value as a contraceptive method.

9.32

Answer: E   Maternal prostaglandin

There are at least four observations that have led researchers to believe that prostaglandins (PGs) play a major regulatory role in the onset of labour:

- the myometrium is exquisitely sensitive to the stimulatory effects of PGs throughout pregnancy
- amniotic production of stimulatory prostaglandins (PGE and PGF) increases in late pregnancy
- administration of inhibitors of PG synthesis (aspirin and indomethacin) causes uterine quiescence and prolongs gestation
- injection of PGF_{2a} precursors into the amnion always induces delivery.

A number of regulatory factors stimulate prostaglandin production: Ca^{2+}/calmodulin, epidermal growth factor, adenylate cyclase and adrenaline. It is believed that both cAMP-dependent and cAMP-independent protein kinases are involved.

9.33

Answer: E   Stimulation of the number of oxytocin receptors in the decidua and myometrium

Oestrogen stimulates prostaglandin (PGE and PGF_{2a} are the most active) output by decidual cells and progesterone inhibits PG output. It is thought that local changes in production of the two hormones near the time of parturition results in oestrogen dominance in some cells, leading to PG production. This may occur locally within the fetal membranes (amnion and chorion) and decidua. However, the chorion appears to be the most important site of such local changes. 3β-Hydroxysteroid dehydrogenase (3β-HSD), necessary for synthesis of progesterone, can be inhibited with oestrone and oestradiol. Local changes in progesterone formation and metabolism, especially in association with rising oestrogen concentrations near the end of pregnancy, might thus affect local progesterone withdrawal, which, in turn, may lead to increased PG output. The decidua contains receptors for oestrogen and progesterone and so hormonal effects are most probably mediated through this tissue. High levels of progesterone before parturition are inhibitory to PG. However, it is possible that high local levels of oestrogen occur near term, which inhibit progesterone locally, leading to a local increase in PG production.

9.34

Answer: C   Formation of Graafian follicles

During the antral phase, the granulosa cells grow and an antrum is formed. Synthesis of oestrogen by the follicle increases in response to increased stimulation by LH and FSH. The higher the levels of LH and FSH, the greater the number of follicles that grow. For unknown reasons a single, dominate follicle, grows much faster than all others. Most of the oestrogen and progesterone is secreted from this Graafian follicle. The other follicles that began to grow regress and become atretic. Toward the end of this phase, a large surge of LH gives a sudden stimulus to the dominant follicle, which now has LH receptors on both granulosa and thecal cells. This preovulatory surge of LH stimulates a burst of oestrogen secretion and then decreases it by rapidly switching off the aromatising activity of the granulosa cells and diverts them to producing progesterone. These dramatic changes culminate in ovulation.

reproductive

9.35

Answer: E   Polycystic ovarian syndrome

Hirsutism (from Latin hirsutus = shaggy, hairy) is defined as excessive and increased hair growth in women in locations where the occurrence of terminal hair normally is minimal or absent. It refers to a male pattern of body hair (androgenic hair) and it is therefore primarily of cosmetic and psychological concern. Hirsutism is a symptom rather than a disease, and may be a sign of a more serious medical indication, especially if it develops well after puberty. The following may be some of the conditions that may increase a woman's normally low level of male hormones:

- polycystic ovarian syndrome
- Cushing's disease
- tumours in the ovaries or adrenal gland
- certain medications
- congenital adrenal hyperplasia.

The woman in this clinical vignette is most likely to have polycystic ovarian syndrome (PCOS, also known clinically as Stein–Leventhal syndrome). It is an endocrine disorder that affects 5–10% of women. It occurs among all races and nationalities, is the most common hormonal disorder among women of reproductive age and is a leading cause of infertility. The principal features are lack of regular ovulation and excessive amounts or effects of androgenic hormones. The symptoms and severity of the syndrome vary greatly between women.

9.36

Answer: B   5α-Reductase

5-Alpha-reductase is an enzyme that converts testosterone, the male sex hormone, into the more potent dihydrotestosterone. There are two isoenzymes, steroid 5α-reductases 1 and 2 (SRD5A1 and SRD5A2). The second isoenzyme is deficient in 5α-reductase deficiency, which leads to a form of intersexualism. The enzyme is produced only in specific tissues of the male human body, namely the skin, seminal vesicles, prostate and epididymis. Inhibition of 5α-reductase results in decreased production of DHT, increased levels of testosterone and possibly increased levels of oestradiol. Gynaecomastia is a possible side-effect of 5α-reductase inhibition.

9.37

Answer: A   Cholesterol

Testosterone is synthesised from cholesterol in the testes. The testis derives about half of the cholesterol required from de-novo synthesis. The other half comes from the plasma pool by receptor-mediated endocytosis of low-density lipoprotein particles. Five enzymatic steps are involved: 20,22-desmolase, 3β-hydroxysteroid dehydrogenase, 17α-hydroxylase, 17,20-desmolase and 17β-hydroxysteroid dehydrogenase. The initial reaction in the process is the side-chain cleavage of cholesterol to pregnenolone. This is the rate-limiting step in testosterone synthesis and is regulated by luteinising hormone. Although testosterone is the major secretory product of the testis, some of the precursors in the pathway as well as very small amounts of dihydrotestosterone (DHT) and estradiol are directly secreted by the testis. However, the major sites of DHT and oestradiol formation are androgen target tissues and adipose tissue.

9.38

Answer: A   2% testosterone circulates as free testosterone

Testosterone circulates in the plasma largely bound to plasma proteins, albumin and testosterone-binding globulin (TeBG). In normal men only about 2% of testosterone is unbound, whereas 44% is bound to TeBG and 54% is bound to albumin and other proteins. Albumin has approximately 1000-fold lower affinity for testosterone than does TeBG. The amount of hormone available for entry into cells depends on capillary transit time in a given organ, dissociation rate from the binding protein and endothelial membrane permeability.

reproductive

9.39

Answer: C   Citric acid

The prostate contributes large amounts of citric acid to seminal fluid; in fact, prostatic function can be diagnosed by the citric acid content of semen (480–2680 mg/100 ml semen). Prostatic secretions are rich in proteolytic enzymes such as acid phosphatases (3950 U/ml semen), which are important in phospholipid metabolism. The secretions are slightly acidic.

9.40

Answer: A   FSH

Menopause occurs when oestradiol secretion no longer occurs. The concentrations of circulating FSH and LH increase markedly because they are no longer suppressed by basal levels of oestradiol.

9.41

Answer: D   Hot flush

A hot flush (sometimes referred to as a hot flash or night sweat) is a symptom of changing hormone levels considered characteristic of menopause. Hot flushes are typically experienced as a feeling of intense heat with sweating and rapid heartbeat and may typically last from 2 to 30 min on each occasion for older women. The event may be repeated a few times each week or up to a dozen times a day, with the frequency reducing over time. Excessive flushing can lead to rosacea. Younger women who are menstruating or expecting to menstruate soon (premenstruation typically lasts 1 or 2 weeks) may encounter hot and/or cold flushes. These episodes do not usually last long. One minute, a woman will feel cold, the next, hot. Hot and cold flushes for younger women occur only during their menstruation or premenstruation. If they occur at other times in a young woman's menstrual cycle, there may be a problem with her pituitary gland. Hormone replacement therapy (HRT) may relieve many of the symptoms of menopause. However, HRT increases the risk of breast cancer, stroke, dementia and has other potentially serious short-term and long-term risks.

9.42

Answer: E   Physiological response

In pregnancy, red cell volume also increases, but this frequently lags behind the plasma volume, resulting in a reduced haematocrit and haemoglobin concentration. This has sometimes been referred to as the physiological anaemia of pregnancy. However, the total amount of haemoglobin is greater during pregnancy and the oxygen-carrying capacity of the blood more than matches the increase in oxygen consumption.

9.43

Answer: A   Progesterone withdrawal

In the absence of a pregnancy and without human chorionic gonadotrophin (hCG), the corpus luteum demises and inhibin and progesterone levels fall. Progesterone withdrawal leads to menstrual shedding (progesterone-withdrawal bleeding) and falling inhibin levels allow FSH levels to rise to raise a new crop of follicles.

9.44

Answer: C   Glucose

The syncytiotrophoblastic cell layer is the limiting barrier to diffusion and active transport. Other components such as connective tissue and endothelium of fetal capillaries may limit diffusion for large molecules and cells. Simple diffusion-exchange is determined by concentration gradient for low-molecular-weight molecules, such as blood gases, sodium, water, urea, non-polar molecules such as cholesterol and steroid hormones. Hexose sugars (eg, glucose) are transported by facilitated diffusion, whereas active transport systems exist for amino acids, conjugated steroids, nucleotides and water-soluble vitamins. Pinocytosis occurs for transfer of plasma proteins, immunoglobulins and lipoproteins.

reproductive

9.45

Answer: D   Explained by failure of testis to descend

Cryptorchidism is a medical term referring to absence from the scrotum of one or both testes. This usually represents failure of the testis to move, to 'descend', during fetal development from an abdominal position, through the inguinal canal, into the ipsilateral scrotum. About 3% of full-term and 30% of premature infant boys are born with at least one undescended testis, making cryptorchidism the most common birth defect of male genitalia. However, most testes descend by the first year of life (the majority within 3 months), making the true incidence of cryptorchidism around 1% overall. A testis absent from the normal scrotal position can be:

- found anywhere along the 'path of descent' from high in the posterior (retroperitoneal) abdomen, just below the kidney, to the inguinal ring

- found in the inguinal canal

- *ectopic,* that is, found to have 'wandered' from that path, usually outside the inguinal canal and sometimes even under the skin of the thigh, the perineum, the opposite scrotum and femoral canal

- found to be undeveloped (*hypoplastic*) or severely abnormal (*dysgenetic*)

- found to have vanished.

About two-thirds of cases without other abnormalities are unilateral; one-third involves both testes. In 90% of cases an undescended testis can be *palpated* (felt) in the inguinal canal; in a minority the testis or testes are in the abdomen or non-existent (truly 'hidden'). Undescended testes are associated with reduced fertility, increased risk of testicular cancer and psychological problems when the boy is grown up. Undescended testes are also more susceptible to testicular torsion and infarction and inguinal hernias. To reduce these risks, undescended testes are usually brought into the scrotum in infancy by a surgical procedure called an orchiopexy.

ANSWERS

9.46

Answer: E   200–500 million

Approximately 200–500 million spermatozoa (also called *sperms*), produced in the testes, are released per ejaculation.

9.47

Answer: D   Occurs after the demise of corpus luteum in the ovary

Menstruation is also called menstrual bleeding, menses or a period. This bleeding serves as a sign that a woman has not become pregnant. (However, this cannot be taken as certainty, as sometimes there is some bleeding in early pregnancy.) Eumenorrhea denotes normal, regular menstruation that lasts for a few days (usually 3–5 days, but anywhere from 2 to 7 days is considered normal). The average blood loss during menstruation is 35 ml, with 10–80 ml considered normal. In the absence of pregnancy, the corpus luteum demises, resulting in fall in progesterone levels. Progesterone withdrawal leads to menstrual shedding (progesterone-withdrawal bleeding).

9.48

Answer: A   Cholestasis of pregnancy

Intrahepatic cholestasis of pregnancy (ICP), also termed obstetric cholestasis, gives rise to troublesome itching during pregnancy, but may lead to possibly serious complications for the mother and very serious outcomes for the fetus. Itching has long been considered to be a common symptom of pregnancy. The vast majority of times, itching or pruritus is a minor annoyance caused by changes to the skin, especially that of the abdomen. However, there are instances when itching is a symptom of ICP. ICP occurs most commonly in the third trimester, but can begin at any time during the pregnancy.

reproductive

9.49

Answer: B   Enhanced motility

Ejaculated sperms are able to swim vigorously and appear structurally mature; however, they require a period of incubation in the female reproductive tract before gaining the potential for fertilisation. Glycoprotein molecules coating the surface of the sperm cell are solubilised by uterine fluid. These molecules were originally acquired in the epididymis and seminal plasma. This process is called capacitation. An oestrogen-dominated uterus is optimal for capacitation. Note that sperm survival is also optimal and that ovulation occurs under these conditions. Capacitation allows: (1) increased energy metabolism; (2) enhanced motility; (3) the acrosome reaction or activation.

9.50

Answer: B   Rh-negative   Rh-positive   Rh-positive

The main difference between the ABO system of blood groups and the Rhesus (Rh) system is the following: ABO antibodies are naturally occurring while a person missing an Rh antigen will not have antibodies against Rh in his serum unless sensitised. Sensitisation of Rh-negative people can occur through massive blood transfusions or through a prior pregnancy with an Rh-positive child. Having a first Rh-negative child does not pose a risk of sensitisation for the mother. However, the second Rh-positive child may still be at risk if the mother was sensitised by other means, for example previous transfusion with Rh-positive blood. Rh-positive mothers do not develop Rh antibodies and there is no risk of haemolytic transfusion reactions due to Rh incompatibility (*see also* answer to 1.58).

reproductive

INDEX

(The number in bold indicates section and the number in italics indicates question number)